AIDS

The Biological Basis

AIDS

The Biological Basis

THIRD EDITION

I. Edward Alcamo, Ph.D.
Professor of Microbiology
State University of New York at Farmingdale

JONES AND BARTLETT PUBLISHERS
Sudbury, Massachusetts
BOSTON   TORONTO   LONDON   SINGAPORE

World Headquarters
Jones and Bartlett Publishers
40 Tall Pine Drive
Sudbury, MA 01776
978-443-5000
info@jbpub.com
www.jbpub.com

Jones and Bartlett Publishers Canada
2406 Nikanna Road
Mississauga, ON L5C 2W6
CANADA

Jones and Bartlett Publishers International
Barb House, Barb Mews
London W6 7PA
UK

Production Credits
Chief Executive Officer: Clayton Jones
Chief Operating Officer: Don W. Jones, Jr.
Executive V.P. & Publisher: Robert W. Holland, Jr.
V.P., Design and Production: Anne Spencer
V.P., Sales and Marketing: William Kane
V.P., Manufacturing and Inventory Control: Therese Bräuer
Executive Editor, Science: Stephen L. Weaver
Managing Editor, Science: Dean W. DeChambeau
Senior Production Editor: Louis C. Bruno, Jr.
Marketing Associate: Matthew Payne
Text Design: Anne Spencer
Illustrations: ANCO-Art
Composition: Circle Graphics
Cover Design: Kristin Ohlin
Printing and Binding: Courier Westford
Cover Printing: Lehigh Press

Library of Congress Cataloging-in-Publication Data

Alcamo, I. Edward.
   AIDS : the biological basis / I. Edward Alcamo.—3rd ed.
     p.cm.
   Includes bibliographical references and index.
   ISBN 0-7637-0238-2
   1. AIDS (Disease) I. Title.
   RC606.6 .A432 2003
   616.97'92—dc21   2002033995

Printed in the United States of America
07 06 05 04 03   10 9 8 7 6 5 4 3 2 1

Contents

7 HIV Testing and Diagnosis 184

8 Treating HIV Infection and AIDS 212

9 An AIDS Vaccine 260

10 AIDS in Perspective 288

Preface

I remember the first AIDS lecture I gave. It was January 1984, and the venue was my local public library. Although my outward purpose was telling people about the new scourge on the horizon, I must admit I was also interested in puffing myself up as someone special—the local guru of germs, so to speak. I vividly remember the title of the lecture: "AIDS—The Cause, the Effect, and the Tragedy." I also recall the size of the audience: seven people.

I suspect most people had better things to do that Wednesday evening. AIDS was something they had heard about but had not witnessed firsthand. In 1983 there had been only several hundred cases in the entire United States, and few people expected the disease to affect them directly or indirectly. But the projections were for much worse. Indeed, I remember showing one particular slide from the Centers for Disease Control and Prevention (CDC) projecting hundreds of thousands of cases by the early 1990s. Secretly, I wondered if it were all a hoax and down deep, I questioned whether the projections would ever come to pass.

Tragically, almost everything the CDC predicted has happened. By the end of 2001, the total number of AIDS cases in the United States passed 800,000—that's more than three-quarters of a million Americans fitting the case definition of AIDS. And over 460,000 had already died! AIDS has become the epidemic of our times, with over 42 million of the world's population currently infected.

For the past 19 years I have been telling the AIDS story, and now I am privileged to be writing it. In this book, I shall be focusing on the biological basis of AIDS, for I am a microbiology educator by training and profession. And you? Perhaps you are a health professional, such as a nurse, dental hygienist, or medical technologist, who is concerned about AIDS. Or maybe you are a biology educator who would like to teach about AIDS with more confidence. Perhaps you need to know more about AIDS because you have tested positive for the human immunodeficiency virus (HIV). You may be a physician, dentist, or researcher who wishes to clarify concepts about AIDS. Or maybe you are taking a one-semester course or doing a term paper on AIDS (it's the hottest term paper topic of this generation). Whatever your profession or needs, you and I share an interest in AIDS, and I look forward to explaining what I know about this dreaded disease in the pages ahead.

Organization and Special Features

AIDS: The Biological Basis contains ten chapters devoted to the biology of acquired immune deficiency syndrome. The book opens with a brief history of the roots and emergence of AIDS. Then, in chapter 2, the human immunodeficiency virus is discussed in the context of other viruses so you can see how it fits into the spectrum of microorganisms. Next comes a chapter on the microbiology of the immune system, because this system bears the brunt of HIV infection. In chapter 4, AIDS is defined by its official case definition, and its development and symptoms are outlined in detail. In chapter 5, the epidemiology and transmission of AIDS are discussed, followed by a chapter on the means for preventing transmission (chapter 6).

The biology of AIDS continues in chapter 7 with focus on the diagnosis and testing methods used for detecting HIV. In chapter 8, the currently available treatments for AIDS and HIV infection are surveyed; then the prospects for an AIDS vaccine are summarized in chapter 9. The book closes in chapter 10 by placing AIDS in a social perspective and describing the multiple ramifications that the epidemic has on day-to-day living.

It is reasonably safe to say that a book can be excellent on facts but less than adequate in its ability to teach. I hope that this book will be a teaching tool for you, and to help your learning efforts, I have incorporated several features:

1. Each chapter has a chapter outline to let you know how the main topic will be approached and what the sequence of subtopics will be.

2. At the beginning of each chapter there is a section entitled Looking Ahead. This section presents five broad objectives that you should be able to achieve by studying the chapter.

3. Pronunciations of difficult terms appear at the end of the book, grouped by chapter, to increase your familiarity with the terms and your confidence in using them.

4. A glossary at the end of the book provides definitions of key terms culled from the text to give you a quick refresher.

5. A series of boxes explores topics allied to the main topic and gives further insight to the information at hand.

6. The Healthline series poses more that 100 questions often asked about AIDS and gives brief answers.

7. At the conclusion of each chapter, a section entitled Looking Back presents a review of the main points and important concepts.

8. The Review section in each chapter is a self-test to assess the extent of your learning. A variety of formats are used for the quizzes. Answers are in Appendix A.

9. Additional readings in each chapter suggest further references that are accessible at most local libraries.

Acknowledgments

Though authors traditionally receive the credit (and sometimes, vilification) for a book such as this, the fact is that many talented individuals contribute to the final product. At Jones and Bartlett Publishers, Clayton Jones saw the wisdom of adding this book to an already impressive list published by the company, and Steve Weaver and Dean DeChambeau handled the editorial phase of the project with professional care and confidence. Lou Bruno lent a deft and experienced hand to the production, and Rebecca Seastrong ensured that every i was dotted and every t was crossed. I especially want to thank my long-time friend John Lennox for his invaluable suggestions and corrections to the final draft of this revision. Numerous other professionals added their expertise to this book, and I extend my kudos to them.

Fall 2002

E. Alcamo

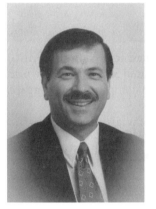

Publisher's Note: Professor Ed Alcamo passed away in December of 2002 after an all-too-brief battle with cancer. Ed was a dedicated educator, prolific author, and a good friend, and his passing leaves a great void in many, many, lives.

The AIDS Epidemic

LOOKING AHEAD

This opening chapter introduces acquired immune deficiency syndrome (AIDS) by exploring the development of its epidemic in the United States and the world and by describing the research to uncover its cause. On completing the chapter, you should be able to . . .

- Understand the conditions that led public health officials to realize that an epidemic of AIDS was in progress.

- Recognize some broad features of AIDS and characterize the individuals at risk for the disease.

- Summarize the research leading to the isolation and identification of the AIDS virus.

- Conceptualize the transmission of the AIDS virus from chimpanzees to humans.

- Discuss some theories for the origin of the AIDS epidemic and its spread in the United States and the world.

- Note the current magnitude of the AIDS epidemic and describe where it is likely to spread in the future.

INTRODUCTION

There is an oft-told fable about six blind men invited to examine an elephant. The first man, falling against the elephant's side, claimed it was a wall; the second, seizing a leg, declared the elephant a tree; another, grasping a tusk, thought the elephant was a spear; the fourth man, grabbing the trunk, decided he was holding a snake; the fifth, touching the ear, believed it to be a fan; and the last blind man, holding the tail, proclaimed the elephant a rope (Figure 1.1).

So it was in the early 1980s with AIDS: The elephant was the disease, and the blind men were the scientists and doctors grappling with its emergence in an epidemic. Without a clear vision of AIDS, they were forced to treat the epidemic piecemeal, to try and explain each bit of knowledge as it came forth.

Physicians were seeing patients whose immune systems were profoundly suppressed, but they had no idea what was causing this problem; public health officers were charting the course of the AIDS epidemic without knowing its cause; manufacturers were searching out new drug therapies, but they were unsure what they were trying to eliminate.

During the first years of the epidemic, the AIDS elephant loomed large. Physicians saw it as a medical problem, economists as a potential disaster to the health care system, employers as a threat to the smooth operation of their businesses, health care workers as a problem requiring personal protection, and politicians as yet another drain on public funds. Until 1984, there was no clear definition of AIDS. No test was available to confirm a diagnosis, and no cure was in sight. Most scientists agreed that a cure would follow only after they found a cause and understood the natural history of the disease.

Despite the pessimism, however, researchers were beginning to unravel the mysteries of AIDS, and a sense of optimism was beginning to surface. In the pages ahead, we shall follow the evolution of the AIDS epidemic over its first two decades, while charting the discoveries made during that period. Although the AIDS elephant remains somewhat elusive, our vision of it has improved considerably.

The Early Years

By 1981, most observers believed that infectious diseases were largely under control in the Western world. There had been no smallpox anywhere since October 1977, and diseases such as typhoid fever, polio, and whooping cough were rarely encountered. Even childhood diseases such as measles, mumps, and rubella appeared to be relics of the past. Indeed, the speed with which an effective therapy for Legionnaires' disease was discovered in 1976 and the success in interrupting the outbreak of toxic shock syndrome in 1978 had strengthened public confidence that scientists could defeat any epidemic.

Moreover, in the early 1980s, American researchers had largely turned away from the negative aspects of microorganisms and were pursuing their practical uses. For instance, bacteria had become mainstays of genetic engineering, which was fast developing as the technology of the future. (A 1981 article in Time magazine described genetic engineering as "the most powerful and awesome skill acquired by man since the splitting of the atom.") Genetically engineered insulin was already in production, synthetic vaccines were in the planning stage, and breathtaking developments in DNA technology were in the headlines daily. The mood of the day was optimism.

The First Observations

On June 5, 1981, the Centers for Disease Control and Prevention (CDC) published a brief but significant article in its weekly bulletin, *Morbidity and Mortality Weekly Report (MMWR)*. The article, appear-

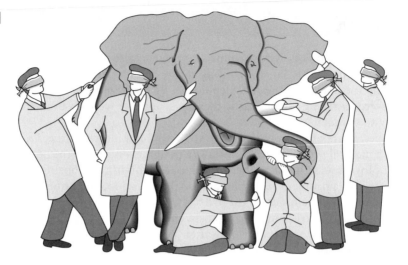

A fable tells of six blind men (seen here as blindfolded) invited to examine an elephant and report what they believed it to be. Each touched the elephant at a different part and reported something completely unlike the others. In the early years of the AIDS epidemic, physicians, researchers, and members of the general public saw disease in different ways, much as different blind men perceived the elephant.

Healthline 1.1

1 **Q** Exactly what is AIDS?

A Defining AIDS can be difficult because AIDS is a complex disease. Basically, AIDS is an infectious disease in which a virus attacks cells of the immune system and thereby renders the body susceptible to microorganisms that otherwise would be held in check. The virus also destroys brain cells. Symptoms of AIDS can be very general (fever, weight loss, night sweats, diarrhea), or they can be more specific (pneumonia, skin cancer). Multiple stages of AIDS are recognized, beginning with infection by the virus, progressing to "early AIDS," and culminating with full-blown AIDS.

2 **Q** Suppose AIDS had been first recognized in 1961 instead of 1981. What might have happened?

A Things would have been considerably different had AIDS made its

ing between discussions of dengue fever and measles, described the case reports of five young men treated at three different hospitals in Los Angeles, California. All five men were sexually active and gay, and all five were suffering from pneumocystosis (also known as *Pneumocystis carinii* pneumonia). This lung disease is caused by the protozoan *Pneumocystis carinii* and is characterized by progressive suffocation as the lungs fill with fluid. By the time of the article's publication, two of the five patients had died.

In the CDC article, the writer observed that three of the patients had "profoundly depressed numbers of thymus-dependent lymphocyte cells and profoundly depressed . . . responses to mitogens and antigens." Because lymphocyte cells are components of the immune system and because responses to mitogens and antigens are among the important functions of the immune system, it was apparent that the patients' immune systems were under stress. Then, in perhaps *the* understatement of 1981, the writer noted: "The occurrence of pneumocystosis in these five previously healthy individuals with underlying immunodeficiency is unusual."

The CDC article of June 5, 1981 is considered a benchmark—the unofficial beginning of the AIDS epidemic in the United States (Healthline 1.1). Statistics were compiled from that date onward, and physicians were alerted to watch for similar cases and report them to their state health departments. The health departments then forwarded the reports to the CDC (Box 1.1).

And such reports arrived quickly. On July 3, 1981, another article appeared in the CDC's *MMWR*, this time describing

Kaposi's sarcoma as well as *Pneumocystis carinii* pneumonia in 26 young homosexual men. Twenty patients were from New York City, and six lived in California. All had been diagnosed during the previous 30 months. Kaposi's sarcoma is normally a relatively mild skin cancer affecting mainly older men of Mediterranean descent, but in these 26 patients, it was aggressive and deadly, with skin and mucous membrane lesions of blue to violet color (Figure 1.2). In ten of the patients, the Kaposi's sarcoma was accompanied by *Pneumocystis carinii* pneumonia. In several others, doctors reported diseases not normally observed in persons with functional immune systems. This article did not comment on the patients' immune systems. It did, however, encourage physicians to continue reporting similar cases.

Because the new disease appeared to be affecting primarily homosexual men, scientists asked what practices might be unique in the homosexual community. They postulated that amyl nitrate, a drug used by some homosexual men to increase sexual pleasure, might be at fault, or perhaps certain disease organisms prevalent in homosexual men might be to blame. One such organism, the cytomegalovirus, was a prime candidate. Another theory was that the immune systems of the homosexual patients had been suppressed by a constant barrage of sexually transmitted diseases. In some publications, the disease was given the pejorative name gay-related immune deficiency (GRID). The idea of a transmissible infectious disease had not yet taken hold.

Then data about further victims began to filter in. Late in 1981, the CDC received reports of heroin addicts and other injection drug users in New York City who were suffering from *Pneumocystis carinii* pneumonia and immune deficiency (Figure 1.3). By early 1982, it appeared that heterosexuals could transmit the disease to one another; and within months, the disease surfaced among blood transfusion recipients and hemophiliacs. By June 11, 1982, the CDC had details on 355 cases from five different states (California, Florida, New Jersey, New York, and Texas). The clustering of cases within several groups and the pattern of spread made it apparent that a transmissible agent, probably a virus, was involved.

On September 3, 1982, the disease was given a new name. In the *MMWR* of that date, the CDC, acting on a recommendation from biologist Bruce Voeller, noted that "the group of clinical entities, along with its specific immune deficiency, is now called acquired immune deficiency syndrome (AIDS)." The thrust of the article, however, was a warning that a hepatitis B vaccine in use at the time might be a possible agent of transmission and should be used with caution. It was a type of warning that was becoming commonplace whenever blood or blood products were involved.

By early 1983, 16 countries were reporting AIDS cases, and more than 1000 Americans from 34 states had been diagnosed with the disease (more than

appearance in 1961. For one thing, knowledge of the immune system was primitive by 1980s standards, and studying the effects of the AIDS virus would have been very difficult. Also, retroviruses were unknown at the time, and the study of viruses was only in its early stages. Moreover, the technology for virology was barely developed. If AIDS had appeared in 1961, investigators would have been able to track the disease but do little more.

Q Suppose AIDS had surfaced in 2001 instead of 1981. What would be different?

A If AIDS had broken out in 2001, the technology for detecting viruses would have been more highly advanced, so the AIDS virus could have been pinpointed more quickly. In 1981, a few antiviral drugs were available; by 2001, drug technology was better developed, so a useful anti-AIDS drug could have been located more quickly. And synthetic vaccines for some diseases were already available by 1987, so AIDS vaccine research would have been more focused in 2001. A useful analogy can be made with Legionnaires' disease, a respiratory illness first detected in 1976. Within a month, scientists located an antibiotic to control the disease, and within six months, they identified the responsible bacterium.

FIGURE 1.2

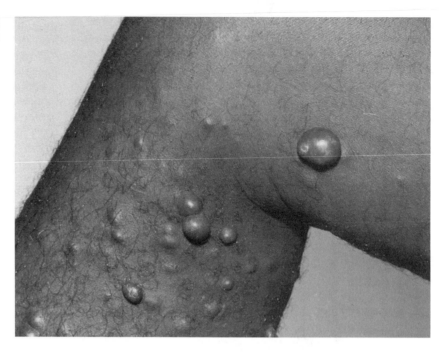

An AIDS patient displaying the skin lesions of Kaposi's sarcoma on his legs. Kaposi's sarcoma is normally a mild skin cancer, but in persons with AIDS, it is aggressive and can be a cause of death.

FIGURE 1.3

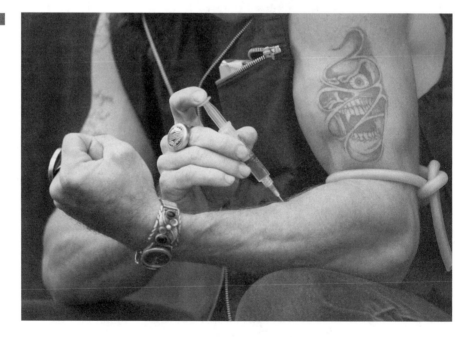

One of the methods by which the AIDS virus is known to spread is through sharing of blood-contaminated syringes and needles. Injection drug users who use contaminated "works" are at risk for AIDS. In this photograph, an unidentified man is injecting heroine.

BOX
1.1

The Centers for Disease Control and Prevention

The Centers for Disease Control and Prevention (CDC), one of six major agencies of the U.S. Public Health Service, has its headquarters in Atlanta, Georgia. Originally established as the Communicable Disease Center in 1946, the CDC was the first governmental health organization ever set up to coordinate a national control program against infectious diseases. At first, it was concerned with diseases spread from person to person, from animals to people, or from the environment to humans. Eventually, though, all communicable diseases came under its aegis. Atlanta was selected as the site for the CDC because it was a convenient central point for the study of malaria, which was then common in the South.

In April 1955, two weeks after release of the Salk vaccine for polio, the CDC received reports of six cases of polio in vaccinated children. Two days later, it established the Polio Surveillance Unit and began collecting data on the occurrence of polio and summarizing it for health professionals. More than 80 percent of vaccine-associated polio cases were related to a single manufacturer, whose vaccine was withdrawn at once. This incident established the role of the CDC in health emergencies, and soon it became a national resource for the development and dissemination of information on communicable diseases. In 1960, the CDC moved its headquarters to a new complex adjoining Emory University. The unassuming appearance of the facility belies its importance.

Reorganized under its current name in 1980 (the words "and Prevention" were added in 1992, but the CDC acronym was retained), the CDC is charged with protecting the public health of the U.S. population by providing leadership and direction in the prevention and control of infectious disease and other preventable conditions, such as cancer. It is concerned with urban rat control, quarantine measures, health education, and the upgrading and licensing of clinical laboratories. The CDC also provides international consultation on disease and participates with other nations in the control and eradication of communicable infections. It employs 3500 physicians and scientists, the largest such group in the world, and processes 170,000 samples of tissue annually. Its publication *Morbidity and Mortality Weekly Report* is distributed each week to over 100,000 health professionals.

half of these patients had died by that time). Also in 1983, physicians in Newark, New Jersey, and New York City reported the first cases of what appeared to be mother-to-child transmission of AIDS. Concern also mounted that the nation's supply of blood in blood banks was contaminated. One public health administrator wrote of a "nightmare time bomb ticking away in the blood supply." Privately, the CDC (Box 1.1) began pressuring blood suppliers to consider ways of protecting the public. But without knowing what the agent was and how it was transmitted, blood banks were unable to take meaningful action.

Alarm climbed a notch higher when a woman in California contracted AIDS through sexual intercourse with her husband, who suffered from hemophilia. The woman then passed the disease to her newborn child. It was becoming apparent

1 Q I've heard that AIDS is caused by a virus. Can you explain what a virus is?

A A virus is one of the smallest microorganisms known. It consists of a segment of nucleic acid (such as DNA) surrounded by a coat of protein and, in some cases, an enclosing membrane. Viruses do not grow, utilize food, or perform any metabolic processes associated with living things. Inside cells, however, they multiply very efficiently.

2 Q Exactly what is the immune system?

A The immune system is a network of cells and a group of chemical compounds largely responsible for the body's defense against infectious disease, cancer, and other maladies. The system is distributed throughout the body, primarily in the spleen and the lymph nodes of the neck, armpits, and groin. Certain cells of the immune system produce highly specific proteins known as antibodies, which interact with and neutralize microorganisms. Other immune system cells attack microorganisms directly.

3 Q Where did AIDS come from?

A No one can be absolutely certain where AIDS originated, but the prevailing wisdom is that the AIDS virus existed in chimpanzees and then crossed the species barrier to infect humans in West Africa, possibly when a human suffered a bite or scratch from a chimpanzee. Movement of individuals from that isolated population to an urban center may have brought the virus into a wider population.

to the general public that anyone could be at risk. Whatever fantasies Americans had that AIDS was exclusively a disease of homosexual men and injection drug users were clearly over.

The Breakthrough

For the first three years of the AIDS epidemic, the number of diagnosed cases doubled about every six months. To many observers, every six months also brought a new theory of the epidemic's cause. As noted above, some scientists initially related the disease to use of amyl nitrate or to immune system depression by a variety of diseases, but these ideas were soon discarded. Certain scientists held to the belief that the agent was the virus that causes African swine fever, since this virus can induce immune suppression in pigs (a temporary alert on undercooked pork was issued); others believed that the agent was a "slow virus," one that apparently multiplies at an extremely low rate in the body and manifests itself after years or more.

At the fringe were a number of other beliefs. One group maintained that the agent was a viral escapee from a genetics engineering laboratory; another attributed it to a failed biological war against Cuba; and still another suggested that AIDS was due to mutations arising from "secret Soviet Union electromagnetic warfare against the United States." Eventually, though, most scientists focused on a virus as the most likely cause of AIDS (Healthline 1.2). Some opponents were quick to point out, however, that such an assumption had been erroneous before. In the previous decade, they noted, scientists had assumed that viruses were responsible for Legionnaires' disease, Lyme disease, and toxic shock syndrome. In each case, the agent was eventually shown to be a bacterium.

By 1982, two cancer research laboratories were involved in the hunt for an AIDS agent. At the Pasteur Institute in Paris, a group led by Luc Montagnier was intrigued by the possibility that the mysterious AIDS agent could also be the cause of Kaposi's sarcoma. In the United States, at the National Cancer Institute, a team headed by Robert C. Gallo was attempting to prove that AIDS was due to a retrovirus similar to certain other viruses related to cancer. In May 1983, both the Gallo and Montagnier groups published reports hinting that they had found the virus responsible for AIDS. There was a sense of excitement in the medical community.

Then, on April 23, 1984, at a press conference in Washington, D.C., Gallo announced that his group had identified a virus in the blood of 48 persons with AIDS. In addition, he and his colleagues found antibodies to the virus in blood samples from 88 percent of all those diagnosed as having AIDS. Gallo recommended that the virus be named human T-cell lymphotropic virus type III (HTLV-III). Four articles in the May 4, 1983 issue of the highly respected magazine *Science* carried the details of the research performed by Gallo's group.

Before the articles in *Science* appeared, however, the Montagnier group rushed to call attention to their work on an AIDS virus. In interviews with the international press, Montagnier described a virus that his team had located in the blood of patients with the early manifestations of AIDS. Like the Americans, the French researchers reported evidence of the virus in more than 80 percent of blood samples from AIDS patients. Montagnier's group suggested that the virus be called lymphadenopathy-associated virus (LAV). The virus appeared to be identical to that isolated by the Americans.

In the months that followed, a rivalry developed between the American and French groups, each claiming to have isolated the virus first. At issue were international awards, research grants, and millions—perhaps billions—of dollars in patent rights for products that might be derived using the AIDS virus, such as an AIDS test. Time did little to sort out the differences between the groups, and the scientific community began referring to the virus as HTLV-III/LAV (in France, it was called LAV/HTLV-III). By February 1985, the American and French teams reported that their viruses were virtually identical. Montagnier and Gallo received much international acclaim (Figure 1.4).

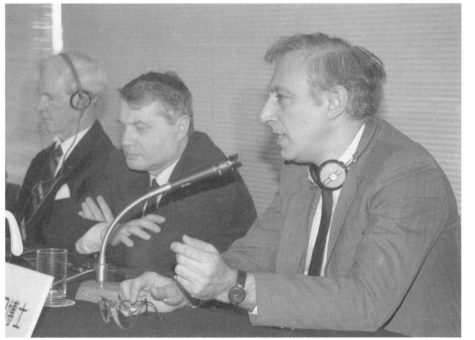

FIGURE 1.4

Robert C. Gallo (right) and Luc Montagnier (center), the American and French researchers who performed much of the seminal work leading to identification of the human immunodeficiency virus. In this 1988 photograph, the two researchers are speaking at a news conference in Japan at which they were jointly honored.

Then, in 1991, Gallo conceded that the virus he identified had originated in tissue samples sent to him by Montagnier. Gallo explained that inadvertent contamination had probably allowed the French virus to enter the tissue samples with which his team was working and from which the American virus was eventually isolated. There followed months of accusation and innuendo, as well as federal charges of scientific misconduct, but Gallo continued to perform high-quality research on AIDS. Indeed, between 1989 and 1993, his name appeared on 191 scientific publications, and his work was cited more than 2000 times by other researchers. In late 1993, all federal charges of scientific misconduct were withdrawn, apparently because the criteria for handling such cases were too restrictive; that is, the accusing agency was required to prove that Gallo's statements made in scientific papers were false, that they were deliberately intended to deceive, and that they had a material effect on the conclusions of the paper. A final chapter in this dispute was written in 1994, when the U.S. government conceded that France's Pasteur Institute deserved a higher percentage of patent royalties from AIDS tests that utilize the virus, since the Pasteur Institute had gained greater recognition for its role in discovering the virus. Under the new arrangement, the French government receives 50 percent of the royalty monies, the U.S. government 25 percent, and the World AIDS Foundation 25 percent. (The World AIDS Foundation funds AIDS research in the developing world.)

Isolation of the AIDS virus had many positive ramifications. One prominent immunologist was quick to proclaim, "What matters is that now we know the face of the enemy." In a more practical sense, it became possible to develop a test to detect the virus in individuals and in the world's blood supply. Indeed, in April 1985, Gallo's group announced development of a blood test for AIDS, and by May 1985, the test was perfected and in use. The test was so effective that over the next five years, only four cases of AIDS were linked to transfused blood.

The year 1986 brought a name change for the AIDS virus. That summer, an international commission of prominent virologists and molecular biologists recommended that the name of the virus be changed from HTLV-III/LAV to the human immunodeficiency virus, or HIV. The commission noted that the new name conforms to common nomenclature for related viruses, that it does not incorporate the term AIDS (because HIV could cause other diseases), that it was chosen without regard to priority of discovery, and that it allows for further names as strains are isolated. Acceptance of the commission's recommendation and confirmation by the scientific community brought one phase of the AIDS saga to an end (Figure 1.5).

Another AIDS Virus

No sooner had HIV been identified than another human immunodeficiency virus emerged. Identified in 1985 by Pasteur Institute scientists led by Luc Montagnier, this virus was designated HIV-2, and the original strain began to be referred to as HIV-1. Blood tests have shown that HIV-2 is rare in the United States but relatively common in parts of Africa, especially West Africa. The virus infects macaque monkeys and baboons, and because its genetic structure and that of HIV-1 match

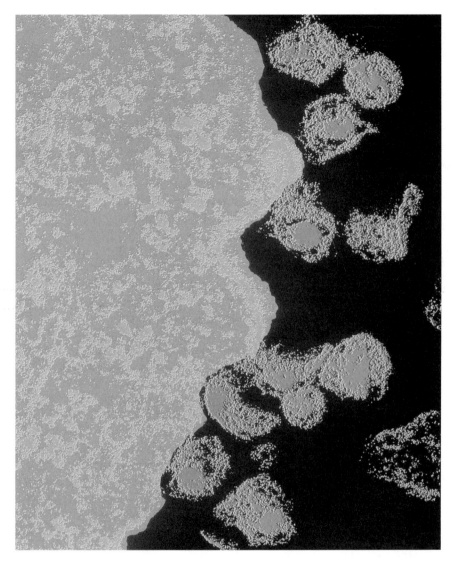

FIGURE 1.5
The human immunodeficiency virus (HIV). This electron micrograph of an infected cell and HIV shows a cross-section of a lymphocyte of the immune system. HIV appears in two stages: the mature stage, having emerged from the cell; and the immature stage, as budding particles in the process of completing their passage out of the cell.

for 40 percent of their makeup, the interaction between HIV-2 and these animals could be used as a model to study the interaction of HIV-1 with human cells.

HIV-2 appears to cause a milder disease than HIV-1, as reported by a Harvard University study. Researchers studied 574 women from Dakar, Senegal, and found that five years after infection, one-third of the women infected with HIV-1 had progressed to AIDS, while none of those infected with HIV-2 had any sign of AIDS. Moreover, the destruction of immune system cells was substantially more extensive in those with HIV-1 than in those with HIV-2. Of course, the possibility exists that HIV-2 could take longer to develop in humans than HIV-1 or that HIV-2 has entered human populations more recently than HIV-1. Either possibility could explain the relative mildness of the disease caused by HIV-2. It is also possible that some form of natural resistance to HIV-2 accounts for the mildness. This possibility has spurred researchers to study closely the interaction between humans and HIV-2.

A Pandemic

In 1985, reports from health officers in Africa indicated that the AIDS epidemic was widespread on that continent. Fearing stigmatization, some African government officials at first sought to distance themselves and to deny that AIDS was occurring in their countries. However, the signs of AIDS were unmistakable: Thousands of men and women were affected with severe weight loss, emaciation, and disrupted immune systems. And the epidemic was spreading; indeed, it had become worldwide—a pandemic.

Within three years, international health officials recognized that Africa was the continent hit hardest by AIDS. The disease was present not only in homosexual men (more specifically, men who have sex with men) and injection drug users but also in heterosexual men and women, where it appeared to spread by sexual contact.

But AIDS was not confined to Africa. By 1988, almost 5000 cases were reported in Europe, and scientists estimated that between 500,000 and 1 million individuals from European countries were infected with HIV. In Asia, the situation was becoming increasingly severe, and in Australia, AIDS was spreading as fast as in the United States and Europe.

Two years previously, in 1986, the World Health Organization (WHO) had established its Global Program on AIDS. Under the direction of Jonathan Mann, the program began carefully to overcome national sensitivities and gain the confidence of the world's health leaders. Soon it was receiving reports from regional offices and the ministries of health of 175 countries. By 1988, 138 of those countries had reported at least one case of AIDS, and many had more than 1000 total cases. Figure 1.6 shows the status of the pandemic ten years later.

As the leader of the world's health community, the WHO continues to chart the development of the AIDS epidemic all over the globe. The WHO also supports the development of national AIDS prevention and control programs in more than 120 countries throughout the world. In addition, it collects information about cases and maintains a virus bank, since HIV strains from different parts of the world can vary somewhat in their biochemistry. Finally, it makes recommendations on international travel and related issues and serves as a forum for discussing the scientific and practical implications of the AIDS pandemic.

Supplementing the WHO's work is the United Nations Programme on HIV/AIDS (UNAIDS), a joint effort of various subdivisions of the United Nations, including the United Nations Children's Fund. Established in 1995 and currently under the direction of Peter Piot, the UNAIDS coordinates the UN's efforts in dealing with the AIDS pandemic. Among other activities, the program works with governments of the world to channel resources, identify directions for global research, and implement educational initiatives.

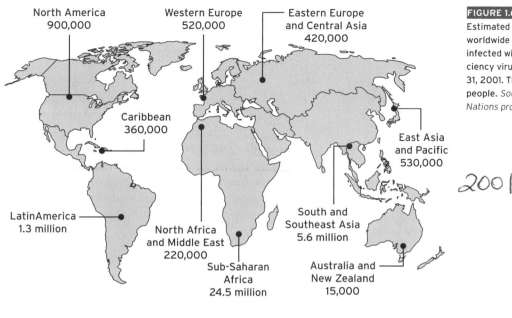

North America
900,000

Western Europe
520,000

Eastern Europe
and Central Asia
420,000

Caribbean
360,000

East Asia
and Pacific
530,000

LatinAmerica
1.3 million

North Africa
and Middle East
220,000

South and
Southeast Asia
5.6 million

Sub-Saharan
Africa
24.5 million

Australia and
New Zealand
15,000

2001

FIGURE 1.6

Estimated numbers of individuals worldwide suffering AIDS or infected with human immunodeficiency virus (HIV) as of December 31, 2001. The total is 40 million people. *Source: Data from United Nations program on HIV/AIDS.*

Origin of the AIDS Epidemic

40,000,000 infected in the world right now

Throughout recorded history, epidemics have sprung up to ravage human populations. In the American swine influenza epidemic of 1918–1919, for example, more than 20 million people died, a figure comparable to mortality during the infamous Black Death in Europe in the 1300s. Although the source of the influenza epidemic was never found, other outbreaks of disease have defined origins. For instance, when the Spanish arrived in the Americas in 1520, they brought smallpox with them. The Aztec population of Mexico was without any immunity to this disease, and the raging smallpox epidemic that followed reduced that population by half. The sources of some other epidemics are also clear. When the first European navigators reached South Pacific islands in the 1700s, they found the people robust, happy, and well adapted to their environment. But the explorers introduced syphilis, tuberculosis, and whooping cough (pertussis), and these diseases swept through the population virtually unchecked. Hawaii was struck especially hard. When Captain Cook landed there in 1778, the island's population was about 300,000; by 1860, it had been reduced to fewer than 37,000.

These examples are somewhat reminiscent of the course of AIDS during the twentieth century. The disease seemed to burst on the scene during the early 1980s and spread out from central foci in major cities of the United States and Africa and other parts of the world. Setting aside claims that HIV is an entirely new virus or the product of a genetic engineering lab, the prevailing hypothesis among scientists is that the virus existed somewhere in nature and emerged at this particular period in history to infect human populations. In this section, we explore where it may have originated and why it came forth at that particular time.

The Origin of HIV

If we assume that HIV existed somewhere in the world prior to its appearance in humans, then the next logical question is "Where?" During the mid-1980s, Max Essex of Harvard's School of Public Health was among the first to provide evidence that HIV originated in African primates such as monkeys, baboons, and chimpanzees. Essex's research resulted in recovery of a virus called the simian immunodeficiency virus (SIV) from African green monkeys (Figure 1.7a). This virus had enough biochemical similarities to HIV to support the notion that the two viruses are related. Essex and his group theorized that SIV may have crossed the species barrier to humans through a primate bite or scratch.

Further evidence for a primate-human transmission was offered by evidence that HIV-2 crossed the species barrier to humans from the sooty mangabey, a type of monkey belonging to the species *Cercocebus atys* (Figure 1.7b). This link was established in the early 1990s by Vanessa Hirsh, a primate researcher at the National Institute of Allergy and Infectious Diseases. Hirsh demonstrated that the SIVsm, the SIV strain from the sooty mangabey, has genes nearly identical to those of HIV-2. Research performed by British scientists indicated that SIVsm from the sooty mangabey monkey may have caused six HIV-2 epidemics, which blended together to give the impression of a single West African epidemic.

The research of Essex and Hirsh was expanded and further developed by a host of other scientists, notably the group led by Beatrice Hahn of the University of Alabama at Birmingham. In 1999, Hahn and her coworkers pieced together

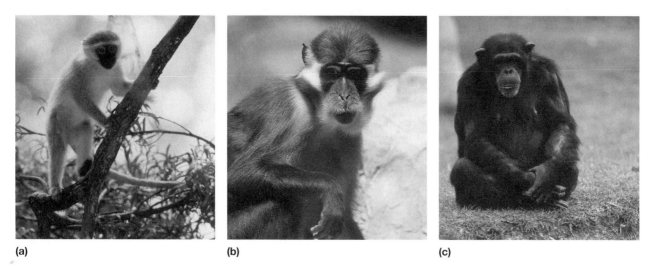

(a) (b) (c)

FIGURE 1.7

(a) The African green monkey. The simian immunodeficiency virus (SIV), a virus similar to the human immunodeficiency virus was recovered from such an animal in the mid-1980s. (b) The sooty mangabey monkey, believed to be the source of HIV-2 in humans. (c) The chimpanzee *Pan troglodytes troglodytes*, which is believed to be the source of HIV-1 in humans.

what was hailed as the best case yet for connecting human HIV to chimpanzees (Figure 1.7c). Their research indicates that different subspecies of chimpanzees harbor different strains of HIV-like viruses and that one particular subspecies is the probable source of the HIV-1 (the "original" HIV) that is causing the current pandemic.

Before Hahn's work, scientists had identified only three chimpanzees infected with simian immunodeficiency viruses (SIVs). The strains of SIV in these animals were designated SIVcpz. Then Hahn's group identified a fourth chimpanzee infected with a strain of SIVcpz. The researchers began an exhaustive and systematic study to carefully examine these SIV strains and the four animals from which they came. The study focused on the nucleic acid of the virus, one of its major chemical components and the substance of which its genes are made. Using sophisticated genetic analyses, Hahn's group compared the nucleic acid content (the genes) of the four SIVcpz strains with that of various samples of HIV obtained from humans.

The results of the research were the key to the origin of HIV: Three of the four SIVcpz strains were found to be closely related (i.e., 70 to 90 percent genetically identical) to HIV particles isolated from humans. All three strains came from the chimpanzee *Pan troglodytes troglodytes*. Significantly, the natural range of the chimpanzee *Pan troglodytes troglodytes* coincides precisely with regions of West Africa where the AIDS epidemic has existed for the longest period of time. The fourth SIVcpz strain had a nucleic acid content (genes) much less similar to that of HIV; importantly, it came from the chimpanzee *Pan troglodytes schweinfurthii* normally found in far-distant East Africa. Hahn's group concluded that chimpanzees living in Gabon, Cameroon, and nearby regions of West Africa were the source of HIV-1 in humans. They surmised that once the virus made its way into humans, it mutated into the existing strains scientists now recognize, while adapting naturally to its new host. We shall discuss when this crossover presumably happened in the next section.

Hahn's research has several key implications, not the least of which is that it apparently resolves the question of HIV's origin. Moreover, the three SIV strains found in *Pan troglodytes troglodytes* are the presumed forerunners of the three groups of HIV-1 now known to exist (Chapter 2 discusses these groups). This finding indicates that chimpanzees have been the starting point for at least three independent crossings to humans. It is reasonable to believe that these cross-species transmissions occurred when humans who hunted and butchered chimpanzees for meat were exposed to their blood via a wound or scratch. Moreover, additional transmissions may have occurred and may still be occurring because the hunting and killing of chimpanzees continues in western equatorial Africa.

The significance of the research is further underscored by the observation that chimpanzees in the wild apparently do not develop AIDS, even though the genetic material of humans and chimpanzees is 98.5 percent identical. Thus, investigators hope to locate a resistance mechanism in the animals that can be applied to humans. It should be noted, however, that strengthening the human-chimpanzee link will require finding SIVcpz in wild chimpanzee populations. To do that, a concerted effort will be launched to save these endangered animals for study.

To further study the human-primate link, researchers began to try to determine whether SIV exists in wild baboons and monkeys of varying species. Results reported in 2001 strengthened that link. Investigators led by Beatrice Hahn and Eric Delaporte collected blood samples from 384 wild primates representing 17 species. They found that 18 percent of the primates harbor SIV antibodies that bind strongly to HIV proteins. The finding indicates that other variants of SIV occur in wild primates and are capable of making the crossover to humans. Thus, many subtypes of SIV could continue to pose risks for humans so long as these animals are hunted for meat or kept as pets.

The Jump to Humans

Scientists now generally agree that a strain of simian immunodeficiency virus (SIV) made the crossing from chimpanzees to humans and later evolved to the current strains of HIV. Exactly when the crossing occurred is uncertain, but an estimate appears to be provided by analysis of the HIV obtained from the oldest documented case of infection. The analysis shows that the passage to humans probably occurred during the late 1940s or early 1950s.

The research leading to this conclusion was performed by Toufo Zhu of the University of Washington and David Ho of New York's Aaron Diamond AIDS Research Center. The scientists began with the insight that about 1 percent of HIV's genetic material mutates each year. Then they analyzed HIV fragments obtained from the blood of a Bantu man who lived in what is now Kinshasa in the Democratic Republic of the Congo. The blood had been drawn in 1959 shortly before the man died.

Although evidence of HIV had been observed in the man's blood in 1986 by Max Essex, the methods for studying HIV's genetic material were not then sophisticated enough to gain much information. But in 1998, Zhu and Ho used state-of-the-art technology to multiply the genetic material of HIV available in the blood many millions of times (thus yielding a sufficient supply to work with). Then, using extensive databases and advanced computers, they compared the genetic material from the 1959 HIV to genetic material from current strains of HIV as well as strains of HIV isolated during many intervening years. The comparisons yielded a "family tree" of HIV showing the progression of changes occurring in its genetic material over a 39-year period. The data indicated that HIV probably entered the human population after World War II had ended, as noted above. This estimate is important because it renders unlikely a hypothesis that the AIDS epidemic originated in the 1950s from contaminated lots of polio vaccine (Box 1.2).

Moreover, the finding is more than a historical footnote. Comparing the 1959 virus with modern forms yields information on how extensively HIV has evolved over the decades and how much it can be expected to evolve in future years. This

BOX
1.2

A Controversy

The controversy apparently began with a 1992 article in *Rolling Stone* magazine by journalist Tom Curtis and gathered momentum with a 1999 book by science writer Edward Hooper entitled *The River: A Journey to the Source of HIV and AIDS*. Both Curtis and Hooper theorized that the AIDS epidemic was ignited when an oral polio vaccine was tested in the late 1950s on hundreds of volunteers in what is now the Democratic Republic of the Congo. Hooper contended that the vaccine was contaminated with simian immunodeficiency virus (SIV), which infects monkeys, chimpanzees, and other primates. The contamination occurred, according to Hooper's research, when kidney cells from infected chimpanzees were used to cultivate the polio virus. In the book, he posits that the earliest cases of AIDS occurred where and when the vaccine was tested.

One of the leaders of the 1950s campaign against polio was Hilary Koprowski from the Wistar Institute in Philadelphia. Answering the hypotheses of Curtis and Hooper, Koprowski maintained that to make the polio vaccine his group used cells from Asian macaque monkeys rather than chimpanzees. He pointed out that samples of the vaccine were preserved in freezers at the Institute and suggested that they be analyzed.

Three independent laboratories were hired to make the analyses. One lab analyzed the DNA in a vaccine sample to determine whether the DNA was from a macaque monkey or a chimpanzee—the results indicated that it was from a macaque monkey. A second lab tested the vaccine sample for genes associated with either HIV or SIV—genes for neither virus were found. A third lab ran tests duplicating those performed by the other two labs—its results confirmed theirs. Augmenting these results were testimonials from 16 of Koprowski's collaborators who stated that they never worked with chimpanzee cells. Moreover, evidence from genetic analyses indicates an origin of HIV in humans that predates the 1950s. These analyses also show that chimpanzees from the region where Koprowski worked do not harbor the SIV that was the ancestor of HIV.

In his book, Hooper made the point of calling for analysis of the archived vaccine samples, as Koprowski offered. However, when the results were reported, and even though they countered his hypothesis, Hooper refused to retract his theory. By contrast, *Rolling Stone* printed a "clarification" in 1993, and Koprowski won a lawsuit against the magazine claiming defamation of character.

data helped in linking HIV to SIV in chimpanzees because Hahn's group could compare the genes of the 1959 virus with those of SIV and search for common features. In addition, identifying when HIV entered the human population puts a time frame on the start of the AIDS epidemic, and by examining social trends of the period, public health officials can understand why the epidemic exploded as rapidly as it did (which we discuss below).

Finally, knowing about the early form of the virus could conceivably help scientists pinpoint the parts of HIV's genetic material that have changed the least, a finding that would assist vaccine researchers. One problem in HIV vaccine research is how to produce a vaccine that can be effective against the multiple strains of HIV known to exist. A vaccine based on features common between ancestral and modern forms might prove more universal in fighting a global epidemic than a vaccine based on a combination of modern types. This and other salient problems associated with vaccine development are explored in Chapter 9.

It is important to note that genetic analyses like this one are used to calculate the dates when strains of an organism mutate and split off from the ancestral strain. At best, this analysis gives an estimate of when the HIV lineage began to diversify, not necessarily when the virus was transmitted to humans. An example of the uncertainty of the data is illustrated by research reported in 2000. A genetic analysis performed by scientists (Chapter 2) indicates that the M group of HIV (the group that causes the vast majority of AIDS cases) came into existence in 1931, with a 95 percent confidence interval of 1915 to 1941. Although this period broadly coincides with the dates deduced in earlier analyses, a slight deviation exists. For this reason, it is important to avoid broad generalizations until the research results have been verified.

Out of Africa

Working on the assumption that HIV made the jump from chimpanzees to Africans somewhere between the 1930s and early 1950s, the next question is "Why did AIDS become such an explosive pandemic in the following years?"

No one knows for sure, but historians point out that the 1960s and 1970s were decades of great turmoil in Africa when the epidemic could have easily gathered momentum. Civil wars were commonplace, national boundaries were redrawn, and population shifts were unprecedented. Demographers note that millions of people in Africa changed from an agrarian lifestyle to an urban lifestyle. It is conceivable that infected people moved from remote areas to the cities and brought the virus to these population centers. Sexual intercourse could then have spread the virus rapidly, especially since those decades saw the emergence of a sexual revolution. Given the roughly ten-year incubation period for the disease, an outbreak in the 1980s appears reasonable. Moreover, a 1988 study indicated that the number of blood samples testing positive for HIV in a city in Zaire increased tenfold in a ten-year span.

Another possibility is that soldiers from Caribbean countries serving as mercenaries in the civil wars could have acquired the virus from remote African populations. The virus may then have made its way to the United States via a Caribbean city. Many people from Haiti, for example, were known to suffer from AIDS early in the epidemic. There is also the possibility that contaminated blood used for transfusion could have been the source of HIV, either by administration to travelers passing through the region or by exportation to other countries.

BOX
1.3

A Much Longer Prologue

Though the "official" beginning of the AIDS epidemic in the United States is considered to be June 1981, there is evidence that AIDS may have made its appearance as early as 1969. The basis for this belief is a report published in October 1987. In the report, researchers related the case of Robert R., a 16-year-old boy from Missouri, who may have died of AIDS-related causes in 1969.

The researchers told of the teenager who came to St. Louis City Hospital in 1968 with substantial swelling of the legs and genital organs and an impaired immune system. A bacterial disease named chlamydia was diagnosed, and Robert was put on a regimen of antibiotics. But the drugs did not work. In the ensuing weeks, his muscles wasted away, his lungs filled with fluid (an unmistakable sign of pneumonia), and he died in May 1969. During the subsequent autopsy, pathologists found in his organs the purplish lesions of Kaposi's sarcoma, a type of cancer now known to be related to AIDS.

Unable to locate a microbial cause for Robert's death, doctors froze samples of his blood and tissues, hoping that some day the mystery could be solved. In June 1986, the samples were sent to Tulane University for analysis for HIV. Virologists at the university found that Robert R.'s blood reacted with all nine chemical markers for HIV. There was little question that the virus had been present in the boy's blood.

Is it possible that the AIDS virus may have been in the United States in a less lethal form in the 1960s? Perhaps so, believe some researchers, but they also question where that virus is today. Did all of that less lethal virus simultaneously mutate to a more lethal form? Not likely, is the opinion of most. What, then, would explain the more than ten-year lapse before the epidemic's breakout? Thus far, there is no answer.

It should be noted that most discussions of Africa as the origin of the AIDS virus are bitterly resented by Africans, who do not wish their continent to be thought responsible for the AIDS epidemic. Such discussions have made many African government officials suspicious of foreign scientists and relief organizations and, in some cases, have impeded the flow of information from that continent. To ease tensions, the World Health Assembly passed a 1987 resolution stating that HIV is a "naturally occurring [virus] of undetermined geographic origin." Writing in 1989, Robert Gallo attempted to further diffuse the sensitivity by suggesting that "tracing the origins of the virus to a particular location doesn't imply blame— we don't blame Lyme, Connecticut, for Lyme disease."

Entry into the United States

The AIDS virus was in the United States well before the first cases of AIDS were identified in 1981. The case of a Missouri boy points up this fact (Box 1.3), as does evidence from blood samples frozen and stored in the late 1970s. During that period, more than 7000 homosexual men came to public health clinics in

San Francisco and New York to participate in a government-sponsored study of hepatitis B. They donated blood samples, and researchers preserved many of the vials for study at a later date. A decade passed before the vials of blood were thawed and tested for evidence of HIV. The results reported in 1987 revealed some interesting patterns: Of 6700 participants in the San Francisco area, at least 70 percent had blood samples positive for exposure to HIV; more than 600 of the participants had AIDS; and about 400 of the 600 had already died.

The results provided substantial evidence that HIV was in the United States well before the first cases of AIDS showed up in 1981. Moreover, the results revealed how rapidly the disease was spreading among men who have sex with men: Of blood samples donated in 1978, 3 percent had evidence of exposure to HIV; of those donated in 1979, 12 percent showed HIV exposure; and by 1981, 45 percent were HIV-positive. It was clear that the epidemic was gathering steam even before public health agencies recognized its existence.

How the AIDS virus entered the United States is still unknown. One possible source is contaminated blood imported from another country (Figure 1.8). Another possibility is sexual contact by Americans with foreigners harboring HIV.

FIGURE 1.8

Although how AIDS entered the United States remains unresolved, one possibility is that the virus was present in contaminated blood imported from abroad. Transfusion of this blood to recipients may have provided a mode of transmission. The young boy pictured here has received hundreds of transfusions since birth to treat a blood disease called Mediterranean anemia.

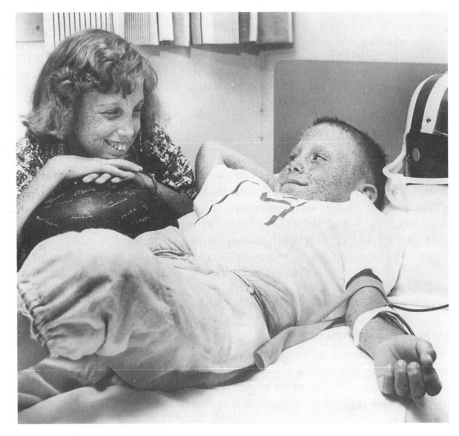

Sharing contaminated syringes and needles with infected injection drug users is a third possibility.

Another possible mode of entry into the United States may involve Haiti. Scientists have theorized that cultural exchanges between Zaire and Haiti, both French-speaking countries, offered possibilities for transporting the virus from Africa. American homosexual men vacationing in Haiti could then have acquired the virus and brought it to the United States. This view is supported by the observation that AIDS was present in Haitians as well as in American homosexual men in the 1980s. It should be pointed out, however, that AIDS may have been introduced to Haiti by North Americans. The evidence that American men were exposed to AIDS before Haitians bolsters this view. Rather than a source, Haiti may have been a recipient of the virus.

The First Decades and Beyond

In late 2000, health officials from the United Nations Programme on HIV/AIDS (UNAIDS) made a startling prediction: They announced that if current trends continued, deaths associated with AIDS could exceed those of the Great Plague of the 1300s (the Black Death) and the catastrophic worldwide influenza epidemic of 1918–1919. AIDS would then become the deadliest contagion in world history. Whether this prediction becomes reality will soon be known. For the time being, however, we close this chapter with a brief summary of the past and future course of the AIDS epidemic.

Two Decades of AIDS

In the twenty years since *MMWR* carried the first report of pneumocystosis in immune-deficient individuals, the statistics attending the AIDS epidemic have reflected the emergence of a major health crisis. One of the first notable benchmarks was reached in the August 18, 1989 issue of *MMWR* when the CDC reported that more than 100,000 cases of AIDS had been diagnosed in the United States through July 1989 (Healthline 1.3). It also noted that AIDS-related deaths had reached about 60,000. The CDC also pointed out that the first 50,000 cases of AIDS were reported from 1981 to late 1987 (six years), and the second 50,000 cases between December 1987 and July 1989 (one and a half years). AIDS had become a major cause of illness and death among children and young adults in the United States; in 1988, it ranked fifteenth among the leading causes of death for Americans.

Healthline 1.3

1

Q How widespread is AIDS in the United States?

A As of December 2000, 774,467 cases of AIDS had been reported to the CDC by physicians through the public health network. Moreover, scientists estimate that perhaps a million Americans are infected with the AIDS virus but show no symptoms and that over 35 million individuals are infected worldwide. Over 440,000 Americans have died of AIDS-associated illnesses.

2

Q Does AIDS occur only in the United States?

A Quite to the contrary, AIDS is a worldwide problem. As of 2000, the disease was reported from 162 of the World Health Organization's 170 member countries. Globally, over 35 million people are living with HIV or experiencing AIDS. AIDS is therefore a worldwide epidemic, or pandemic.

3

Q When did AIDS enter the United States?

A Although the first cases of AIDS were reported in the summer of 1981, AIDS was probably in the United States as early as the mid-1970s and possibly before then. Blood samples taken in the late 1970s and frozen until tested for AIDS in the late 1980s provide evidence for this hypothesis. The number of those samples testing positive for exposure to the AIDS virus was substantial.

By 1989, homosexual and bisexual men were still accounting for most reported AIDS cases, but injection drug users, their sexual contacts, and their children represented an increasing proportion of all cases. For example, 63 percent of AIDS cases occurred in homosexual men before 1985, but only 56 percent of new cases did in 1989. By contrast, injection drug users accounted for 18 percent of cases in 1985, but this percentage rose to 23 percent by 1989. The number of females involved was also rising: Before 1985, only 7 percent of AIDS cases were in females, but in 1989, the number rose to 11 percent.

In the January 25, 1991 issue of *MMWR*, the CDC updated its figures. By that time, more than 100,000 persons had *died* of AIDS (compared to 100,000 *cases* in 1989). Among American men aged 25 to 44 years, AIDS had become the second leading cause of death, surpassing heart disease, cancer, and suicide. For women aged 25 to 44, AIDS was projected to be among the top five causes of death. By 1995, the prediction had become reality, and AIDS was the leading cause of death in women in fifteen U.S. cities.

Things began to change in 1996, however. That year, new optimism surfaced with the news that protease inhibitors, a class of drugs that complement AZT (azidothymidine), could be used to reduce blood concentrations of HIV to undetectable levels (Chapter 8). Also that year, investigators uncovered striking new clues on how HIV binds to host cells, clues that kindled hopes for new therapies, especially since a genetic defect that prohibits binding apparently makes some individuals immune to AIDS (Chapter 2). These advances in therapeutic and basic research were augmented by development of a new test, the viral load test, that uses state-of-the-art biotechnology to measure precisely the number of HIV particles in a sample of blood (Chapter 7). This direct measurement of infection is far superior to measurements of host cell destruction for gauging a patient's response to drugs or predicting long-term survival. The optimistic mood of 1996 marked a turning point in the battle against AIDS and persuaded the editors of *Science* magazine to name the collection of advances as the Breakthrough of the Year.

By December 1999, the AIDS epidemic had been affecting the United States for over two decades. As the world celebrated the closing of the twentieth century, the CDC reported that there had been a total of 733,374 AIDS cases in the United States since the first case was recorded in 1981. Of this total, 81 percent of cases had occurred in men, 18 percent in women, and 1 percent in children. Statisticians noted that the epidemic was shifting toward a growing percentage of cases in women, African-Americans, and Hispanic-Americans and that a decreasing percentage was occurring in homosexual men. Despite this statistic, homosexual men continue to remain the largest single exposure group, as we discuss in Chapter 5. In addition to the confirmed cases, almost a million individuals were living with HIV in 1999 but remained undiagnosed. Over 425,000 had died of AIDS-associated illnesses.

In the United States, the good news at the end of the century was the steep decline in AIDS in newborns. AIDS cases in newborns reached a peak in 1992, leveled off during 1993, then began a dramatic dropoff in 1994, as Figure 1.9 shows. The most apparent reason was improved diagnosis of HIV infection in pregnant women combined with rapid implementation of therapy with AZT to prevent transmission from mother to child. AZT interferes with the replication of HIV in infected cells, as Chapter 8 explores in detail. Improved treatment of HIV-infected newborns is another notable reason for the decrease because the treatment delays the progression from HIV infection to AIDS, as Chapter 4 describes.

But in the rest of the world at the end of the century, the news was much more grim. Worldwide, the UNAIDS reported that over 35 million adults were living with HIV or experiencing AIDS, and that an astounding 5 million had become infected in the year 2000 alone. Already, over 20 million individuals had died from AIDS-related causes since the beginning of the pandemic, over 3 million in the year 2000. And 90 percent of infected individuals were from sub-Saharan Africa, Southeast Asia, and Latin America. The toll of AIDS had vastly exceeded the most pessimistic report of two decades earlier. AIDS was a worldwide firestorm.

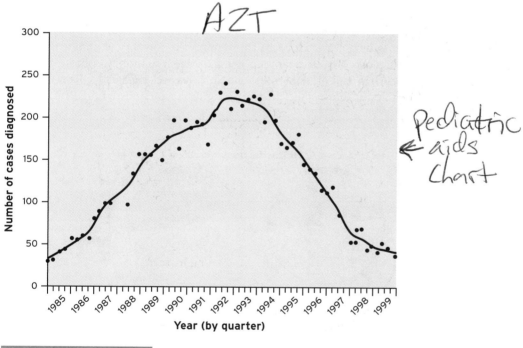

FIGURE 1.9

Cases of AIDS diagnosed in newborns in the United States reported quarterly for the period 1985-1999. The dropoff is related to the detection of HIV in pregnant women and the use of AZT to interrupt the replication of HIV.

AIDS in the Twenty-First Century

As the new century opened, the AIDS crisis in the United States had lessened. To some observers, the disease had practically dropped off the proverbial radar screen. Many people infected with HIV were living almost normal lives thanks to a sophisticated combination of anti-HIV drugs (which we discuss in Chapter 8). Moreover, the infection rate had leveled off and even declined for some groups (although it was rising for others), and the public was becoming somewhat complacent about the epidemic. Public health officials were hoping to accelerate the decline in HIV infection in newborns during the twenty-first century by encouraging improved counseling and testing of pregnant women, by increasing prenatal care among high-risk women, and by using vigorous public information campaigns.

But, as we have noted, the situation was much different in Africa: AIDS was threatening to be more devastating than civil wars and famines put together. Each day, between 6000 and 7000 people in sub-Saharan Africa were dying of the effects of AIDS, and public health scientists estimated that HIV had infected over 35 million adults. Figure 1.10 shows some of the alarming projections related to the AIDS epidemic.

Referring to the African problem, activists were writing of a dying continent as they exhorted the United States and other countries to be more aggressive in fighting the spread of AIDS. They implored drug companies to lower the price of anti-HIV drugs; they lobbied for increased funding of AIDS education programs; and they pleaded for wealthy countries to lower or eliminate the backbreaking debts owed by African countries so that the money could instead be used to fight AIDS and other serious epidemic diseases such as Ebola fever. And they warned about the social upheavals, economic collapses, and political insta-

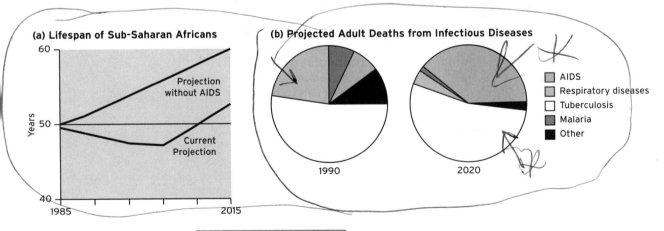

FIGURE 1.10

The devastating long-term effects of AIDS on sub-Saharan Africa. (a) The projected lifespan of people in sub-Saharan Africa if there were no AIDS epidemic and the current projection taking the AIDS epidemic into account. (b) The projections of adult deaths from various infectious diseases between 1990 and 2020. All statistics courtesy of UNAIDS.

bilities of disease-ravaged countries—effects that would almost surely spill over and engulf the rest of the world.

Meanwhile, in the United States, public health officials warned that in the foreseeable future, AIDS will continue to affect homosexual men, while becoming more prevalent among poor, African-American, and Hispanic-American heterosexuals living in the inner cities. Contributing to this prediction is the observation that the rate at which homosexual men contract AIDS has reached a plateau, whereas the rate has risen dramatically among injection drug users, particularly those of minority groups. In New York City, for instance, in a recent year, four out of five AIDS cases attributed to sharing needles occurred among African-American and Hispanic-American individuals. Public health officials stress that fighting the spread of AIDS among drug addicts and their sex partners will require significant increases in drug treatment programs as well as education programs that target poor urban areas.

In the early 1980s, AIDS was an unknown entity, shrouded in uncertainty and conjecture. But the disease began to reveal itself through the mid- and late-1980s when the scientific base of information expanded (Table 1.1). Now, in the twenty-first century, our vision of AIDS is clearer, although far from perfectly in focus. The first two decades of research brought hopes of great advances, but the sad fact is that scientists have not provided reliable therapies, nor is an effective vaccine in sight. Our society's ability to alter risk-taking behaviors is still limited, and we do not understand major aspects of the interaction of HIV with the infected individual, nor do we fully comprehend the nature of the host response. And we do not know how AIDS will fit into the total spectrum of public health in the future.

Writing in 2001, Peter Piot of the UNAIDS and Stefano Vella, president of the International AIDS Society, highlighted some of the questions still lingering: Why does AIDS predispose an HIV-infected individual to certain diseases, but not others? What route does HIV take after it enters the body to reach the immune system? How exactly do the genes of HIV work? What is the nature of the immune response against HIV? Which of the many combinations of HIV therapies will work best? Why do most babies born to HIV-infected women escape infection? And what new strategies can be effective in modifying behavior patterns and changing risks for acquiring HIV?

Can Africa avert the catastrophe of the AIDS pandemic? Public health officials wonder what hope the poorer nations have and what the economic impact of the pandemic will be. And, they question, can the United States keep HIV from broadening its net? As you read the pages ahead, try to bear in mind that the history of AIDS is being written minute-by-minute. Answers to some of these questions are probably emerging as you read.

LOOKING BACK

In the early 1980s, AIDS was compared to an elephant being examined by blind men, because scientists and public health officials were ignorant of the disease's

TABLE 1.1	A Brief Chronology of the AIDS Epidemic
June 5, 1981	Five cases of *Pneumocystis carinii* pneumonia reported in the COC's *MMWR*
December 1981	*Pneumocystis carinii* pneumonia reported in New York City drug addicts
June 11, 1982	365 cases of immune deficiency reported from five states in United States
September 3, 1982	The name acquired immune deficiency syndrome (AIDS) coined
Early 1983	16 countries reporting AIDS; 34 states in United States with AIDS cases
April 1983	Research groups led by Gallo and Montagnier independently report discovery of AIDS virus
May 1985	Blood test for AIDS antibody made available
August 1986	AIDS virus named human immunodeficiency virus (HIV)
1987	Azidothymidine (AZT) licensed for use in AIDS patients; AIDS vaccine research ongoing
1988	138 countries reporting AIDS
July 1989	100,000 cases of AIDS in United States; 60,000 deaths in United States from AIDS and complications
January 1991	501,310 cumulative cases of AIDS in United States; 311,381 deaths
November 1991	202,843 cases of AIDS in United States; 130,687 deaths in United States from AIDS and complications; estimated 1 million Americans infected with HIV; estimated 6 to 8 million people worldwide infected with HIV
October 31, 1995	100,000 deaths associated with AIDS in United States
1996	Protease inhibitors licensed for use in United States; new discoveries on HIV binding to host cells; new HIV detection tests approved; declining number of cases in newborns
1999	Over 900,000 cases of AIDS in United States with over 425,000 deaths; over 35 million worldwide infected with HIV; 28.5 million deaths from sub-Saharan Africa pandemic.

cause, transmission, symptoms, and other characteristics. Reports beginning in June 1981 made it clear that suppression of the immune system was occurring in homosexual men and that diseases not ordinarily considered dangerous had led to death in many of these men. Similar symptoms were later observed in injection drug users, blood transfusion recipients, hemophiliacs, heterosexual individuals, and newborns.

Many theories purporting to explain the cause of AIDS existed in the early 1980s, but in April 1984, a virus was identified as the agent. The discoverers were members of a group headed by Luc Montagnier of France. Though initially called HTLV-III/LAV, the virus was renamed human immunodeficiency virus, or HIV, in 1986 on the recommendation of an international commission. Another AIDS virus called HIV-2 has been identified in people from West Africa. The disease it causes seems to be milder that that caused by the original HIV, now known as HIV-1.

AIDS was recognized as a global problem as early as 1985. The African continent has been particularly hard hit, with high infection rates in sub-Saharan Africa. Researchers believe that HIV-1 originated in chimpanzees of the species *Pan troglodytes troglodytes* and was probably passed to humans via a scratch or bite from one of these animals. The crossover to humans occurred at least three times, probably in the late 1940s or early 1950s, although some dispute remains about the exact timing. The possibility that HIV was introduced to human populations through tests of polio vaccines has been discounted. Decades of turmoil in Africa encouraged the virus to spread to the remaining world.

By the beginning of the twenty-first century, more than 700,000 cases of AIDS had been reported in the United States. But there was hope of forestalling the epidemic since a cocktail of drugs used since 1996 has been shown to decrease the number of deaths associated with AIDS. Moreover, studies indicate that when AZT is used in HIV-infected pregnant women, the transmission of HIV to their newborns can be interrupted. Furthermore, the percentage of AIDS cases in sexually active homosexual men was dropping, but the percentage in injection drug users and women was rising. The AIDS elephant is becoming visible after two decades of discoveries, but some of its features, such as its susceptibility to a preventative vaccine, remain obscure.

As members of the health community gather for the annual international conferences on AIDS, they continue to confront the implications of the AIDS epidemic. Two worrisome issues move to center stage: how to stem the spread of HIV and how to provide sophisticated and expensive medical care to vast numbers of people who are likely to develop AIDS-related illnesses, particularly in Africa. Moreover, many questions remain regarding HIV's route into the body, how its genes work, and which drug combination is most effective. We shall encounter these problems again in later chapters.

REVIEW

This chapter has explored the development of the AIDS epidemic during two decades, touching on its, origin, method of spread, and magnitude. To test your knowledge of these concepts, consider the following statements. Write T for "True" if a statement is correct as it stands. If the statement is false, change the underlined word or phrase to correct the statement. The correct answers are listed in Appendix A.

___F___ **1.** Although the agent responsible for AIDS was probably in the United States during the 1970s, the "official" beginning of the AIDS epidemic in the United States occurred in ~~1991.~~ 1981

___F___ **2.** Two diseases that physicians commonly observe in AIDS patients are *Pneumocystis carinii* pneumonia and a form of skin cancer known as ~~adenocarcinoma.~~ Kaposi's sarcoma

___T___ **3.** It is now generally recognized that AIDS is caused by a <u>virus</u>.

___F___ **4.** One of the important modes of transmission for the human immunodeficiency virus (HIV) is contaminated ~~food.~~ blood

___T___ **5.** AIDS is a disease that occurs in homosexual men as well as in <u>injection drug users</u>.

___F___ **6.** In France, the research team that confirmed the identity of the AIDS virus was led by ~~Bernard Schwartlander.~~ Luc Montagnier

___T___ **7.** The AIDS virus, originally designated <u>HTLV-III/LAV</u>, is now known by the acronym HIV.

___F___ **8.** Since the introduction of blood tests for AIDS, the number of transfusion-linked cases of AIDS has ~~increased~~ decreased sharply.

___F___ **9.** Because of its global involvement, the AIDS epidemic is more properly termed an AIDS ~~endemic.~~ pandemic

___F___ **10.** By 1989, the number of cases of AIDS diagnosed in the United States had passed ~~1 million.~~ 100,000

___T___ **11.** A global program to combat the spread of AIDS has been established by the <u>World Health Organization</u>.

___F___ **12.** One theory relating to the origin of the AIDS virus suggests that it may have existed in African ~~birds~~ monkeys before being transmitted to humans.

___F___ **13.** The form of AIDS caused by HIV-2 appears to be ~~deadlier~~ milder than the form caused by HIV-1.

___T___ **14.** The current research thinking is that epidemics of AIDS due to HIV-2 originated from SIV in the <u>sooty mangabey monkey</u>.

___F___ **15.** At the beginning of the twenty-first century, the AIDS pandemic was particularly severe on the continent of ~~Asia.~~ Africa

FOR ADDITIONAL READING

Altman, L. K. 1998. "Study places HIV origins a decade earlier." *New York Times*, February 4.

Anonymous. 1999. "The man who lives to defeat AIDS." *Discover*, June.

Balter, M. 1998. "Virus from 1959 sample marks early years of HIV." *Science* 279: 801.

Fee, E., and N. Krieger. 1993. "Understanding AIDS: historical interpretations and the limits of biomedical individualism." *J. Public Health* 83: 1477–1486.

Fox, J. 2000. "Specimens from wild chimpanzees, mangaby monkeys yield clues on HIV origins." *ASM News* 66: 716–717.

Hahn, B. H., et al. 2000. "AIDS as a zoonosis: scientific and public health implications." *Science* 287: 607–614.

Pennisi, E. 1999. "AIDS virus traced to chimp subspecies." *Science* 283: 772–773.

Richman, E. 1996. "The once and future king." *The Sciences*, November/December.

Schwartlander, B., et al. 2000. "AIDS in a new millennium." *Science* 289: 64–67.

Weiss, R. 1994. "Of myths and mischief." *Discover*, December.

Weiss, R. 1999. "Is AIDS man-made?" *Science* 286: 1305–1306.

CHAPTER 2

Viruses and HIV

LOOKING AHEAD

This chapter explores the structure of viruses and how they replicate, focusing on the human immunodeficiency virus (HIV). On completing the chapter, you should be able to . . .

- Understand how viruses relate to other microorganisms in structure and replication patterns.
- Describe the general components of a virus and the specific components of the human immunodeficiency virus (HIV).
- Outline the replication process in viruses and explain how the process occurs with HIV.
- Summarize the effect of HIV on the cells of the body's immune system.
- Discuss some general principles of viral inactivation and inhibition and identify methods for treating viral disease.

INTRODUCTION

Every science has its borderland where the known and visible merge with the unknown and invisible. Startling discoveries often come from this hazy, uncharted realm of speculation, and certain objects loom large. In the borderland of biology, at the fringe of our understanding, are curious and puzzling objects known as viruses.

Scientists have always had an awkward time fitting viruses into the scheme of living things. Viruses do not grow, nor do they move or adapt to their environment. They display few of the biochemical structures or processes we find in living things. Strictly speaking, they are not microorganisms, but in practical terms they are more like microorganisms than like any other group of living things.

In this chapter, we shall explore the structure and replication patterns of viruses, with emphasis on the human immunodeficiency virus (HIV), the cause of AIDS. We shall study the properties that make viruses unique and that put them at the threshold between living organisms and inert molecules. To illustrate the uncertain status of viruses as organisms or molecules, one virologist has whimsically suggested that they be called "organules" or "molechisms," depending on one's preference.

Structure of Viruses and HIV

Viruses are among the smallest objects that can cause disease in plants, animals, and humans (Figure 2.1a and b). Indeed, some viruses are so tiny that 10 million laid end to end might stretch across the period at the end of this sentence. Counting these 10 million viruses nonstop at a rate of one per second would consume close to four months.

Using the electron microscope, scientists have been able to magnify viruses many millions of times and photograph them. These photographs reveal that viruses occur in a variety of shapes. Certain viruses, for example, appear as a tightly wound coil known as a helix. The rabies virus is a typical helical virus. Other viruses have the shape of an icosahedron, that is, a geometric figure with 20 triangular faces and 12 points. The chickenpox, herpes simplex, and human immunodeficiency viruses can take this form. The shapes of several viruses are depicted in Figure 2.2.

All viruses consist of two basic components: a core of nucleic acid, called the genome, and a surrounding layer of protein, known as the capsid. The nucleic acid of the genome may be either deoxyribonucleic acid (DNA) or ribonucleic acid (RNA), but not both. DNA is familiar to most of us as the hereditary material found in the chromosomes and genes of cells. RNA, by contrast, is a nucleic acid used by cells for several purposes, including the production of proteins. The chickenpox and herpes simplex viruses contain DNA in their genomes, while the measles, mumps, and polio viruses contain RNA. HIV is also an RNA-containing virus. It contains two identical molecules of this type of nucleic acid.

The second viral component, the capsid, encloses the genome and gives the virus its helical or icosahedral symmetry. The capsid also provides protection for the genome, because its protein can resist certain changes in the external environment, such as drying or increasing acidity. This resistance varies among viruses and is relatively low for HIV. The combination of genome and capsid is referred to as the nucleocapsid. Special proteins may line the inner surface of the capsid and coat the genome, as we discuss for HIV below.

Careful examination of the viral capsid with the electron microscope has revealed subunits called capsomeres. Capsomeres are relatively simple proteins. They are joined to one another like patches of a quilt to make the capsid. The number of capsomeres varies among viruses of different types.

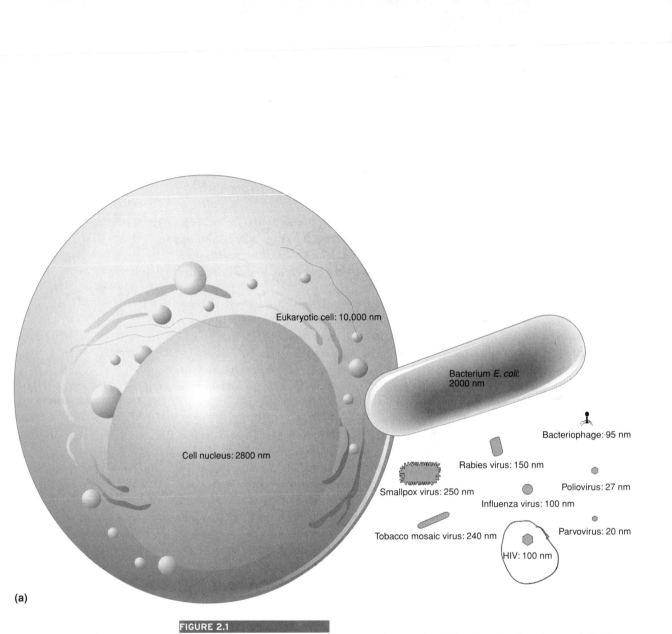

(a)

(a) A comparison of size relationships among microorganisms. The sizes of various viruses relative to a eukaryotic cell, a cell nucleus, and the bacterium *E. coli.*

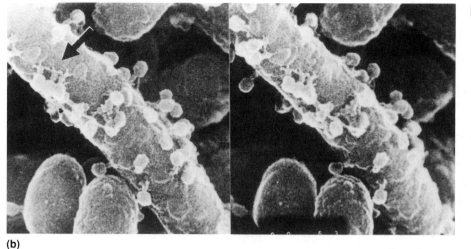

(b)

FIGURE 2.1 CONTINUED
(b) Numerous bacteriophages are attached to the surfaces of the host cells. The arrow indicates the tail fibers (x 70,000).

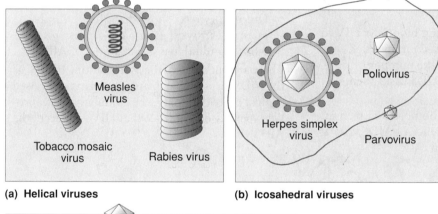

(a) Helical viruses

Measles virus

Tobacco mosaic virus

Rabies virus

(b) Icosahedral viruses

Poliovirus

Herpes simplex virus

Parvovirus

(c) Complex viruses

Bacteriophages

Smallpox virus

Influenza virus

FIGURE 2.2
Viruses exhibit numerous variations in symmetry. (a) The capsid has helical symmetry in the tobacco mosaic, measles, and rabies viruses. The helix resembles a tightly coiled spiral. (b) Certain viruses, such as herpesviruses, polio viruses, and parvoviruses, exhibit icosahedral symmetry in their capsids. The icosahedron is a polyhedron having 20 triangular faces and 12 points. (c) In other viruses, neither helical nor icosahedral symmetry exists exclusively. A bacteriophage, for example, has an extended icosahedral "head" and a helical tail with extended fibers. The smallpox virus has a series of rodlike filaments embedded within the membranous envelope at its surface. And the influenza virus consists of a series of helical segments enclosed by an envelope.

But How Do They Know?

It is generally accepted by the scientific community that the human immunodeficiency virus (HIV) is the cause of AIDS. But, critics say, the final proof demands inoculation of pure virus into a human volunteer and development of AIDS in that individual. Such an experiment is ethically unthinkable.

How, then, do scientists associate HIV with AIDS? Consider the following:

- Almost every case of AIDS has occurred in someone who has been shown to harbor HIV.

- In no country where AIDS is present is HIV absent.

- In no country where HIV is present is AIDS absent.

- Blood banks began testing blood for HIV in 1985 and removing HIV-contaminated blood from circulation; the number of transfusion-associated AIDS cases then declined sharply.

- In a long-term study of homosexual men in San Francisco, the incidence of AIDS rose as the rate of HIV infection rose.

- In a study of blood transfusion recipients, 19 recipients developed AIDS; in each of the 19 cases, the donor of the blood was located and found to be positive for HIV.

- In every country of the world studied so far, AIDS has appeared only after HIV has appeared.

- All HIV-positive hemophiliac patients have died from symptoms resembling AIDS; put another way, not a single HIV-negative hemophiliac is known to have died from symptoms resembling AIDS.

- Using highly sophisticated technology, HIV can be located in almost 100 percent of individuals who have AIDS.

- Laboratory tests show that HIV multiplies in and destroys the very T-lymphocytes whose gradual loss is a signpost of AIDS.

These are but a few of the data pointing to HIV as the AIDS virus. Though arguments may be raised against individual data, the cumulative data provides persuasive evidence that HIV is, indeed, the AIDS virus.

Many viruses, including HIV, have an envelope. The envelope is a flexible lipid-bilayer membrane outside the capsid. Though similar to the surface membrane of a cell, the envelope contains virus-specified chemical components. It is acquired by the virus when the virus leaves the cell at the conclusion of a replication cycle, as we shall see presently. In certain viruses, the envelope has projections known as spikes. These spikes are composed of chemical substances that assist the union of viruses with cells, as we discuss below. Influenza viruses are well known for their spikes, and researchers have found that the envelope of HIV also has spikes.

To summarize, viruses are noncellular particles consisting of either DNA or RNA enclosed in a coat of protein (Box 2.1). Essentially, each virus is a genome plus a capsid. In some viruses, an envelope with spikes is also present. In HIV, the genome consists of RNA, and the capsid is initially icosahedral (before restructuring itself into the shape of a bullet, as we shall see). Surrounding the capsid of HIV is an envelope with spikes (Figure 2.3). The virus has a diameter of about 0.1 micrometer (one ten-millionth of a meter); 0.1 micrometer can also be expressed as 100 nanometers (one hundred billionths of a meter).

Two features of HIV are worthy of note: First, different HIV particles may have slightly different chemical components in their spikes. This fact has presented substantial problems for vaccine researchers because a vaccine must take into account all possible forms of the virus (Chapter 9). The second unique feature is the presence of a dual enzyme called reverse transcriptase. (An enzyme is a protein that catalyzes a biochemical conversion while itself remaining unchanged.) Molecules of reverse transcriptase are found among the strands of RNA in HIV. The function of reverse transcriptase is to synthesize DNA, using the viral RNA as a template, after cell infection has occurred (Figure 2.4). We shall examine the practical significance of reverse transcriptase later in this chapter. Molecules of the enzymes integrase and protease are also found beneath the capsid, as we shall note presently.

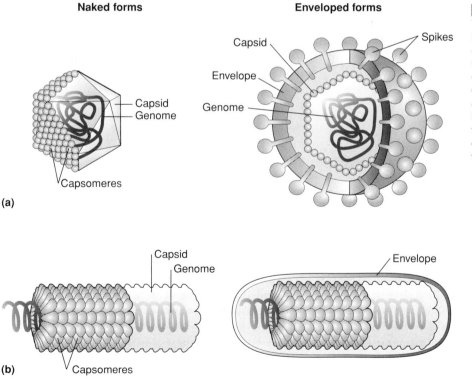

Naked forms

Capsid
Genome
Capsomeres

(a)

Enveloped forms

Capsid
Envelope
Genome
Spikes

Capsid
Genome
Capsomeres

Envelope

(b)

FIGURE 2.3

The components of viruses. (a) An icosahedral virus in both naked and enveloped forms. Capsomere units are shown on one face of the capsid. The genome consists of either DNA or RNA and is folded and condensed. (b) A helical virus in both naked and enveloped forms. The genome is in the form of a helix. The capsomeres are protein subunits that form the capsid.

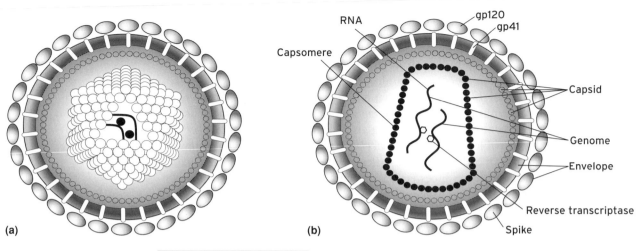

FIGURE 2.4

Stylized and diagrammatic representations of the human immunodeficiency virus (HIV). (a) HIV is shown with icosahedral symmetry and multiple capsomeres composing the capsid. Two strands of RNA are shown within the capsid. The two dots represent molecules of reverse transcriptase. The envelope is illustrated with projecting spikes. (b) In diagrammatic form, the parts of HIV are highlighted. Note that the icosahedral capsid has collapsed to form a bullet-shaped capsid.

Compared with other microorganisms and cells, viruses are structurally very simple (Healthline 2.1). Their chemistry is equally simple. Viruses perform no energy-generating chemical reactions, nor can they synthesize proteins on their own. They consume no food, do not grow, and produce no waste products. Because of their unusual characteristics, many scientists hesitate to refer to viruses as "alive." Viruses replicate, however, and they perform this function efficiently. Replication takes place within a living cell, at the cell's expense.

Replication of Viruses and HIV

The process of viral replication is among the more remarkable of natural phenomena. A virus penetrates a living cell thousands of times its size and uses the chemical compounds and structures of the cell for its own purposes. In doing so, the virus produces hundreds (in some cases, thousands) of copies of itself and leaves behind a poorly functioning or dead cell. On its own, a virus cannot replicate, but within a cell, the process occurs with extraordinary efficiency. Such a relationship, in which one object uses and often destroys another, is known as parasitism. For viruses, parasitism is a necessary prerequisite for replication.

Adsorption

The first step in viral replication is the union between the virus and its host cell, a step called adsorption. Such a union is highly specific, and certain viruses interact only with certain cells. Hepatitis viruses, for instance, unite with liver cells; influenza viruses unite with respiratory tract cells; and polio viruses unite with brain cells. For HIV, a primary target cell is a cell of the immune system called the T-lymphocyte (also known as the T-cell). This cell contains on its surface a series of proteins called CD4 molecules (Box 2.2). Each CD4 molecule contains 433 amino acids. The CD4 molecules are also located on macrophages (microbe-engulfing white blood cells) and on brain cells, which is why HIV can infect macrophages and the brain. (We discuss T-lymphocytes and macrophages extensively in Chapter 3.) Biologists refer to chemical points of interaction, such as the CD4 molecules, as receptor sites. Other sites called coreceptors are also found on T-lymphocytes, as we shall see presently.

The union between the HIV particle and the CD4 receptor site involves a molecule on the spikes of HIV called glycoprotein 120, or gp120. This molecule is so named because it is a carbohydrate-containing ("glyco") protein with a molecular weight of 120 kilodaltons (*kilo* means "thousand"; *dalton* is a unit of weight equal to the mass of a hydrogen atom). Both CD4 and gp120 molecules play significant roles in virus-cell interaction. They also have practical importance: CD4 molecules have been investigated for their therapeutic value (Chapter 8) and gp120 is used in vaccine preparations (Chapter 9).

The gp120 molecule extending out from a viral spike is a complex structure containing at least five areas (or domains) that can vary in their amino acid content. Near the midpoint of the molecule, scientists have identified one domain, a loop of amino acids called the V3 loop, that helps HIV lock tightly to the CD4 site, possibly by uniting with another molecule on the T-lymphocyte surface. This finding bears significance because vaccine-induced antibodies produced against the V3 loop could conceivably prevent HIV's union with T-lymphocytes. Moreover, drugs that destroy the V3 loop could be used to prevent virus-cell union and bring infection to an end. A disquieting note was sounded in 1998, however: Researchers determined the crystalline structure of the gp120 molecule and reported that the amino acid loops of the molecule are shielded from antibodies and drugs by a screen of complex carbohydrates. Moreover, the loops and carbohydrates render the gp120 molecule flexible enough to further avoid antibody molecules, a problem that impacts on vaccine development. Figure 2.5 shows the bonding that takes place.

Healthline 2.1

1 Q Are viruses a type of microorganism?

A Viruses are generally considered to be microorganisms. However, they are not alive in the true sense of the word because they do not grow, use food, produce waste products, or perform any other metabolic activities we associate with living things. Inside cells, however, they replicate themselves very efficiently.

2 Q Can viruses multiply outside the body in things like food or water?

A No, viruses multiply only within the cells of a living organism. Outside an organism, they are inert particles of matter, unable to replicate themselves. Some viruses, such as those of hepatitis A, can resist environmental pressures and remain active, but other viruses, such as HIV, are extremely fragile and quickly disintegrate when exposed to the environment.

3 Q How do viruses compare with other microorganisms in size?

A Viruses are the smallest known agents able to cause infectious disease. Some viruses are so small that several hundred can fit inside a bacterium. And a thousand bacteria, lying side by side, would extend only a millimeter.

BOX
2.2

On the Trail of CD4

For every lock there is a key, or so it appeared to Steven McDougall, immunologist at the Centers for Disease Control (CDC). If HIV is the key, then there must be a lock on the T-lymphocyte where the two fit together. Even if the virus should subtly change its envelope structure (as HIV is known to do), the part that binds with the lymphocyte must remain constant because the binding between the virus and host cell is an essential element in HIV infection. But how could McDougall prove the existence of a lock-and-key arrangement, and how could he identify the lock on the T-lymphocyte?

Two papers published in 1985 provided a provocative clue for McDougall. They indicated that when lymphocytes attacked by HIV were treated with highly specific antibodies, the lymphocytes resisted HIV attachment. By reacting with the cells, the antibodies were apparently blocking the binding site. This finding suggested to McDougall that the molecules that identify a lymphocyte cell are also the binding sites of the virus.

To test this hypothesis, McDougall and his colleagues began by "painting" a radioactive substance onto the surface of lymphocytes. Then they exposed the cells to HIV. The radioactive material concentrated where the HIV bound to the cells. Next, they dissolved the lymphocytes with a detergent and mixed the fragments with beads coated with antibodies against HIV. The antibody-coated beads combined with fragments of lymphocytes where HIV was clinging, because HIV antibodies unite specifically with HIV. By analyzing the fragments for radioactivity, the researchers could locate the viruses and, hence, the receptor sites.

The next step was to pass the fragments through a sievelike gel to separate the fragments according to size. The gel was then placed against special paper sensitive to radioactivity. The researchers analyzed the paper to see where the radioactivity (and, hence, the receptor sites) came to rest. McDougall and his group found that the radioactivity corresponded to molecules weighing 58 kilodaltons. It was clear that one molecule of the lymphocyte had been recognized as the lock by the viral key. Although the molecule's weight was elucidated, little else was known about it at that time. McDougall's group gave the molecule the name CD4 (CD for "complementary determinant" or "cluster of differentiation" or "cluster designation," depending on one's interpretation and recollection). Now the real work on analysis could begin.

Since the early days of AIDS research, scientists were aware that the T-lymphocyte's CD4 site is an important key to viral binding, but their research evidence indicated that other molecules called coreceptors were involved as well. Then, in 1996, the mystery of the identity of these other coreceptors was partially resolved by Edward Berger and his colleagues at the National Institute of Allergy and Infectious Diseases. These investigators reported that one of the elusive coreceptors is a protein molecule they called fusin. Fusin molecules are embedded in the membrane of the T-lymphocyte.

Shortly thereafter, the coreceptor fusin was found to be leading a double life—apparently, it is also a receptor for a chemokine. A chemokine is a hormonelike

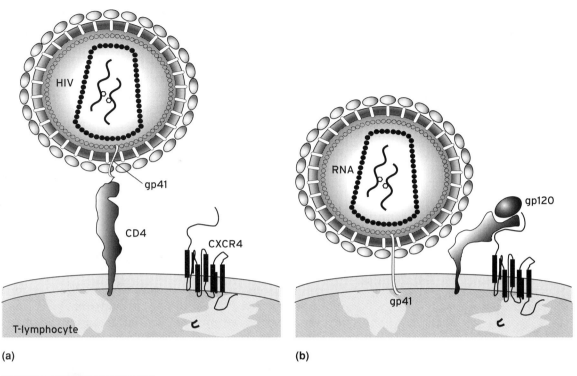

FIGURE 2.5

The union between the human immunodeficiency virus (HIV) and its host T-lymphocyte. (a) The HIV envelope makes contact with the surface of the T-lymphocyte and a gp120 molecule on HIV's spike binds to a CD4 receptor site of the T-lymphocyte. (b) The gp120-CD4 complex then bends down, and a portion of the gp120 molecule binds to the CXCR4 coreceptor site. This action releases the gp41 molecule, which pierces the membrane of the T-lymphocyte. Penetration of the HIV capsid into the T-lymphocytes cytoplasm follows.

small protein secreted by certain body cells such as phagocytic cells. Chemokines latch onto the surface of immune system cells at so-called chemokine receptors (*kinesis* is Greek for "motion," a reference to the attraction). One effect of the binding is to attract phagocytic cells to body cells that have been infected (such as T-lymphocytes), so the cells can be engulfed and destroyed. Another effect is to induce inflammation; after binding to the chemokine, the immune system cell is transported to a site of injury. Because of its second function, fusin was renamed CXCKR-4 (abbreviated CXCR4). (CXC refers to "canonical" amino acids at a specific site in the protein, two cysteines separated by another amino acid. R4 refers to the fourth receptor in the CXC.) Researchers discovered that CXCR4 functions primarily to link T-lymphocytes and HIV (since brain cells, macrophages, and other host cells do not have the coreceptor in abundance). Its activity is shown in Figure 2.5.

The sensation over the discovery of CXCR4 had barely subsided before another coreceptor was pinpointed by five research teams working independently.

The second coreceptor is a protein named CC-CKR-5 (abbreviated CCR5). It snakes through the cell membrane of macrophages and is also a chemokine receptor. Investigators found that the CCR5 coreceptor on the macrophage docks with HIV in the following way: After the gp120 molecule has united with the CD4 receptor site (via the V3 loop), the gp120 changes shape, peels back several loops of shielding amino acids, and exposes a portion of its structure that drops down and snugly binds to the CCR5 coreceptor. Thus, the gp120 molecule binds twice to the macrophage: once at the CD4 site and once at the CCR5 site.

We should pause and note that much of the biochemistry of HIV's binding to its host cell is still under investigation. For example, the CCR5 coreceptor seems to predominate on macrophages, while the CXCR4 coreceptor works primarily on T-lymphocytes. Although the significance of this observation is not completely understood, it may give insight as to why the infection cycle of HIV proceeds as it does; that is, scientists have noted that early in the infection, macrophages bear the brunt of the HIV infection (the virus is "M-tropic"), while later on, the T-lymphocytes are the most heavily involved (the virus is "T-tropic"). Perhaps HIV uses the CCR5 coreceptor in the initial stages of infection and then shifts its biochemistry and develops the ability to unite with the CXCR4 coreceptor on the T-lymphocyte surface. The pathology would thus fit the biochemistry. But, as always in science, we must be cautious about drawing hasty conclusions until the experimentation is complete. For example, as of 2002, researchers had identified more than a dozen molecules on host cells that could act as coreceptors. Moreover, they were postulating that HIV may undergo a genetic shift to change its coreceptor allegiance. Still, even at these early stages, the research on coreceptors has provided a clue as to why certain individuals appear to enjoy genetic resistance to HIV (Box 2.3).

After the CD4 receptor and a coreceptor have bound to the gp120 molecule, another glycoprotein in the HIV spike is uncovered. This molecule is glycoprotein 41, or gp41 (molecular weight of 41 kilodaltons). The gp41 molecule looks somewhat like a harpoon or pointed spring. Triggered into action by the gp120 attachment to the cell surface, the gp41 molecule darts out and pierces the cell membrane of the macrophage or T-lymphocyte and encourages fusion of the viral envelope with that membrane. The crystalline structure of the gp41 molecule has been known since 1997, a factor that may assist understanding of its binding to the host cell. Penetration of the HIV nucleocapsid into the host cell's cytoplasm follows.

Penetration and Infection

Once a virus has united with its specified host cell, the viral genome and capsid enter the cellular cytoplasm. This is the penetration step. In the cytoplasm, the protein capsid is stripped away by cellular enzymes (the uncoating phase) and the genome is released. For many viruses (HIV excluded), the viral nucleic acid provides genetic codes for the synthesis of viral parts. Cellular compounds are used in this synthesis. For example, cellular amino acids are used to synthesize viral pro-

BOX
2.3

Immune to AIDS

June 1996 was a very hot period for AIDS researchers. During that month, scientists from five different laboratories were working to identify the CCR5 coreceptor and within a two-week period, all five labs crossed the finish line almost simultaneously.

But then a new issue emerged. Biochemist Richard Koup of New York's Aaron Diamond AIDS Research Center had been investigating the mysterious cases of two sexually active homosexual men who were not infected with HIV despite their high-risk sexual behavior that doubtlessly exposed them to the virus. In all probability, the men should have been infected. But Koup had found that T-lymphocytes from the two men were not attacked by HIV. Could it be that the men's T-lymphocytes lacked coreceptors?

Koup and his colleague Ned Landau accelerated their research from zero to warp speed and began an exhaustive search for a genetic basis for HIV (specifically HIV-1) resistance. They examined the nuclear material from cells of the two men, and within 2 months, they discovered a gap of 32 missing bases in the DNA of the gene that encodes CCR5 coreceptors. Apparently, the resulting CCR5 protein was so badly deformed that the T-lymphocytes destroyed it instead of placing it on their surface as a coreceptor. And without the CCR5 coreceptor, HIV could not dock on the cell's surface.

The discovery was a bombshell. But it immediately precipitated questions about whether the immunity of the two men was an unusual happenstance of nature or was authentic and prevalent. Thousands of blood samples would be needed to test the theory. It just so happened that 10,000 samples were in the freezer at the lab of Stephen O'Brien of the National Cancer Institute. In the late 1970s, O'Brien had observed a gene that protected mice against a leukemia virus by denying entry of the virus to the host cell. Then, when the AIDS epidemic began in 1981, he was struck by the possibility that such a gene might exist in human cells. Over a 15-year period he had collected from physicians thousands of blood samples from patients at high risk for contracting HIV. His research had been fruitless, however.

The discovery of the CCR5 coreceptor put a new spin on O'Brien's search. Now, in 1996, he and his collaborators tested the blood sample for evidence of the defective genes. Their results were surprising: Two copies of the defective genes apparently exist in 1 percent of Caucasian Americans of Western European descent, and fully 20 percent have one copy of the gene. Although members of the latter group can be infected by HIV, they remain healthy up to 3 years longer than those with no copies of the gene (possibly because they have half the number of coreceptors on their T-lymphocytes). Further, the gene seems to be much rarer in Africans, Native Americans, and Asians. This could indicate that the gene originated after the Caucasian line split off from the others. It is therefore of rather recent evolutionary origin.

The research has opened several new directions for additional research. For example, understanding the normal gene's activity may lead researchers to methods for mutating it to a defective form to protect patients. Providing defective genes to patients via gene therapy could be used to develop another avenue of treatment. And other researchers are hunting for different HIV-blocking mutations in other groups, mutations that might help explain why some prostitutes in Africa and Thailand have managed to avoid AIDS despite repeated exposure to HIV.

At the very least, these new discoveries remind us that a genetic mutation deemed a "defect" can prove to be a blessing in disguise, that is, can confer surprising benefits on those lucky enough to inherit it.

teins (such as capsomeres), and raw materials in the cellular cytoplasm are used to build viral nucleic acids. Cellular enzymes are then engaged to fit together the new viral genomes and capsids in the assembly phase. Soon, complete viral particles appear in the cytoplasm (Figure 2.6). The process for HIV is somewhat different and more complex, as we discuss below.

The parasitism of the host cell continues as hundreds, sometimes thousands, of viruses are manufactured within the cytoplasm. For certain viruses, the replication process is measured in minutes; for other viruses, the cycle may take several hours or days. Eventually, the cytoplasm of the cell swarms with viruses, and in many cases, the cell begins to disintegrate. Viruses are thus set free to infect nearby cells in the release phase. Disease symptoms arising from the destruction of vital tissues can appear soon thereafter (Healthline 2.2).

Lysogeny of HIV

What we have just explored is a general replication cycle in which viruses utilize a cell to produce copies of themselves. In biochemical jargon, the process is called the lytic cycle, from *lysis,* meaning "to break." For HIV, the replication pattern varies slightly. The essential difference is that HIV remains in its host T-lymphocyte, becoming part of the cell and programming the synthesis of additional HIV particles during an extended period of time.

The HIV replication cycle begins with fusion of the virus to the cell's surface membrane, using the interaction between gp120 and gp41 molecules and the CD4 receptors and coreceptors, as described above. Penetration of the HIV genome and capsid into the cell cytoplasm follows. Cellular enzymes now remove the capsid, releasing the RNA and two proteins: the p24 protein that coats the HIV genome and the p17 protein that lines the inside of the capsid (Healthline 2.2).

Also released is the dual enzyme known as reverse transcriptase. One of the enzymes in this complex is DNA polymerase. It synthesizes a single-stranded copy of DNA, using one of the viral RNA molecules as a template (model). The second enzyme of the complex, ribonuclease, then destroys the original RNA molecules. During this period, the DNA polymerase also synthesizes a DNA strand complementary to the first strand, using the first DNA strand as a template. This activity results in a double-stranded DNA molecule.

The process associated with HIV is unique because in most known cellular biochemistry, DNA is used as a template for the synthesis of RNA in the process of transcription that is part of protein synthesis. By utilizing RNA as a template for DNA synthesis, reverse transcriptase reverses the flow of biological information (hence, the enzyme's name "reverse transcriptase"). Moreover, HIV is known as a *retro*virus because of this enzyme's activity (*retro-* implies reverse). Within the retrovirus family of viruses, HIV belongs to a subgroup called lentiviruses.

Once the double-stranded DNA molecule has been formed, it migrates to the nucleus of its host T-lymphocyte, macrophage, or other cell. The distance the DNA molecule must travel is formidable (up to 20 micrometers), and research

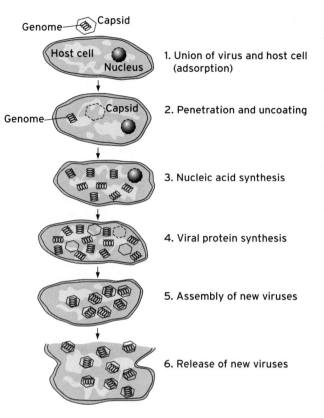

Genome — Capsid

Host cell
Nucleus

1. Union of virus and host cell (adsorption)

Genome — Capsid

2. Penetration and uncoating

3. Nucleic acid synthesis

4. Viral protein synthesis

5. Assembly of new viruses

6. Release of new viruses

FIGURE 2.6
A generalized schematic of viral replication in a host cell. In this representation, the virus unites with the host cell. Then the capsid and genome penetrate into the cytoplasm of the cell, and the synthesis of viral enzymes begins. Nucleic acid and protein molecules for the virus are synthesized next. After assembly, the mature viruses are released. This generalized scheme of viral replication should be compared with the replication process for human immunodeficiency virus in Figure 2.7.

reported in 1998 suggests that the molecule may use the actin filaments of the cell's cytoskeleton as an ultramicroscopic highway. The data from experiments using green fluorescent proteins indicate that DNA molecules move along fairly linear paths in bursts somewhat like stop-and-go traffic on a busy street. The entire trip appears to take a few minutes to complete.

On arriving at the nucleus, the DNA molecule is incorporated into the cell's DNA at a random site by a viral enzyme named integrase. Researchers indicate that incorporation is most efficient while the cell is dividing because the nuclear envelope has broken down at this time and need not be penetrated. (How the DNA molecule gets through the nuclear envelope of nondividing cells such as macrophages is still uncertain.) The incorporated DNA molecule thus becomes part of one of the cell's 46 chromosomes. Within the nuclear material, the DNA molecule is termed a provirus (Figure 2.7). A phenomenon like this is not often observed in biology. It is referred to as lysogeny, and the cycle of events is called the lysogenic cycle. The process implies that a person carries HIV as a provirus in the T-lymphocytes. With HIV in this latent form, the person is perfectly healthy, even though a carrier of HIV. In medical terms, this person does not have AIDS; rather, the individual has a condition known as HIV infection.

1 Q How do viruses multiply?

A Viruses do not multiply by the method of cell division that we associate with most living things. Instead, viruses invade a living cell and release their nucleic acid, and the latter directs the synthesis of new viruses utilizing structures and chemical components of the cell. No other object studied in biology multiplies in this manner. The process results in hundreds or thousands of copies of the virus as well as a poorly functioning or dead cell.

2 Q I've noticed that the incubation period for AIDS is unusually long. Why is that so?

A The human immunodeficiency virus (HIV) that causes AIDS follows the general pattern of viral replication, with an important exception. Once released in a host cell, the viral nucleic acid (RNA) serves as a template for the synthesis of a DNA molecule that incorporates itself into one of the cell's chromosomes. HIV remains in this DNA form in the infected cell, and it may be many months or years before enough viruses are encoded to overwhelm the body's immune system. Therefore, the incubation period tends to be very long in some individuals.

3 Q Can you get rid of HIV once it has invaded your cells?

A Once an individual is infected with HIV, the virus will probably remain for life. This is because HIV in its DNA form becomes part of a chromosome in the cell and is duplicated with the chromosome when the cell undergoes division. Thus, all the progeny of the originally infected cells will contain the DNA derived from HIV. It is unknown at this time whether a person can be infected for life without developing the symptoms of AIDS.

Public health specialists at the Centers for Disease Control and Prevention (CDC) estimate that as of 2002, close to 1 million Americans had HIV infection. Though in good health, these individuals could transmit the provirus if their infected T-lymphocytes are transferred to another person. And since blood and semen carry T-lymphocytes, it is clear that blood and semen can transfer HIV in its provirus form.

The passage of HIV among healthy individuals is but one consequence of HIV's residing in T-lymphocytes in its DNA form. Another consequence is that the virus escapes body defenses because it is inside a cell. The body's antibodies cannot reach the provirus (antibodies do not enter cells), nor can the provirus be attacked by the body's white blood cells (phagocytes) that normally engulf and destroy microorganisms. Moreover, any drug developed against HIV must penetrate living cells and eliminate the provirus without killing the cell, a formidable task. It is also unlikely that a vaccine against AIDS will be able to protect the 1 million Americans who carry HIV, because they are already infected.

HIV Activation and Release

Researchers are certain that the DNA provirus continues to encode new HIV particles within T-lymphocytes or other host cells. As new viruses are encoded and synthesized, the injured T-lymphocytes are able to replace themselves and the body defenses continue their response, but the virus eventually overwhelms the cells by a number of mechanisms we explore in Chapter 3.

The synthesis of HIV components appears to depend on the activity of sections at the end of the nucleic acid molecules of the viral genome. These regions are believed to direct cellular enzymes to form RNA, using the genetic code provided by the proviral DNA. Certain of the RNA strands are used to construct a new generation of HIV genomes, while other RNA strands carry genetic instructions for the capsid proteins and reverse transcriptase molecules of the new viruses. The genomes, capsid proteins, and enzyme molecules are then assembled at the edge of the cell. Here they form a somewhat circular structure that binds to the cell membrane.

At this point, an enzyme called protease comes into play. Protease is a protein-cleaving enzyme (and the objective of anti-HIV drugs discussed in Chapter 8). It snips out enzyme molecules and capsid proteins from preliminary protein molecules, then sections the capsid proteins into capsomere segments. The

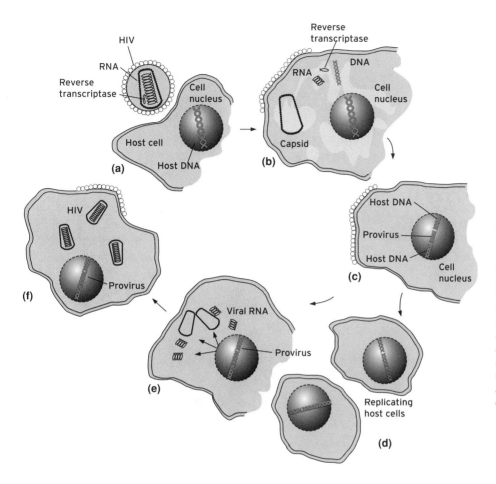

FIGURE 2.7

The replication cycle of human immunodeficiency virus (HIV). (a) The virus unites with the host cell as the viral envelope contacts the cell's surface membrane via the gp120, gp41, and CD4 molecules. (b) After union, the capsid is stripped away and the RNA of HIV is released. Reverse transcriptase uses the RNA as a template and synthesizes a double-stranded DNA molecule. (c) The new DNA migrates to the cell nucleus and is integrated into one of the host cell's chromosomes as a provirus. (d) The host cell may divide indefinitely with the provirus in position. (e) The provirus provides the genetic code for the enzymes that will mediate the production of capsid proteins plus RNA genomes. This is the stage of active HIV production. (f) After assembly of viral components, the new HIV particles move to the cell's surface membrane and bud through, thereby acquiring their envelopes. The cycle is now ready to repeat itself.

capsomeres unite and form an icosahedral capsid. This icosahedron then collapses to yield a bullet-shaped capsid surrounding the RNA genome and enzymes. Now the virus encloses itself in a portion of the host cell's surface membrane, which will become the envelope. Before forming the envelope, however, the patch of membrane unites with the virus-specified glycoproteins, gp120 and gp41. These glycoproteins then extend from the membrane as spikes.

While HIV is acquiring an envelope, it is also leaving the cell. In this process, known as budding, the virus moves through the cell membrane, surrounds itself with the envelope, and is released to the extracellular environment (Figure 2.8). The cycle of HIV replication is now complete. When the virus combines with a neighboring T-lymphocyte, macrophage, or other cell, the cycle is repeated.

Cell Destruction

The release of HIV from the cell appears less explosive than for many other types of viruses. How then do the HIV particles destroy the cell? One possibility is that

FIGURE 2.8

This sequence shows the formation of an HIV particle at the surface of an infected lymphocyte. The first appearance of the virus (top left) is as a small bump on the surface of the cell. The virus then buds out (top right) and is eventually cut off from the cell membrane. The newly released virus particle is at the bottom left, and the mature virus is at the bottom right.

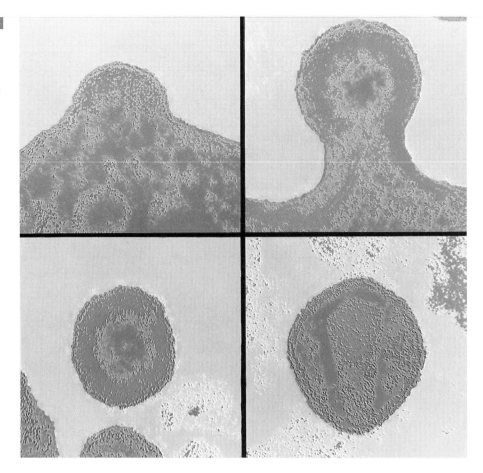

as the virus buds through the cell membrane, it tears holes in the membrane. Cytoplasmic leakage through the holes may bring on cell destruction.

Another possibility is that HIV induces T-lymphocytes to cling together in a giant, multinucleated cell mass called a syncytium. Syncytial formation is possible because an HIV-infected cell manufactures gp120 molecules and deposits the molecules on its surface membrane. When an infected cell later encounters a healthy cell, the gp120 molecules of the infected cell bind to the CD4 molecules of the healthy cell. The two cells then continue to fuse with other cells, until as many as 500 cells have combined to yield a huge, functionless syncytium (Figure 2.9). The supply of useful T-lymphocytes is thus depleted, and the efficiency of the immune system is impaired.

The deleterious effects of syncytia were shown in 1998 experiments conducted at the University of Iowa. Researchers led by David R. Soll showed that mobile syncytia can disrupt membranes containing collagen, membranes similar

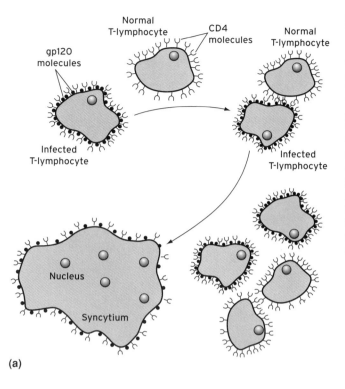

(a)

FIGURE 2.9

Syncytium formation. (a) An infected T-lymphocyte displays gp120 molecules on its surface as a result of infection with HIV. It unites with an uninfected T-lymphocyte having CD4 receptor sites on its surface. The union results in a fused T-lymphocyte. Additional uninfected T-lymphocytes unite with this fused cell (shown below the fused cell). The result of multiple fusions is a giant multi-nucleated cell mass known as a syncytium. (b) An electron micrograph of an HIV-infected syncytium on a bed of collagen fibers.

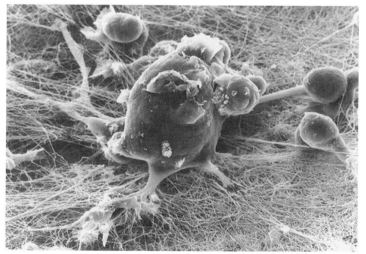

(b)

to those found in lymph nodes. The syncytia can also destroy the tissues lining blood cells and open microscopic holes in the blood vessels. These tendencies may explain why AIDS patients often experience disrupted lymph nodes and leaky blood vessels.

Still another possible mechanism of cell destruction is that the provirus is triggered to direct the synthesis of an unusually large number of new HIV particles. This pulse of activity rapidly uses up cellular components and leads to cell disintegration. The viruses of many other diseases also induce this destruction. T-lymphocyte depletion by this process and others (Chapter 3) will soon manifest itself in low immune system efficiency.

Before we continue, we should note that HIV also infects brain cells and depletes their numbers. Brain cell destruction leads to a form of AIDS called HIV encephalopathy. Although studied less thoroughly than T-lymphocyte infection, HIV encephalopathy is an equally serious form of AIDS. The ramifications of HIV encephalopathy are explored more completely in Chapter 4.

The HIV Genome

The genetic information for the replication of HIV is contained in a genome consisting of 9747 nucleotides. These nucleotides are known to exist as nine units of genetic activity, or genes (a human cell, by contrast, is currently estimated to have approximately 50,000 genes).

Nine Genes

The nine genes of HIV consist of segments of DNA, observed in HIV in its proviral form. Three genes providing genetic information for HIV's structural components are termed *gag, pol,* and *env.* These genes contain the genetic codes for the capsid proteins, viral enzymes, and envelope proteins, respectively. At one point in the genome, the genetic codes for *gag* and *pol* overlap, a situation observed with many genetic codes in nature.

The remaining six genes of HIV appear to be regulatory genes that control such things as penetration of the host cell, uncoating of the HIV genome, production of viral DNA, and integration of the provirus. One regulatory gene is the transactivator gene (*tat*). Research evidence indicates that this gene is responsible for the burst of HIV replication that occurs when infected T-lymphocytes are stimulated. Such a stimulation can be caused by the chemical components of microorganisms or other foreign molecules known as antigens (Chapter 3). The *tat* gene is unique in that it is composed of two separate segments of DNA within the genome (Figure 2.10). Mutant strains of HIV that lack this gene react far less actively when antigens stimulate the T-lymphocytes. The gene apparently encodes a protein that increases the expression of HIV genes, thus leading to increased synthesis of new viruses.

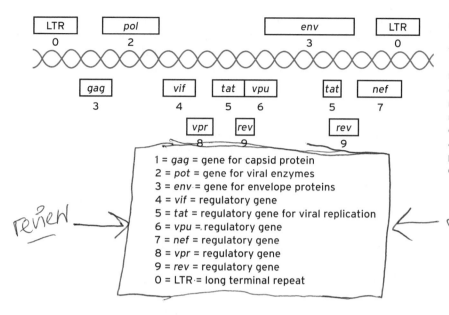

FIGURE 2.10

A diagrammatic representation of the genome of HIV, displaying nine known genes. The genes have been numbered because portions of two genes (*tat* and *rev*) occur in separate segments. The long terminal repeat (LTR) segments at the ends of the genome are not genes, but are shown for orientation purposes. Activities encoded by the genes are summarized in the text.

1 = *gag* = gene for capsid protein
2 = *pot* = gene for viral enzymes
3 = *env* = gene for envelope proteins
4 = *vif* = regulatory gene
5 = *tat* = regulatory gene for viral replication
6 = *vpu* = regulatory gene
7 = *nef* = regulatory gene
8 = *vpr* = regulatory gene
9 = *rev* = regulatory gene
0 = LTR = long terminal repeat

Another regulatory gene is the "*regulator of expression of viral protein*" gene, or *rev*. This gene, also composed of two separate DNA segments, enables the provirus to encode regulatory proteins or viral components, depending on proviral needs at the time. When the provirus lies dormant, for example, *rev* encodes proteins that prevent viral replication (the infection remains silent); but when a pulse of viral reproduction is to take place, *rev* encodes proteins to be used for new viruses (the infection is activated). In the latter case, *rev* apparently acts by increasing the efficiency with which the genetic code in the proviral DNA is translated to make proteins for producing new viruses. Once replication is under way, *rev* may interact with *tat* to produce the slow and controlled level of viral production that characterizes HIV.

Still another regulatory gene is the "*negative regulatory factor*" gene, or *nef*. This gene encodes a protein that remains near the nuclear membrane and enhances the movement of genetic messages into the cytoplasm of the host cell. From this position, the protein can also influence biochemical messages to other genes within the nucleus. Apparently these messages profoundly suppress all further gene expression, leading to a dormant provirus. A high concentration of proteins encoded by *rev* apparently can suppress *nef* activity and thereby switch on viral replication.

The function of another regulatory gene is to encode *viral protein R,* and hence it is called *vpr*. This protein assists the transport of viral DNA into the nucleus, where it will integrate into a chromosome. The protein also appears to assist the assembly and release of new HIV particles from the cytoplasm of the host cell.

The regulatory gene *vif* is necessary for the reverse transcription of RNA to DNA. The protein encoded by this gene acts at the end of the process and may function in the correct winding of the new proviral DNA molecule.

Still another regulatory gene called *vpu* encodes *v*iral *p*rotein *U*. This protein breaks down the CD4 receptor protein normally produced within the cytoplasm before it is transported to the cell surface. Unless destroyed, this CD4 protein would inhibit the budding of HIV out of the cell. The activity of the *vpu* gene is thus essential to continued HIV production.

The genome of HIV also contains at its opposite ends two stretches of DNA called long terminal repeats (LTRs). These LTRs are not genes as such, but they apparently direct host cell enzymes to transcribe the biochemical information of proviral DNA into RNA during viral replication. This activity is performed by defining the initiation site for RNA production. Thus, the LTRs play a key role in the activation of the process leading to new HIV particles.

Biochemical and genetic analyses have made it clear that the physiology of HIV is quite complex. The elaborate set of genetic controls reflects a well-adapted virus that carries out its activities in a carefully coordinated manner. In the practical sense, a knowledge of these activities can provide possible bases for drugs to control HIV replication, as we explore in Chapter 8.

Three Groups of HIV

Analysis of the HIV genome has made it clear that permanent genetic changes called mutations occur often during the replication of HIV. Indeed, one researcher has estimated that at least one mutation takes place in the HIV genome each time a round of replication occurs. Compounding the likelihood of mutation is the presence of two RNA molecules per virus, either of which can mutate. Moreover, mutation is possible in the biochemical step in which RNA is used to synthesize DNA. Most mutations have no effect on the virus, but sometimes the genetic flexibility leads to drug resistance or encourages the virus to escape the body's immune response; it also increases the difficulty of producing an effective vaccine.

Mutations in the HIV genome have probably led to the three groups of HIV-1 now known to exist. The first group is the "main" or M group. Viruses in this group are responsible for 99 percent of all AIDS cases in the world. The M group contains ten subgroups (also called clades) based on variations in the *gag* and *env* genes. The subgroups, lettered A to J, are present on all continents. Their presence makes developing a universal vaccine difficult because the vaccine must take all subgroups into account. Subgroup B predominates in North America.

The second group of HIV-1 is the "outlier" or O group. Viruses in this group have been found in West African countries such as Gabon and Cameroon. They cause less than 1 percent of AIDS cases, and their RNA shows less than a 50 percent watch with the RNA of the M group. Group O viruses were not detected in the United States until 1996, and fewer than five cases of AIDS have been related to viruses in the group. For this reason, tests for group O viruses are not routinely performed in the United States. Figure 2.11 shows how the O group is related to the M group.

The third group, the N group, was discovered in 1998 by French researchers led by François Simon. Appropriately named the "new" group, the viruses are genetically distinct from those in the M and O groups. They were isolated from a small population of individuals in Cameroon. Like the O group viruses, the N group viruses are not routinely sought in the HIV tests. Their similarity to SIV found in chimpanzees suggests that the N group's ancestors might have been transmitted to humans from nonhuman primates (Chapter 1).

Inhibiting Viruses

Viruses have a structure and replication pattern not found elsewhere in the natural world. However, viruses are composed of chemical compounds, and many of the principles of destruction that apply to all the microorganisms apply to viruses (Healthline 2.3). Viruses, for example, may be inactivated by many of the physical and chemical agents routinely used for other microorganisms. Heat and ultraviolet (UV) radiation are typical of the physical agents. Heat alters the structure of proteins and nucleic acids, and the heat of boiling water destroys most viruses in a matter of seconds. Ultraviolet radiation affects nucleic acids by binding together adjacent portions of their molecules. Germicidal lamps that emit UV radiation thus eliminate viruses after a few seconds of exposure.

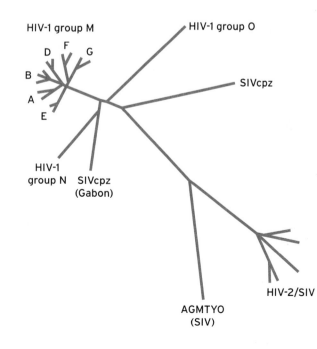

FIGURE 2.11

Genetic relatedness among strains of HIV. The M, N, and O groups originate from a common ancestor. Note that N group viruses are closely related to a strain of SIV, and both may have originated from a common ancestor. HIV-2 is distant from the three strains of HIV-1, showing that it is poorly related to HIV-1. However, it is closely related to an SIV strain. The various lettered subgroups of HIV-1 are included in group M.

1 **Q** Why is it not possible to use antibiotics against viruses?

A Antibiotics interfere with metabolic processes in bacterial cells. Because viruses do not show any metabolic processes, there is nothing to interfere with. Consider bacteria, for example. They are surrounded by cell walls, and penicillin interferes with the production of cell walls. Viruses perform no such activity.

2 **Q** Can viruses be controlled with antiseptics and disinfectants?

A Very definitely. Viruses are particles of nucleic acid, proteins, and other organic substances. As such, they are susceptible to the destructive effects of myriad antiseptics and disinfectants. In broad terms, any agent useful against bacteria will be equally useful against viruses.

3 **Q** How are vaccines useful for the prevention of viral disease?

A Vaccines contain altered forms of viruses, either weakened viruses that multiply slowly in the body or inactivated viruses that are unable to multiply at all. When introduced into the body, a vaccine stimulates the immune system to produce highly specific antibody molecules. The antibody molecules react with and destroy the active form of the virus if it should appear at a later date in the body. Destruction of the virus prevents the disease.

Among the antiviral chemical agents are compounds of chlorine, iodine, and silver, as well as phenol, formaldehyde, and detergents. Each has a different effect on viruses, as Figure 2.12 illustrates, and most are available commercially. We shall explore their uses in Chapter 6, but for the present it is worth remembering that viruses, including HIV, are no more difficult to destroy than any other microorganisms, when they are outside living cells. Indeed, for fragile viruses such as HIV, destruction is rather swift.

By contrast, destroying viruses with drugs is very difficult. Viruses lack complex structures, chemical reactions, or any biochemical activity, so there is little for drugs to interfere with. Penicillin destroys the cell wall of a bacterium, but viruses have no cell wall; therefore, penicillin is useless.

Nevertheless, certain antiviral drugs are available for treating people infected with viruses. Acyclovir, for instance, is a drug that interferes with the synthesis of nucleic acids by herpes simplex viruses, and azidothymidine (AZT) works similarly with HIV. Useful drugs such as these are rare because drugs often exhibit toxic side effects and can interfere with essential chemical reactions in the body. For HIV, the problem is compounded because the virus remains inside infected T-lymphocytes and brain cells. Still, molecular biologists have identified several steps in the replication cycle of HIV that may yield to interference by antiviral drugs. Among these steps are the binding of HIV to the CD4 receptor site of the host cell, the shedding of the viral coat in the host cell's cytoplasm, the activity of reverse transcriptase (the point at which AZT works), the assembly of viral components into new viruses, and the budding of new HIV particles from the host cell. These approaches to drug therapy are discussed in Chapter 8.

The major public health approach to viral diseases is through prevention, rather than treatment, and the major weapon for prevention is vaccines. In contemporary medicine, vaccines exist for such viral diseases as measles, mumps, and rubella (the MMR vaccine); hepatitis B; rabies; and some strains of influenza. Certain vaccines contain attenuated viruses, that is, viruses that multiply at a low rate; other vaccines contain inactivated viruses, that is, viruses that cannot multiply any longer but are structurally integrated; still others contain laboratory-produced viral fragments. Vaccines stimulate the body's immune system in various ways, one of which is to induce the system to produce protein molecules called antibodies. These antibodies then circulate and provide surveillance against the active virus, should it enter the body.

It is conceivable that a vaccine may hold the key to interrupting the AIDS epidemic. Many problems are associated with producing such a vaccine, how-

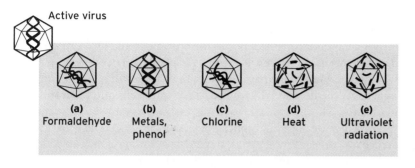

FIGURE 2.12

Six methods of inactivating viruses. (a) Formaldehyde combines with free amino groups on nucleic acid bases. (b) Metals and phenol react with the protein of the viral capsid. (c) Chlorine combines chemically with nucleic acids in viruses. (d) Heat denatures proteins of the capsid. (e) Ultraviolet radiation binds together thymine molecules in the genome and distorts the nucleic acid.

ever. Among the problems that must be resolved are deciding which form the vaccine should take (attenuated, inactivated, or fragmented virus), dealing with the various components of the envelope spikes, locating an animal model for testing purposes, and measuring the vaccine's effectiveness in field trials. There is also the possibility that many forms of HIV are causing AIDS in multiple overlapping epidemics. If so, then the usefulness of a single vaccine would be reduced. Chapter 9 of this book addresses these issues and describes how researchers are dealing with them. For the time being, it is well to note that the pessimism of the early 1980s has been replaced with cautious optimism for the new century. In many circles, the question is no longer "If?" but rather "How soon?"

LOOKING BACK

Viruses appear to be transitional forms between inert molecules and living organisms. They are extremely small particles of nucleic acid surrounded by a protein coat and, in some cases, an envelope with spikes. The human immunodeficiency virus (HIV) has a genome of RNA, a capsid that is first icosahedral and then bullet-shaped, and an envelope containing spikes. Molecules of the enzyme reverse transcriptase exist among the strands of RNA in the HIV genome.

Viruses begin their replication process by uniting with host cells. They then penetrate to the cytoplasm of the cells, where the viral nucleic acid is released. Next, the nucleic acid molecule directs the synthesis of new viruses, usually destroying the cell in the process. For HIV, the union between virus and T-lymphocyte involves the glycoproteins gp120 and gp41 of HIV and the CD4 receptor site of the cell as well as several coreceptors. Once the RNA has been released in the cell's cytoplasm, reverse transcriptase uses the RNA as a template to synthesize DNA. The resulting DNA then takes up residence in the chromosomal DNA of the cell, where it is called a provirus. From this location, the provirus encodes the synthesis of new HIV particles. Membrane tearing, syncytium formation, and rapid viral replication may lead to the death of T-lymphocytes. Brain cells and macrophages may also be involved.

The genetic information for HIV replication is contained in nine genes, three of which are structural genes. These genes, named *gag, pol,* and *env,* encode the viral capsid proteins, enzymes, and envelope proteins, respectively. The remaining six genes appear to be regulatory genes that oversee such processes as HIV replication, the rate of protein production, and the ability to remain latent in the host cell. Three major groups, the M, N, and O groups, have been identified for HIV-1 based on genetic relatedness. The M group occurs worldwide and is responsible for 99 percent of AIDS cases in the world.

Like other viruses, HIV can be inactivated with physical and chemical agents such as heat and chlorine. However, drug therapy for viruses is difficult because of the structural and biochemical simplicity of viruses and the toxicity of antiviral drugs to body cells. The fact that HIV resides in cells as a provirus adds to the difficulty. However, antiviral drugs are useful in halting the synthesis of DNA and in retarding the formation of the capsid. Vaccines against viruses can contain weakened or inactivated viruses or viral fragments. For HIV, however, multiple problems must be resolved before a vaccine becomes available.

REVIEW

The major thrust of this chapter has been to survey the structure and mode of replication of the viruses, with particular reference to the human immunodeficiency virus. To gauge the extent of your learning, select the letter that corresponds to the best answer for each of the following. Answers are listed in Appendix A.

_e_   **1.** All viruses consist of two basic components known as
  a. cytoplasm and a cell membrane.
  b. an envelope and a protoplast.
  c. a genome and an envelope.
  d. a cell membrane and a protoplast.
  e. a capsid and a genome.

_e_   **2.** Which of the following is true regarding the genome of a virus?
  a. The genome contains both DNA and RNA.
  b. An envelope is found within the genome.
  c. The genome contains complex carbohydrates.
  d. Only DNA viruses have a genome.
  e. None of the above is true.

b

3. Different forms of human immunodeficiency virus (HIV) are possible because
   a. the capsomeres vary among strains of HIV.
   b. chemical components of the spikes vary among HIV strains.
   c. the envelope is present in some strains of HIV but absent in others.
   d. not all strains of HIV have reverse transcriptase.
   e. capsid proteins vary among strains of HIV.

a

4. The human immunodeficiency virus (HIV) is able to replicate
   a. only within a living cell.
   b. only if the enzyme amylase functions effectively.
   c. only after the envelope has entered the cytoplasm of a cell.
   d. in either brain cells or liver cells.
   e. in media normally used to cultivate bacteria.

c

5. The CD4 molecule is a protein that
   a. is located on the surface of T-lymphocytes.
   b. reacts with an envelope glycoprotein of HIV.
   c. serves as a receptor site for HIV.
   d. All the above are true.
   e. None of the above is true.

d

6. For HIV to replicate within a host cell,
   a. the envelope must enter the host cell's cytoplasm.
   b. the viral capsid must be converted to carbohydrate.
   c. the virus must be engulfed by a white blood cell.
   d. the viral nucleic acid must be released from the capsid.
   e. the cytoplasm of the host cell must contain CD4 receptor sites.

a

7. Reverse transcriptase, a key enzyme found in HIV, is so named because it
   a. reverses the generally accepted flow of biological information.
   b. converts DNA to RNA, a reversal of the expected bio-chemistry.
   c. reverses the replication cycle of HIV and yields broken viruses.
   d. changes capsid proteins into nucleic acids for viral synthesis.
   e. reverses the pathway of HIV from inside the host cell to outside.

d

8. In its proviral form within the host cell, HIV
   a. can remain for an undetermined period of time.
   b. can escape body defenses such as antibodies.
   c. can be passed from one individual to another.

d. All of the above are true.

e. None of the above is true.

9. Which of the following pairs is mismatched?

a. spikes/envelope

b. reverse transcriptase/T-lymphocytes

c. provirus/DNA

d. protein/capsid

e. HIV/retrovirus

10. Blood and semen are able to transmit AIDS because

a. antibodies do not react with HIV in blood or semen.

b. blood or semen may contain viral capsids.

c. drugs are too toxic for use in blood or semen.

d. viruses do not replicate in blood or semen.

e. blood or semen may contain infected T-lymphocytes.

11. HIV may destroy its host cell in the body by

a. inducing the cell to multiply without control.

b. blocking the passage of important nutrients into the cell.

c. preventing the cell from uniting with other body cells.

d. tearing holes in the cell membrane as the virus buds through.

e. inhibiting the cellular production of reverse transcriptase.

12. Syncytium formation takes place

a. when HIV particles cling together.

b. after the transactivator gene has been activated.

c. when infected and uninfected T-lymphocytes unite to form a mass of cells.

d. only in uninfected T-lymphocytes.

e. only when a virus contains DNA in its genome and gp41 in its spikes.

13. The drug AZT acts against HIV by

a. interfering with the construction of viral nucleic acid.

b. precipitating the protein in the HIV capsid.

c. altering the structure of the HIV envelope so as to induce precipitation.

d. All of the above are true.

e. None of the above is true.

14. Compared to other viruses, HIV is generally

a. more resistant to acid and heat.

b. more resistant to UV radiation and drying.

c. more susceptible to physical and chemical treatments.

    d. more susceptible to treatment with drugs such as penicillin.

    e. more susceptible to acyclovir.

_a_   **15.** The genetic information for HIV replication is contained in

    a. nine genes.

    b. the capsid of the virus.

    c. the reverse transcriptase of the virus.

    d. the envelope protein molecules in the genome.

    e. 9000 protein molecules in the genome.

FOR ADDITIONAL READING

Alcamo, I. E. 2000. *Fundamentals of Microbiology*, 6th ed. Sudbury, MA: Jones & Bartlett.

Balter, M. 1998. "Revealing HIV's passkey." *Science* 280: 1833–1835.

Benditt, J. M., and B. R. Jasney, eds. 1993. "AIDS: the unanswered questions." *Science* 260: 1253–1293.

Blattner, W., R. C. Gallo, and H. M. Temin. 1988. "HIV causes AIDS." *Science* 241: 515–519.

Duke, R. C., et al. 1996. "Cell suicide in health and disease." *Scientific American,* December.

Emerman, M., and M. H. Malim. 1998. "HIV-1 regulatory genes: keys to unraveling viral and host cell biology." *Science* 280: 1880–1883.

Evans, A. 1989. "Does HIV cause AIDS? An historical perspective." *Journal of AIDS* 2: 107–111.

Gallo, R. C. 1987. "The AIDS virus." *Scientific American* 256(1): 47–56.

Hoffman, M. 1994. "AIDS: solving the molecular puzzle." *American Scientist* 82(2): 171–177.

Hu, D. J., et al. 1996. "The emerging genetic diversity of HIV." *JAMA* 275: 210–215.

Levine, A. J. 1992. *Viruses.* New York: Scientific American Library, distributed by W. H. Freeman.

Moore, J. P. 1997. "Coreceptors: implications for HIV pathogenesis and therapy." *Science* 276: 51–53.

The Immune System and HIV

LOOKING AHEAD

Because it provides a specific defense against infectious disease, the immune system is one of the key systems of the body. This chapter explores how the immune system functions and how the human immunodeficiency virus (HIV) interacts with it, resulting in AIDS. On completing the chapter, you should be able to . . .

* Describe the fetal development of the immune system and understand which cells are central to the system's formation and operation.
* Explain how T-lymphocytes provide specific defense against certain microorganisms, such as fungi and protozoa.
* Summarize the process by which stimulation of B-lymphocytes results in antibodies against viruses, bacteria, and other microorganisms and describe how antibodies act in body defense.
* Conceptualize how HIV depresses the functions of the immune system by interacting with two types of T-lymphocytes.
* Summarize the features of AIDS that make it a unique disease, accompanied by phenomena that do not occur in other infectious diseases.

INTRODUCTION

The human body is shaped like a doughnut. Just as the hole passes through the doughnut, the gastrointestinal tract passes through the body. Being in the hole does not mean being in the doughnut; nor does being in the gastrointestinal tract mean that an object is in the body. The respiratory tract and urinary tract technically lie outside the body as well. One is led to conclude that the body is a closed container (Figure 3.1).

The construction of the body is of more than passing interest. Indeed, it is essential to the body's resistance to disease: If a microorganism is to invade the body tissues, it must pass the cellular barrier separating the interior of the body

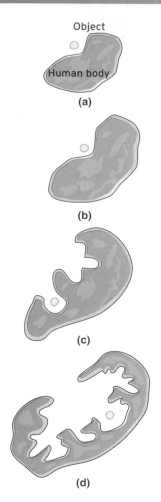

Object

Human body

(a)

(b)

(c)

(d)

FIGURE 3.1

The body as a closed container. (a) An object is clearly outside the body. (b) The object remains outside the body as the outer surface bulges inward. (c) Despite additional inward bulging, the object remains outside. (d) The object continues to be outside the body, even though many surface alterations have occurred. Being within a body cavity such as the gastrointestinal tract or lung does not necessarily imply that an object is in the body's internal environment.

from the exterior. Resistance like that provided by the cellular barrier is said to be nonspecific because it operates against all forms of microorganisms, not just one or more specific forms. Other forms of nonspecific resistance include powerful enzymes in the tears and saliva, which help resist infection in the eyes and mouth, respectively; the high acid content of the stomach, which presents a chemical barrier to the intestine beyond; the sticky mucus that traps microorganisms in the respiratory tract; and phagocytosis, the complex process by which the body's white blood cells engulf and destroy microorganisms.

But, sometimes, nonspecific resistance needs to be supplemented. The cells of the skin, for example, may be penetrated during an arthropod bite (the microorganisms causing Lyme disease, plague, and malaria are introduced this way); microorganisms may be able to resist the body's protective enzymes; or microbial toxins may injure or destroy the white blood cells dispatched to eliminate the microorganisms. In cases such as these, the body responds with a second major type of resistance called specific resistance.

Specific resistance is resistance mounted against a single species of microorganism or a single type of chemical compound. The resistance is stimulated by that microorganism or compound and is directed solely at the stimulant. The specific resistance that arises during an attack of measles, for instance, helps rid the body of the measles virus only. The resistance then remains in the body for many years (often for life), so that should the measles virus return, it cannot gain a foothold in the body. Ultimately, specific resistance prevents serious injury and death (Figure 3.2).

The body system that provides specific resistance is the immune system. The term "immune" is derived from the Latin *immuno,* meaning "to be free from"; the immune system frees the body of foreign microorganisms and chemicals and keeps it free of them. The system is a complex series of cells, chemical factors, and processes in which white blood cells, called lymphocytes, respond to and eliminate foreign agents. The agents that elicit the response are called antigens. Elimination of the antigens can occur through direct destruction by lymphocytes or through indirect destruction by specialized protein molecules called antibodies. As we shall discuss presently, the antibodies destroy the antigen directly and target it for destruction by other cells.

The immune system bears the brunt of attack in most individuals infected by HIV. Thus, to fully comprehend the nature of HIV infection and AIDS, it is important to have a clear idea of the workings of the immune system. Indeed, the very name "acquired *immune deficiency* syndrome" refers to a poorly functioning immune system.

We shall study the immune system by first exploring its origin in the fetus. We then investigate the substances that stimulate its operation and outline the two major branches of the system. Once a firm foundation on the mechanics of the system has been set, we shall study the effects of HIV on the system's cells and explore how AIDS comes about.

Development of the Immune System

During the third month after conception, the developing individual in the uterus is unmistakably human and is termed a fetus. The fetus is about 2 inches long, and all its organ systems are present in various stages of development. Its head is large, its nose is flat, its eyes are far apart, and its reproductive organs are distinguishable. The fetus is quite active, bending its arms and legs and pivoting its head. Like an astronaut floating in a weightless environment, the fetus waves and kicks as it tumbles in slow motion in its sac of uterine fluid.

At this period in fetal development, cartilage is being replaced by bone, and within the bone marrow is a set of primitive cells called stem cells. For two weeks or so, stem cells have been forming red blood cells through a complex process. Now, certain of the stem cells begin forming forerunners of the immune system, called lymphopoietic cells (Figure 3.3).

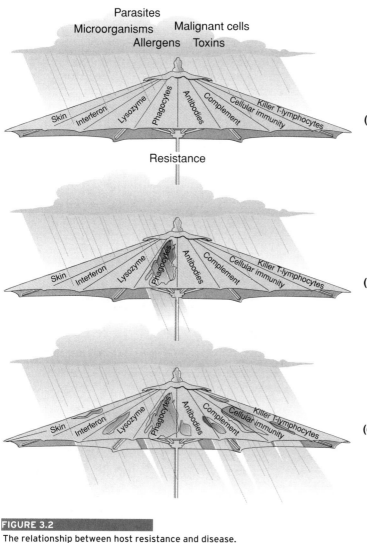

Parasites
Microorganisms Malignant cells
Allergens Toxins

Resistance

(a) Host resistance to microorganisms and other agents depends on many factors that must function well in the individual. The factors on the left side of the umbrella are nonspecific factors; those on the right are specific factors.

(b) Resistance may begin to break down when one or more factors is inoperable. When phagocytosis fails to take place, for example, some infectious agents penetrate the umbrella of defense.

(c) Disease develops when many host defenses are compromised. Under these conditions, the body cannot defend itself. Even when defenses are not compromised, the aggressiveness and toxicity of the pathogen may lead to infection.

FIGURE 3.2

The relationship between host resistance and disease.

Lymphopoietic cells follow either of two courses of development. Certain lymphopoietic cells pass through an organ near the thyroid gland called the thymus. Here they are modified to form T-lymphocytes (or T-cells; T for thymus). This modification includes insertion of receptor molecules on the cell surfaces; the receptor sites will unite with substances foreign to the body. The T-lymphocytes then migrate through the circulatory system and come to rest at the spleen, tonsils, adenoids, and lymph nodes. Lymph nodes are pockets of white blood cells prevalent in the armpits, neck, groin, and other body locations (Figure 3.4). They form the "swollen glands" one sometimes experiences during illness.

FIGURE 3.3

The origin of the immune system.

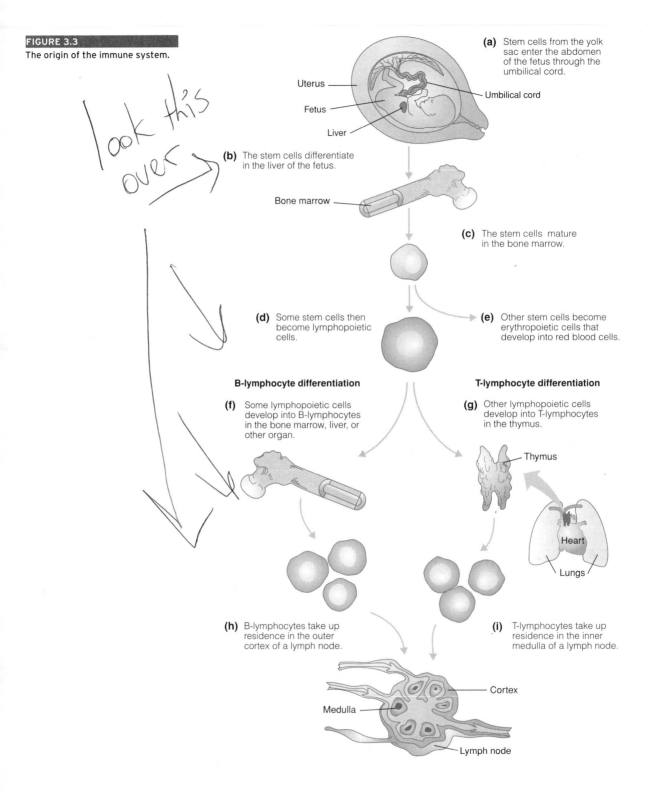

(a) Stem cells from the yolk sac enter the abdomen of the fetus through the umbilical cord.

Uterus

Fetus

Liver

Umbilical cord

(b) The stem cells differentiate in the liver of the fetus.

Bone marrow

(c) The stem cells mature in the bone marrow.

(d) Some stem cells then become lymphopoietic cells.

(e) Other stem cells become erythropoietic cells that develop into red blood cells.

B-lymphocyte differentiation

(f) Some lymphopoietic cells develop into B-lymphocytes in the bone marrow, liver, or other organ.

T-lymphocyte differentiation

(g) Other lymphopoietic cells develop into T-lymphocytes in the thymus.

Thymus

Heart

Lungs

(h) B-lymphocytes take up residence in the outer cortex of a lymph node.

(i) T-lymphocytes take up residence in the inner medulla of a lymph node.

Cortex

Medulla

Lymph node

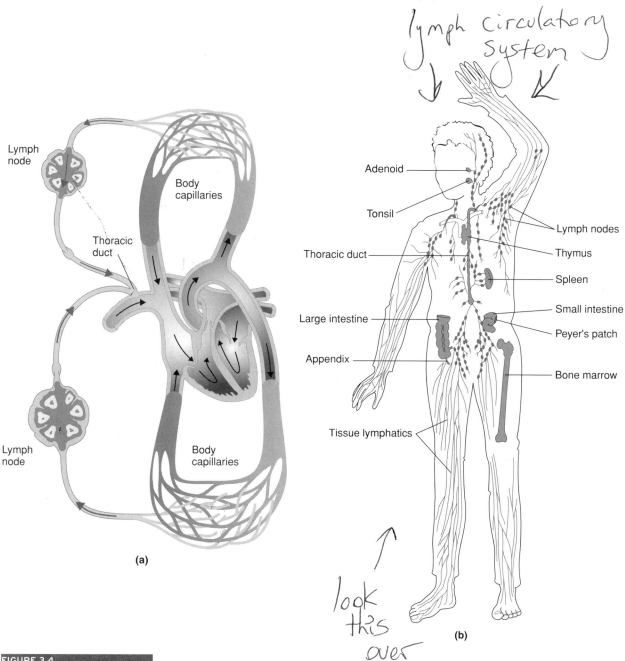

lymph circulatory system

Adenoid

Tonsil

Thoracic duct

Large intestine

Appendix

Tissue lymphatics

Lymph nodes

Thymus

Spleen

Small intestine

Peyer's patch

Bone marrow

Lymph node

Body capillaries

Thoracic duct

Lymph node

Body capillaries

(a)

(b)

look this over

The interrelationship of the circulatory system and the lymphatic system. (a) Fluid passes out of the blood from the arteries in the upper and lower parts of the body. It enters a system of lymphatic ducts that arise in the tissues. The fluid, called lymph, passes through lymph nodes and on the right side makes its way back to the general circulation via the thoracic duct. The thoracic duct enters a main vein just before the vein enters the heart. A similar system exists on the left side. (b) The human lymphatic system consists of lymphocytes, lymphatic organs, lymph vessels, and lymph nodes located along the vessels. The lymphatic organs are illustrated, and the preponderance of lymph nodes in the neck, axilla, and groin is apparent.

The remainder of the immune system also develops from the lymphopoietic cells. Certain of these cells pass through an organ, not yet identified in humans, to form B-lymphocytes (Figure 3.4). In the embryonic chick, the organ is the bursa of Fabricius, hence, the name B-lymphocyte (or B-cell; B for bursa). The human organ corresponding to the bursa of Fabricius may be the bone marrow, liver, or lymph node tissues of the gastrointestinal tract. During formation, B-lymphocytes synthesize antibody molecules and position these molecules on their cell membranes. These antibody molecules will later act as receptor sites and react with foreign substances during the immune process. Thousands of different types of B-lymphocytes synthesize an equally diverse variety of antibodies. For example, one group of B-lymphocytes has measles antibodies on their cell surface, one group has influenza antibodies, one group has chickenpox antibodies, and so on. Once formed, the B-lymphocytes enter the circulation and, like the T-lymphocytes, migrate to the spleen, tonsils, adenoids, and lymph nodes.

When the immune system becomes functional after birth, B-lymphocytes and T-lymphocytes play a central role in the system and dominate its two main branches. From their vantage point in the lymph nodes and other lymphoid organs, the B-lymphocytes and T-lymphocytes encounter most microorganisms that enter the systems of the body. These encounters occur because lymph vessels contact or penetrate most body organs, and the fluid they drain passes through the lymph nodes on its way to the general circulation. The two types of lymphocytes are thus positioned to provide an immune response.

Antigens

B-lymphocytes and T-lymphocytes can be stimulated by specific molecules called antigens. An antigen is a substance, usually a large protein or polysaccharide, that stimulates the immune system. It may be part of a viral capsid or a bacterial flagellum or a mold spore, or it may be a chemical substance such as a cytoplasmic macromolecule. The list of antigens is enormously diverse and includes over a million agents. Such things as bee venom, penicillins, and animal hairs may act as or contain antigens. When antigens stimulate the immune system, a specific form of resistance results.

Normally a person's own proteins and polysaccharides do not stimulate an immune response because they are interpreted as "self." Research evidence suggests that before birth, the proteins and polysaccharides of body cells contact and paralyze immune system cells that might later respond to them. Thus, the individual becomes tolerant of "self" and remains able to respond only to antigens interpreted as "nonself," or foreign. The paralysis of responsive cells must continue throughout life for tolerance to self to persist.

Antigens may be described as any parts of a microorganism or chemical substance interpreted as foreign (nonself). These substances enter the body through a variety of portals, including tiny openings in the mucous membranes of the respiratory tract and openings in the skin when it is penetrated by arthropod bite or wound. Before the immune system is mature, antigens cannot elicit an immune response, but once the system has attained maturity, antigens are potent stimulators of the system (Healthline 3.1).

The Immune Process

The immune system reaches maturity several months after a person's birth and continues to function until a person's death. As antigens enter the body, either as free chemical substances or in association with microorganisms, the immune process begins in earnest. To initiate the process, the organisms are approached by phagocytes, the white blood cells that specialize in engulfing and destroying foreign materials (Figure 3.5). Chief among the phagocytes are large, amoeboid cells called macrophages.

Macrophages set the immune process into motion by taking microorganisms into their cytoplasm and digesting them. However, the organism's antigens are preserved and displayed on the surfaces of the macrophages. Macrophages also have on their surfaces a set of proteins called MHC (major histocompatibility complex) proteins. These proteins are present on all the body's cells and are unique for a particular person. In effect, the MHC proteins distinguish the macrophages as normal body cells. With both MHC proteins and foreign antigens on their surfaces, the macrophages move off toward the lymph nodes.

When a macrophage enters the lymph node, it encounters a T-lymphocyte called a helper T-lymphocyte (also called a CD4 cell because it possesses the CD4 receptor sites). As the two cells meet, the antigens and the MHC proteins on the macrophage react with receptor sites on the surface of the helper T-lymphocyte (Figure 3.6). This reaction activates the helper cell to produce and release a series of highly reactive proteins called lymphokines. Lymphokines then stimulate either the B-lymphocytes or the T-lymphocytes, depending on the nature of the antigen that began the process. The immune system therefore diverges at this point into two major functional branches. One branch is dominated by the T-lymphocytes, and the immunity that results is called cell-mediated immunity; the other branch is dominated by the B-lymphocytes, and the resulting immunity is called antibody-mediated immunity. In the following paragraphs, we shall discuss each type of immunity in turn, beginning with cell-mediated immunity.

Cell-Mediated Immunity

Cell-mediated immunity (CMI) is so named because the defense imparted by this branch of the immune system involves a direct

Healthline 3.1

1 **Q** I often hear the term "lymphocyte" used in connection with AIDS. What is a lymphocyte?

A A lymphocyte is a type of white blood cell functioning in the body's defense. Certain lymphocytes produce antibodies, which are specialized protein molecules that neutralize foreign substances or microorganisms. Other lymphocytes attack foreign microorganisms directly. Still other types of lymphocytes attract engulfing cells to an infection site and encourage them to rid the body of microorganisms.

2 **Q** Exactly where in the body is the immune system?

A The immune system is a complex series of cells distributed throughout the body, mainly in pockets of tissue called lymph nodes. Lymph nodes are prominent in the neck, armpits, and groin. Immune system cells are also found in the spleen, a long triangular organ near the stomach, and in the tonsils in the rear of the mouth.

3 **Q** How does the AIDS virus weaken a person's immunity to disease?

A The AIDS virus targets cells of the immune system for destruction and, in so doing, diminishes a person's ability to react to disease. Organisms normally held under control by the body then invade the tissues and bring on the symptoms of AIDS. These organisms are called "opportunistic organisms" because they seize the opportunity to invade. Death often results from their effects.

Phagocytosis. In this scanning electron micrograph, a phagocytic cell called a macrophage is engulfing old, misshapen red blood cells. Macrophages also engulf bacteria and other microorganisms and set the immune process in motion.

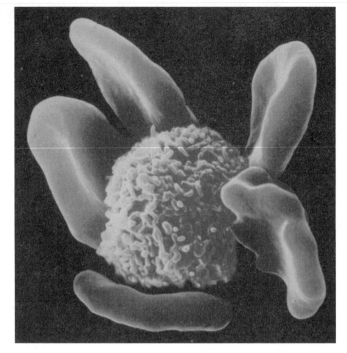

A scanning electron micrograph of lymphocytes observed in the human circulatory system. It is not possible from a photograph such as this to distinguish B-lymphocytes from T-lymphocytes, but both types play central roles in the immune system.

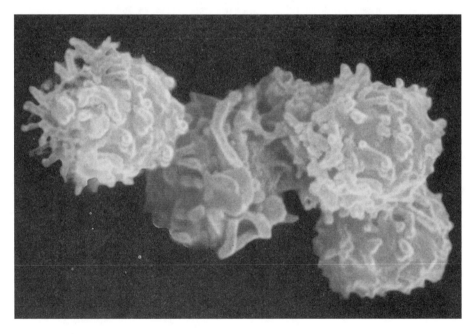

assault by cells on microorganisms or foreign molecules. The lymphokines released by the helper T-lymphocytes begin the process of CMI by stimulating other T-lymphocytes, called cytotoxic T-lymphocytes, to multiply rapidly (Figure 3.7). Cytotoxic T-lymphocytes then enter the circulatory system and search for body cells displaying the antigens that sensitized the lymphocytes. Fungi, protozoa, and certain virus-infected or bacteria-infected cells can also be the targets of the cytotoxic cells. A cytotoxic T-lymphocyte interacts with a microorganism by recognizing the MHC proteins and foreign antigens, then

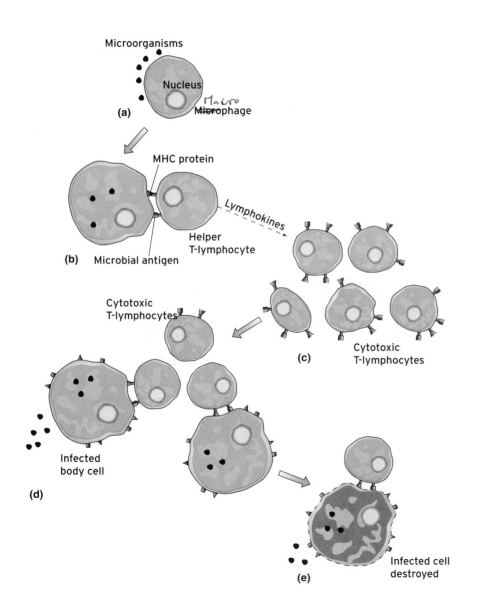

FIGURE 3.7

Cell-mediated immunity. (a) Microorganisms are engulfed by a macrophage, and microbial antigens are displayed on the surface of the macrophage together with MHC proteins. (b) Receptor sites on a helper T-lymphocyte react with the microbial and MHC proteins. This reaction stimulates the helper cell to release lymphokines. (c) The lymphokines activate cytotoxic T-lymphocytes and induce them to react with antigen-marked infected cells. (d) The lethal hit by a cytotoxic cell on an infected cell leads to cell death for the latter. (e) Lymphokines also stimulate cytotoxic T-lymphocytes to multiply and attack other infected cells, thereby continuing and expanding the immune process.

attacking and destroying the microorganism. This "lethal hit," as it is called, is assisted by a protein released from the cytotoxic cell and inserted into the surface membrane of the infected cell. The protein appears to open holes in the microbial cell membrane, and the cell's cytoplasm leaks out, resulting in death.

Cytotoxic T-lymphocytes are also the source of additional lymphokines. Secreted at the site where the antigens were first detected by macrophages, the lymphokines draw a host of fresh macrophages to the infection site and stimulate them to destroy the microorganisms (Healthline 3.2).

Another kind of T-lymphocyte we should note is the natural killer cell. This cell also attacks microorganisms and infected cells, but it is less specialized than the cytotoxic T-lymphocyte. Natural killer cells appear to be a primary mechanism of defense by the body against tumor cells, which are regarded as foreign. Together with cytotoxic T-lymphocytes, the natural killer cells provide an important line of defense in the body (Figure 3.8). The immunity they offer is called cell-mediated, because cells are the actual modes of defense.

To prevent the immune process from becoming too exaggerated and destroying normal body cells, another T-lymphocyte comes into play. This is the suppressor T-lymphocyte (also called a CD8 cell because it possesses the CD8 receptor sites). The suppressor T-lymphocyte dampens the activity of cytotoxic T-lymphocytes and natural killer cells and slows the immune process as the antigen stimulus lessens. With the gradual elimination of microorganisms and the antigens they carry, the process of cell-mediated immunity comes to a halt.

Antibody-Mediated Immunity

The second major branch of the immune system depends on the activity of B-lymphocytes and results in antibody-mediated immunity (AMI). To begin this process, B-lymphocytes are stimulated by helper T-lymphocytes after the latter have interacted with the antigen-bearing macrophages. As before, the helper T-lymphocytes produce lymphokines to activate the B-lymphocytes and stimulate their division. But there is also a second stimulant, the antigens on the macrophages' surfaces. As a macrophage moves among the hundreds of thousands of different types of B-lymphocytes, it eventually encounters one type that has surface antibody molecules corresponding to its antigens. The binding of the antigen and

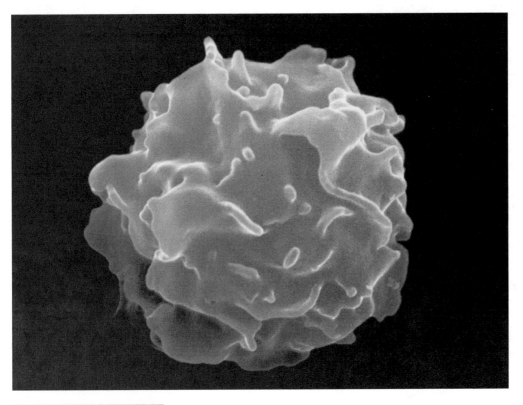

A scanning electron micrograph of a natural killer cell. Natural killer cells, although less specialized than cytotoxic T-lymphocytes, are an important component of the body's defensive capabilities.

antibody molecules, along with the helper T-lymphocytes' intervention, activates or "commits" the B-lymphocytes.

Once committed, B-lymphocytes undergo cell division and give rise to a colony (or clone) of cells programmed to produce antibodies. Antibodies designed to react with the antigen pour forth from the B-lymphocytes at a rate of more than 2000 molecules per second. Within hours, other biochemical signals convert many of the B-lymphocytes into plasma cells, a group of highly active antibody-producing cells (Figure 3.9). The antigens initiating process of antibody-mediated immunity are found primarily in viruses and bacteria. Other substances such as milk protein, bee venom, food molecules, and ragweed proteins can also stimulate the process.

Antibody molecules are proteins. There are five types of antibodies, the most common of which is composed of four chains of amino acids arranged as two long chains and two small chains. Such an antibody molecule has a hinge point where

FIGURE 3.9

Antibody-mediated immunity.
(a) The process of antibody-mediated immunity begins with the reaction between the receptor site of a helper T-lymphocyte and a macrophage bearing MHC proteins and microbial antigens. This process activates the helper cells. (b) The activated helper T-lymphocytes produce lymphokines and stimulate uncommitted B-lymphocytes. At the same time, the macrophage "searches" among uncommitted B-lymphocytes until it locates a B-lymphocyte with surface antibody receptors that match both the microbial antigen and the MHC protein. (c) The binding of macrophage and helper T-lymphocyte commits the B-lymphocyte, which now undergoes proliferation and differentiation to plasma cells. Lymphokines assist the process. (d) Plasma cells produce highly specialized antibody molecules to lend immunity.

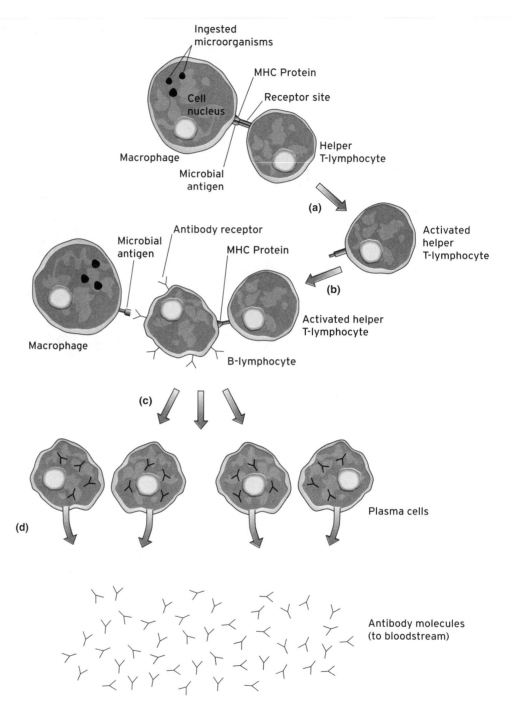

the chains diverge, and the molecule is therefore depicted as a Y. One end of the molecule is highly specific for the antigen that elicited its production. This implies that the antibody will interact with that antigen only. The immune system has the capacity to produce perhaps a million different kinds of antibodies, one for each different antigen. Thus, a measles antibody will react only with proteins in a measles virus, a chickenpox antibody only with a chickenpox virus, and so forth.

Antibodies circulate through the body and soon encounter the microorganism whose antigens stimulated their production. They then chemically combine with the antigen molecules and neutralize the microorganism by any of several mechanisms. For example, some antibodies bind to viral capsids and prevent the viruses from entering cells by covering their receptor sites. Other antibodies combine with antigens on the surface of bacteria and bind the bacteria together in a meshlike pattern that can easily be phagocytized. Still others form a bridge between microorganisms and macrophages to encourage phagocytosis, and others set off a cascading series of reactions that tear apart microbial membranes (Figure 3.10). The antigen-antibody reaction usually results in destruction of the microorganism.

From the foregoing, we can see that the immune system is the source of specific resistance originating with T-lymphocytes or B-lymphocytes. The common thread between the two branches of the system is the helper T-lymphocyte. This cell can stimulate either branch to function, depending on which antigens are delivered by macrophages. As we have noted, antigens primarily from fungi, protozoa, and certain types of bacteria and viruses stimulate the T-lymphocytes, whereas antigens primarily from bloodborne bacteria and viruses set the B-lymphocytes into action. Once activated, the T- or B-lymphocytes serve as the underpinning for the immune response that provides specific defense for the body. Should that defense be compromised, the results can be extraordinarily detrimental. Herein lies the basis for AIDS.

HIV and the Immune System

In its most simplified form, the general pattern of infectious disease is one in which the body and a population of microorganisms compete for supremacy. It is a battle of sorts, with each side trying to outdo the other. Some microorganisms attempt to overwhelm the body with sheer numbers, while consuming nutrients needed by the body; some microorganisms produce toxins that interfere with critical cellular processes such as nerve transmission; some synthesize enzymes that interfere with body defenses (e.g., some bacteria produce enzymes that destroy white blood cells). The body, in turn, responds via its immune system. Though some diseases, such as malaria, plague, and typhoid fever, often terminate in death, most diseases have a favorable prognosis because the specific resistance provided by the immune system is substantial. For example, we do not fear death from measles, chickenpox, or a common cold.

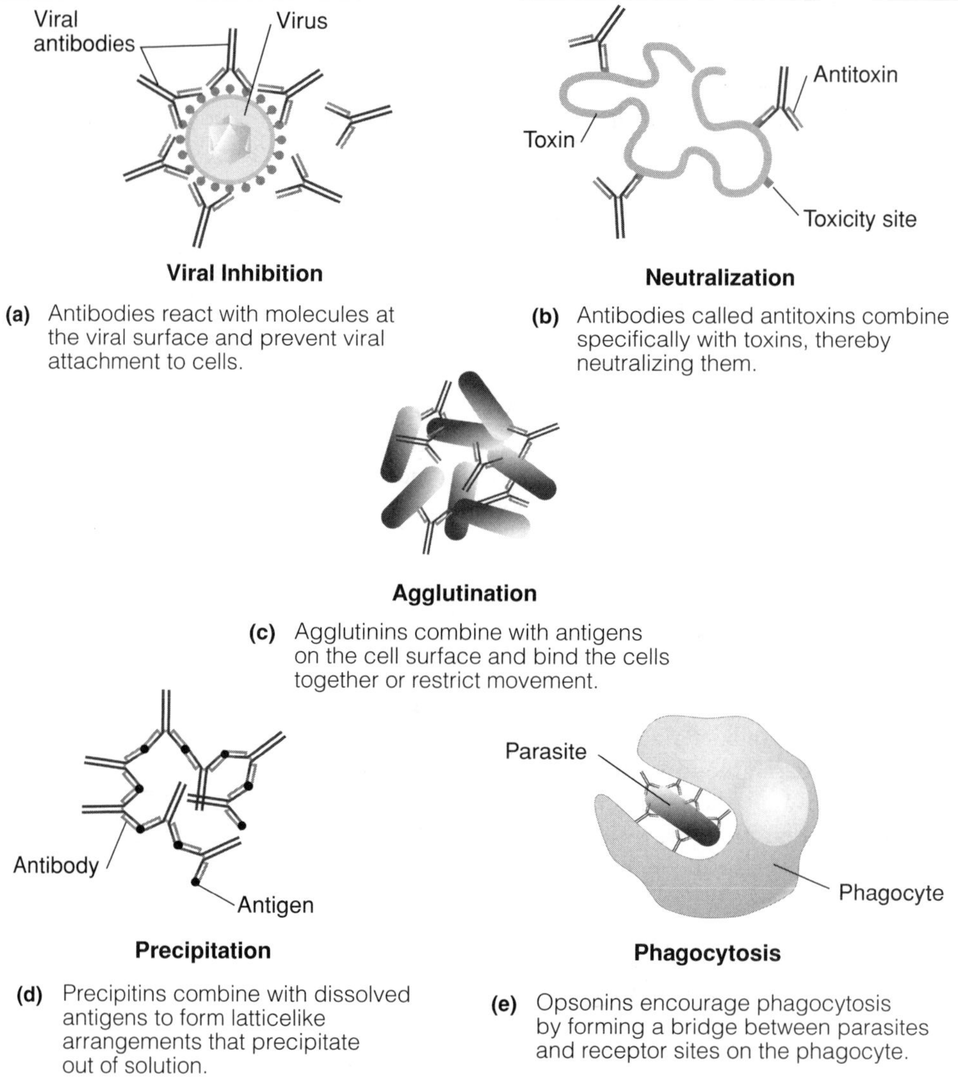
Viral antibodies
Virus
Viral Inhibition
(a) Antibodies react with molecules at the viral surface and prevent viral attachment to cells.
Antitoxin
Toxin
Toxicity site
Neutralization
(b) Antibodies called antitoxins combine specifically with toxins, thereby neutralizing them.
Agglutination
(c) Agglutinins combine with antigens on the cell surface and bind the cells together or restrict movement.
Antibody
Antigen
Precipitation
(d) Precipitins combine with dissolved antigens to form latticelike arrangements that precipitate out of solution.
Parasite
Phagocyte
Phagocytosis
(e) Opsonins encourage phagocytosis by forming a bridge between parasites and receptor sites on the phagocyte.

FIGURE 3.10

Five mechanisms by which antibodies interact with antigens.

It is now generally accepted that the human immunodeficiency virus (HIV) is the causative agent of AIDS. This virus was first isolated in 1984 by Luc Montagnier and his group at the Pasteur Institute (Chapter 1). It is a retrovirus containing RNA in its genome as well as the enzyme reverse transcriptase, which synthesizes the DNA provirus using RNA as its template (Chapter 2). Although a number of critics disagree (Box 3.1), most scientists and public health officials are convinced that HIV infection in the body cells leads to AIDS.

BOX
3.1

The Duesberg Phenomenon

In 1988, Peter Duesberg, a respected retro-virologist and cancer researcher at the University of California, published a paper arguing that HIV is not the cause of AIDS. Duesberg suggested that factors such as illicit drug use and AZT, the anti-HIV compound, cause the disease. In the years that followed, most mainstream AIDS researchers dismissed Duesberg's idea as unsupportable, but his challenge to the conventional wisdom continued to win converts. International symposia addressed Duesberg's theories, and news media occasionally presented his arguments for the reading public. Duesberg guest-edited scientific journals devoted to alternative AIDS hypotheses, and prominent scientists came out in his support. In 1995, *Science,* the journal of the American Association for the Advancement of Science (AAAS), devoted a special news report to his theories.

What, then, is the basis for Duesberg's objection? Duesberg points to evidence in studies with hemophiliacs. He says that contaminants in blood obtained from donors are the cause of AIDS and that HIV is a "harmless passenger." He describes data suggesting that noninfected hemophiliac patients show T-lymphocyte variations similar to those in AIDS patients. However, other researchers explain that the variations are not necessarily characteristic of AIDS and may not indicate an immune deficiency. Moreover, they argue that hemophiliacs receiving larger doses of donated blood products should be more likely to develop AIDS (since they would receive more "contaminants"), but studies indicate no association between dose levels received and the likelihood of developing AIDS.

Second, Duesberg notes that HIV has never been given to a healthy host, who then developed AIDS. An experiment such as this is part of a series of procedures known as Koch's postulates, whereby a particular agent is related unquestionably to a particular disease. However, Duesberg's critics point out that in three separate and tragic laboratory accidents, a pure strain of HIV infected researchers, who then developed AIDS symptoms. In the first case, the researcher developed *Pneumocystis carinii* pneumonia, an AIDS-defining opportunistic disease, within five years; the second worker had a depressed T-lymphocyte count after six years; and the third had depressed counts after two years. No other risk factors (such as injection drug use) were involved.

Third, Duesberg points out that in Thailand a predicted epidemic of AIDS did not materialize in the late 1980s, even though a great number of people tested positive for HIV. His critics argue that there was a dramatic rise in HIV infection (even though the typical symptoms of AIDS have not yet been observed), and, subsequently, the number of AIDS cases rose from 143 in 1990, to 603 in 1991, to 2088 in 1992, and to 8114 during 1993. The critics maintain that the Thailand statistics do in fact support the notion that HIV is the cause of AIDS.

Finally, Duesberg argues that heroin, cocaine, and amphetamines, as well as AZT, can be the causes of AIDS, particularly because they are widely used among AIDS patients (e.g., injection drugs among users and AZT among patients). The critics counter that T-lymphocyte counts are normal among HIV-negative drug users, while HIV-positive individuals have severely reduced T-lymphocyte counts. In addition, heroin causes immune system abnormalities but not the type experienced by HIV-infected persons. Only these individuals display the type of abnormalities associated with AIDS.

1 Q Why does HIV attack cells of the immune system and brain but not other cells?

A HIV and its host cell bear a resemblance to a key and a lock. The virus is the key, and whichever cell contains the lock is the cell that will be attacked. In humans, certain cells of the immune system and certain cells of the brain have the necessary "lock" in the form of receptor protein molecules called CD4 and coreceptors. Other body cells lack CD4 molecules, and these cells do not attach to HIV. Therefore, they do not become infected by the virus.

2 Q Once HIV invades a cell, how does it kill the cell?

A After an HIV particle penetrates a cell, it uses the cell as a living factory to produce hundreds or thousands of copies of itself. The cell's biochemicals are used up in viral replication, and many essential structures are broken down to supply building blocks for viral parts. The cell cannot sustain itself under these conditions, and it disintegrates. Chapter 2 suggests other possible consequences of viral invasion.

3 Q Do any symptoms arise directly from the destruction of immune system cells?

A There are no specific symptoms that point to destruction of the immune system cells. An affected individual may experience general symptoms, however. These include swollen lymph nodes in the neck, armpits, and groin; extended periods of headache, mild fever, or diarrhea; and a general feeling of fatigue. The symptoms are usually of long duration and can resemble those of mononucleosis or influenza. They should encourage a visit to a doctor.

AIDS is a particularly insidious disease because HIV attacks the immune system (Healthline 3.3). The virus does not compete with the immune system; instead, it targets the system for destruction. HIV does not multiply in some remote body tissue and wait for elements of specific resistance to arrive; rather, it multiplies in and destroys the cells that are responsible for specific resistance. Left with no defenses, the body suffers infection from microorganisms that are normally not considered pathogenic. As far as we know, this pattern of infectious disease has no parallel.

The Focus of HIV

A key focus of HIV is the collection of helper T-lymphocytes. These T-lymphocytes have on their surface protein molecules called CD4. (The T-lymphocytes are therefore called CD4 cells, CD4+ cells, or CD4 T-lymphocytes.) These CD4 molecules provide the receptor sites for HIV, as Chapter 2 explains. When these cells are experimentally infected with HIV, they are observed to be distorted, with numerous cytoplasmic projections and a tendency toward disorganization (Figure 3.11). Photographs such as those shown in Figure 3.11 also reveal the extremely small size of HIV relative to a T-lymphocyte.

The competition between HIV and helper T-lymphocytes is intense. The virus accumulates in the lymph nodes of the infected individual and multiplies at an extraordinarily high rate (by mechanisms discussed in Chapter 2) yielding more than 100 billion new viral particles per day. At the same time, the helper T-lymphocytes multiply at a high rate, yielding 1 to 2 billion new cells per day, and a race is on between these cells and the viruses. To retain its edge, the body inactivates an estimated billion viral particles per day, but also loses about a billion helper T-lymphocytes per day.

Research reported in 1995 indicates that during the struggle, every one of the body's helper T-lymphocytes is replaced within fourteen days, but that HIV counteracts this by replenishing its numbers every three days. The research conducted by David Ho and his associates apparently contradicts the notion that HIV kills by gradually undermining the immune system's ability to produce helper T-lymphocytes. Rather, the virus outlasts the immune system (the so-called "empty sink" model) and overwhelms it because its regenerative capacity is finite. Insight into how the virus exhausts the immune system was offered by mathematical biologists Robert May and Martin Nowak of Oxford University. These investigators postulated that AIDS is triggered when the infecting virus mutates and

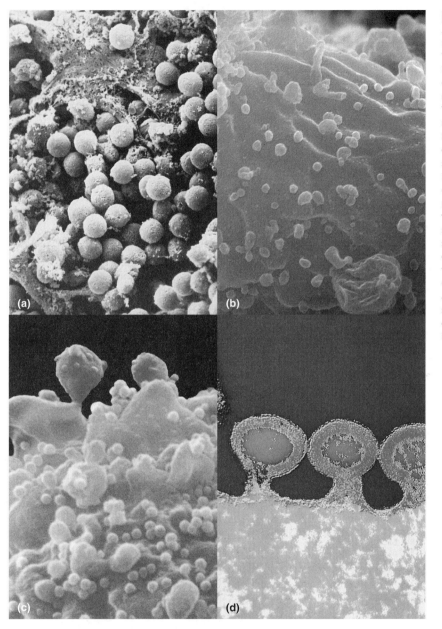

FIGURE 3.11

A sequence of scanning electron micrographs showing host T-lymphocytes and the human immunodeficiency virus (HIV). (a) T-lymphocytes are seen at low magnification. (b) A single infected T-lymphocyte. Note the disorganized appearance of the cell membrane and the long extensions of cytoplasmic material at the cell surface. These hairlike extensions indicate cell infection. The small dots at the cell surface are HIV particles. (c) Close-up of one section of a T-lymphocyte. Viruses are seen at the cell surface and, in some cases, emerging from the cell. The icosahedral shape of the viruses is somewhat evident. (d) An even closer view of HIV and its host cell. The icosahedral symmetry of the viruses is more evident, and budding from the cell is clear.

diversifies into so many different strains that the immune system is suddenly overwhelmed. The diversification of HIV introduces new strains different enough from the original to elude the immune system. This imaginative theory was based on observations that the number of viral strains in HIV-infected men kept escalating until the men developed AIDS. Thus, viral diversity is a possible cause of degenerating immune systems. HIV is not a subtle intruder, as many believed, but a raw aggressor.

At odds with the theory of destroying established cells (the "empty sink" model) is an alternative theory that HIV interferes with the production of new cells (the disease "turns down the tap," rather than empties the sink). This theory was first proposed in 1997. It is based on the study of telomeres, the extreme ends of chromosomes that shorten slightly each time a cell divides. Dutch researchers found that the telomeres from helper T-lymphocytes of infected patients were not shorter than telomeres from cells of uninfected patients, indicating that the turnover rate of the cells was the same. Thus, it did not appear likely that established cells were being lost; rather, destruction of new cells was the key to understanding the pathology of HIV. Another group, also working with telomeres, found that the lengths of telomeres in lymphocytes from HIV-infected patients are equivalent to those in 100-year-old individuals, a sign that immune system cells were replicating so often that they were becoming worn out. Research on both of these approaches is continuing.

In 1999, a team of researchers from the University of California at Berkeley added to the notion that HIV affects the production of new T-lymphocytes more than it induces destruction of mature T-lymphocytes. Using innovative methods in which patients were infused with isotope-containing nucleic acid precursors, the biochemists found that the rate of T-lymphocyte production was no higher in HIV-infected patients than in uninfected individuals. Moreover, the average T-lymphocyte lifespan in untreated patients was a third of that in uninfected individuals, a factor consistent with a certain level of T-lymphocyte death due to HIV; antiretroviral therapy encourages the immune system to boost its production of new T-lymphocytes above normal levels. Taken together, these data appear to support the "turn down the tap" model of HIV pathogenesis.

Research first reported in 1995 indicates that HIV is probably carried from the initial infection site to the brain and lymph nodes by macrophages, the cells that function in normal immune processes discussed earlier. In the lymph nodes, cells called follicular dendritic cells then come into play. These cells are found within the germinal centers of the lymph nodes (the follicles) and have treelike branches (they are dendritic). The cells remove the HIV from the macrophages and "trap" the viruses. Virtually every other cell in a lymph node is touched by the branches of the follicular dendritic cells, and it is only a matter of time before T-lymphocytes come in contact with these cells and are activated by receiving the HIV particles. In 2000, Dutch researchers found that molecules of a protein extending like fingers on the branches of the follicular dendritic cells act like an adhesive to bind the cells with T-lymphocytes and pass HIV into the lymphocytes. Later in the infection, the follicular dendritic cells dissolve, die, and become part of the general destruction taking place in the lymph nodes. The activated T-lymphocytes appear to be ones not previously stimulated by any type of antigen. These so-called naive T-lymphocytes are different from those previously committed to destroying a particular microorganism.

But what happens when the activated T-lymphocytes have been destroyed by replicating HIV particles? Will the virus run out of suitable host cells and itself be destroyed? Apparently not. In 1998, researchers at Boston's Dana-Farber Cancer Institute reported that the *tat* gene of HIV (Chapter 2) encodes a protein (the *tat* protein) that activates naive T-lymphocytes and transforms them into host cells suitable for HIV infection. Their evidence came in part from observations that naive cells exposed to *tat* protein display a set of properties consistent with those of activated cells. Also, *tat*-activated cells were more supportive of HIV replication than untreated cells. It did not escape the researchers that a drug directed at the *tat* protein could conceivably slow down HIV replication in cells.

In addition to transporting HIV, macrophages represent another important focus of infection, especially in late stages of infection, where they probably contribute to the high blood level of HIV seen in patients at this point. Indeed, while helper T-lymphocytes die within a few days of HIV infection, macrophages appear to persist for months, while continuing to release HIV (we note the relationship of the CCR5 coreceptor to this activity in Chapter 2). Of significance is the finding that the brain's macrophages, called microglia, are related to HIV encephalopathy, the brain infection that characterizes AIDS (Chapter 4). Perhaps, scientists say, the infected macrophages produce and release a number of neurotoxic substances that induce inflammation. Thus, the macrophage that normally helps rid the body of deadly foes has turned into a foe itself, an HIV-harboring "Trojan horse."

The Effects of HIV

HIV has a profound effect on macrophages (Figure 3.12) as well as helper T-lymphocytes. By destroying helper cells, HIV affects the entire immune system because helper cells set into action both the cytotoxic T-lymphocytes and the B-lymphocytes. Since helper T-lymphocytes are also known as T4 cells (from CD4) in the jargon of immunology, it is not uncommon to hear scientists speak of "T4 cell destruction."

The effect of HIV on suppressor T-lymphocytes is much less severe, partly because they contain CD8 receptor sites to which HIV does not bind easily. While this factor may appear advantageous at first glance, the effects work against the body because suppressor T-lymphocytes dampen the activity of the immune system's cytotoxic T-lymphocytes. Normally a person has twice as many helper cells (T4 cells) as suppressor cells (also known as T8 cells). However, as the helper cells disappear, the relative number of suppressor cells climbs. Put another way, the ratio of T4 to T8 cells (helpers to suppressors) is normally 2 to 1, but with a reduction in the helper cell population, the ratio of T4 to T8 cells gradually reverses and eventually becomes 1 to 2. As that occurs, the effects of cytotoxic T-lymphocytes are dampened.

Research reported in 1999 indicates that properly functioning suppressor T-lymphocytes may be critical to controlling HIV in the body. Scientists depleted

FIGURE 3.12

The association of HIV with macrophages. (a) At least 20 HIV particles (many indicated by arrows) are associated with the cell membrane of the macrophage (×25,000). (b) Two HIV particles have budded from an extension of the macrophage cell (×130,000). (c) Five HIV particles are intermixed with membranous vesicles (×50,000). (d) HIV particles are observed within membranes of the macrophage's Golgi body (×66,000).

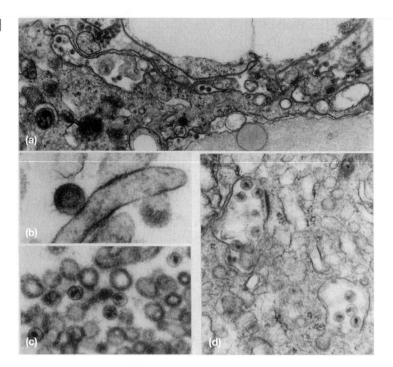

the population of suppressor cells in the blood and lymph tissues of monkeys and found that increased viral replication took place and the disease progressed more rapidly. Furthermore, the level of HIV in the bloodstream increased significantly. However, the suppressor cells reappeared, the level of HIV in the bloodstream declined, and the disease regressed. The results appeared to confirm the importance of cell-mediated immunity in controlling HIV infection, while pointing up the role of suppressor T-lymphocytes in HIV destruction.

HIV also multiplies in and destroys the cytotoxic T-lymphocytes as well as the natural killer cells. With the loss of these cells, an entire branch of the immune system is first depressed, then eliminated. Now the affected individual cannot mount a defense against fungi, protozoa, and various viruses and bacteria. Persons with AIDS often suffer serious bouts of illness from protozoa such as *Pneumocystis carinii* and *Toxoplasma gondii* and from fungi such as *Candida albicans* and *Cryptococcus neoformans*, as we discuss in Chapter 4. Before the advent of AIDS, the names of these organisms were largely unfamiliar to most people because T-lymphocytes normally kept them and their diseases under control. In the HIV-infected individual, however, the populations of helper and cytotoxic T-lymphocytes diminish, and the microbial populations increase dramatically. Disease and death may follow. Chapter 4 explores these effects in greater depth.

The actual mechanisms of T-lymphocyte destruction are surveyed in Chapter 2, but they bear repeating here. In many cases, the multiplication of HIV within the lymphocyte literally "uses up" the lymphocyte's nutrient molecules to construct new viruses. This intense level of parasitism leaves the T-lymphocyte in such a damaged state that it undergoes lysis and disintegrates.

T-lymphocytes can also be destroyed during the release phase of the HIV replication cycle. In this case, the virus moves through the cell membrane (a process called budding), thereby altering the membrane and causing cellular leakage. Moreover, T-lymphocytes infected with HIV are marked at their surfaces with virus-specified molecules that induce the infected T-lymphocytes to cling to uninfected T-lymphocytes. As molecular cross-bridges form, there develops a giant multinucleated cell mass, called a syncytium. The syncytium is functionless, which implies that all the T-lymphocytes in it are essentially useless. Another effect of being marked with virus-specified molecules is that normal cytotoxic T-lymphocytes will attack and destroy the infected T-lymphocytes as if the latter were foreign to the body. Thus, we see the unusual and ironic phenomenon of body cells destroying other body cells.

There is also the effect of apoptosis. Apoptosis is programmed cell death, that is, the natural mechanism whereby a cell dies at the end of its normal life cycle. Apoptosis is believed to be an altruistic phenomenon, one in which the body rids itself of "old" cells as new ones are produced through mitosis and cell division. In the case of the normal immune system, between 10 billion and 20 billion T-lymphocytes are produced daily, and an equal number undergo apoptosis to make room for the new cells.

When a virus infects a cell, the body seeks to get rid of that cell as quickly as possible in order to eliminate the viral infection. Examples of this phenomenon are seen in cells infected with cowpox virus, cytomegalovirus (Chapter 4), and Epstein-Barr virus. To get rid of the infected cell, one mechanism the body apparently uses is speeding up the process of apoptosis. However, when the infected cells are T-lymphocytes, their elimination brings about a loss of immune function at a time when the body most needs it. Thus, the body must confront a dilemma: Encouraging apoptosis eliminates HIV but also lowers the body's resistance to HIV.

There are some complex applications of the apoptosis theory. For example, some researchers believe that the binding of gp120 molecules to the CD4 receptor sites "misactivates" the helper T-lymphocytes, rendering them unable to respond to further stimulations and speeding up their programmed death. Another possibility is that gp120 molecules bind to uninfected T-lymphocytes and trigger their apoptosis, while the combination of gp120 molecules with host cells actually inhibits apoptosis via a gene-encoded protein of HIV. While the evidence for these theories is not persuasive, they are intriguing.

Nor are the effects of HIV limited to the T-lymphocytes. The evidence is substantial that HIV also infects brain cells. This is because brain cells, like T-lymphocytes, have CD4 receptor sites on their surfaces. Thus, the devastating effects on the immune system are often compounded by impairment of neural function. To be sure, AIDS is a very complex disease, with many facets and implications. Many researchers and physicians feel that nothing like it has ever been experienced in medicine.

LOOKING BACK

The body depends on two types of resistance—nonspecific and specific—to protect itself from disease. Nonspecific resistance operates against all foreign organisms and is centered in the body's enzymes, its covering structure, and the process of phagocytosis, among other mechanisms. Specific resistance operates only against the organism that elicited it; it involves the immune system.

The immune system arises during fetal development from bone marrow cells called stem cells. These cells become T-lymphocytes or B-lymphocytes, depending on where they are modified in the body. Both T- and B-lymphocytes carry highly specific receptor sites and accumulate in the lymph nodes, spleen, and similar tissues. The lymphocytes respond via their receptor sites to chemical components of microorganisms interpreted as foreign. The foreign chemicals, usually large proteins or polysaccharides, are called antigens.

One branch of the immune system, cell-mediated immunity, is based in the cytotoxic T-lymphocytes. Antigens from macrophages stimulate these cells, using helper T-lymphocytes as intermediaries. The cytotoxic T-lymphocytes travel to the antigen site, where they promote phagocytosis via the activity of lymphokines. Moreover, they attack microorganisms directly and kill them. Natural killer cells provide additional defense by destroying foreign cells. B-lymphocytes are also stimulated by antigens. The B-lymphocytes remain in the lymphoid tissues and produce antibodies, and some are converted to plasma cells that produce additional antibodies. Antibodies are protein molecules that neutralize microorganisms by reacting with their antigens.

The human immunodeficiency virus (HIV) attacks both helper T-lymphocytes and cytotoxic T-lymphocytes, destroying them in the process. As cell-mediated immunity is depressed and the whole immune system is compromised, minor organisms that are normally of minor consequence can cause life-threatening illnesses. The destruction of T-lymphocytes by HIV is a unique phenomenon in medicine. So far as is known, AIDS has no parallel in any other infectious disease. We examine some of its symptoms and effects on the body in Chapter 4.

REVIEW

Having completed this chapter, you should be familiar with the structures and activities of the human immune system and how HIV affects it. To review your knowledge, match the term on the right side with the description or characteristic listed on the left side by placing the appropriate letter in the space. (A letter may be used more than once.) The correct answers are listed in Appendix A.

K 1. Forerunners of the immune system

J 2. Large, amoeboid cells that function as phagocytes to initiate the immune process

N 3. Type of immunity resulting from activity of B-lymphocytes

O 4. Prevents the immune process from becoming too exaggerated

O 5. Also known as T8 cell

H 6. Products of B-lymphocytes and plasma cells

L 7. Organ in the embryonic chick where B-lymphocytes are modified

M 8. Type of immunity involving a direct assault on microorganisms by body cells

D 9. Site where T-lymphocytes and B-lymphocytes are found

P 10. General class of body cells to which lymphocytes belong

Q 11. Attacks microorganisms but is less specialized than cytotoxic T-lymphocyte

B 12. Antigens present on all body cells that define an individual's uniqueness

C 13. Also called a CD4 cell

M 14. Type of immunity resulting from activity of cytotoxic T-lymphocytes

G 15. Exerts a "lethal hit" on fungus-infected and protozoa-infected cells

A. Thymus

B. MHC proteins

C. Helper T-lymphocyte

D. Spleen

E. Antigen

F. Lymphokines

G. Cytotoxic T-lymphocyte

H. Antibodies

I. Phagocytes

J. Macrophages

K. Lymphopoietic cells

L. Bursa of Fabricius

M. Cell-mediated immunity

N. Antibody-mediated immunity

O. Suppressor T-lymphocyte

P. White blood cells

Q. Natural killer cells

_H_ **16.** Composed of four chains of amino acids

_A_ **17.** Organ in which cells are modified to form T-lymphocytes

_O_ **18.** Type of T-lymphocyte unaffected by HIV

_E_ **19.** A substance, usually a protein or polysaccharide, that stimulates the immune system

_H_ **20.** Located on the surface of unstimulated B-lymphocytes

_C_ **21.** Normally twice as common as suppressor T-lymphocyte

_I_ **22.** White blood cells that specialize in engulfing and destroying foreign materials

_C_ **23.** First lymphocyte encountered by an antigen-bearing macrophage

_F_ **24.** Highly reactive proteins from helper T-lymphocytes that stimulate other lymphocytes

_N_ **25.** Type of immunity involving activity of antibodies

FOR ADDITIONAL READING

Alcamo, I. E. 2000. *Fundamentals of Microbiology,* 6th ed. Sudbury, MA: Jones & Bartlett.

Balter, M. 1997. "How does HIV overcome the body's T cell bodyguards?" *Science* 278: 1399–1401.

Barinaga, M. 1995. "Scientists air alternative views on how HIV kills cells." *Science* 269: 1044–1046.

Bottomly, K. 1999. "T cells and dendritic cells get intimate." *Science* 283: 1124–1126.

Chicurel, M. 2000. "Probing HIV's elusive activities within the host cell." *Science* 290: 1876–1880.

Christensen, D. 1999. "Why AIDS? The mystery of how HIV attacks the immune system." *Science News* 155: 204–207.

Cohen, J. 2000. "Novel protein delivers HIV to target cells." *Science* 287: 1567.

Cowley, G. 1995. "HIV's raw aggression." *Newsweek,* January 23.

Decker, J. M. 2000. *Introduction to Immunology.* Malden, MA: Blackwell Science.

Duesberg, P. 1988. "HIV is not the cause of AIDS." *Science* 241: 514–515.

Jaret, P. 1986. "The wars within." *National Geographic,* June.

Jaroff, L. 1988. "Stop that germ." *Time,* May 23.

Kimball, J. W. 1990. *Introduction to Immunology,* 3rd ed. New York: Macmillan.

Lawrence, J. 1985. "The immune system in AIDS." *Scientific American* 253: 84–93.

Nowak, M. A., and A. J. McMichael. 1995. "How HIV defeats the immune system." *Scientific American* 273(1): 58–65.

Richardson, S. 1995. "The race against AIDS." *Discover,* May.

Travis, J. 1997. "HIV protein prepares virus' next victim." *Science News* 152: 53.

Weiss, R., and H. Jaffe. 1990. "Duesberg, HIV, and AIDS." *Nature* 345: 649–653.

Defining and Recognizing AIDS

LOOKING AHEAD

AIDS is a very complex disease, with multiple phases and symptoms. This chapter discusses how public health officials define AIDS and points out the symptoms associated with various phases of HIV infection and AIDS. On completing the chapter, you should be able to . . .

- Understand the case definition for AIDS and appreciate why it is important to spell out the definition clearly.
- Describe how AIDS develops through multiple phases.
- Define the key symptoms that accompany HIV infection, AIDS-related complex, and AIDS.
- Identify the different regions of the body affected by the human immunodeficiency virus.
- Describe the important elements of HIV wasting syndrome and AIDS-dementia complex.
- List several opportunistic diseases that accompany AIDS, identify the agents that cause these diseases, and discuss the nature of each disease.

INTRODUCTION

Physicians and researchers are often asked to provide a clear and precise definition for AIDS. After a few tries, they realize that defining AIDS is a difficult task because AIDS is a very complex disease. They must ask themselves: Does a person infected with human immunodeficiency virus (HIV) have AIDS? And what about the HIV-positive individual who has swollen lymph nodes and vague flulike symptoms, but is in generally good health? Does that person have AIDS? If so, then what do we call the condition where patients are wracked with pneumonia and reduced almost to skeletons?

One might suggest that these distinctions are merely semantics and that "AIDS" is a label we can apply to any stage of the disease and still be correct. Perhaps so, but in public health matters it is important to define terms carefully. One reason is that AIDS is an extremely volatile issue in our society, and we must be very cautious before stigmatizing an individual. For instance, a person who has tested positive for HIV antibodies does not have AIDS; rather he or she has HIV infection.

Defining AIDS is also important from the viewpoints of record-keeping and public health. Since 1981, the Centers for Disease Control and Prevention (CDC) has been tracking the AIDS epidemic in the United States by asking physicians to report cases they have treated. The statistics generated from such reports are only as reliable as the physicians' ability to recognize AIDS when they see it. Physicians must therefore have a clear definition at their disposal.

Finally, it is important to define AIDS so that we can understand the disease more fully. As we shall see, there are many phases to the disease, and only in the final stages does the patient truly have AIDS. In the earlier stages, the virus may be present, but the disease is not (Healthline 4.1).

The Case Definition

In 1981, officials at the CDC spelled out a relatively simple case definition for AIDS: (1) A person with AIDS was suffering from Kaposi's sarcoma (a rare cancer) or an infectious disease that occurs only when the immune system is impaired; and (2) there was no other reason except AIDS for the impaired immune system (if a person were taking an immune-suppressing drug after organ transplant surgery, for example, that would be a reason for an impaired immune system not related to AIDS).

In the early years of the epidemic, this case definition for AIDS worked well (Table 4.1), and the CDC was able to follow the epidemic's development based on reports from physicians. Then, in 1984, the human immunodeficiency virus was identified, and soon thereafter scientists developed a blood test for antibodies produced by the body when infected with this virus. Physicians could now test their patients to see whether they were harboring HIV. In doing so, they discovered that a number of conditions accompany HIV infection. It was clear that a spectrum of AIDS-related conditions exists. The CDC therefore revised its case definition for AIDS, and in conjunction with physicians, it promulgated an updated version in 1987 (Table 4.2). The new definition took into account the presence of HIV and 23 conditions that can accompany infection with HIV.

Then, on January 1, 1993, the CDC revised the case definition once again. The latest definition (Table 4.3) took into account the number of helper T-lymphocytes (CD4 cells) present in the patient and added three new conditions to the previous 23. According to this case definition, a person infected with HIV had AIDS if the count of helper T-lymphocytes fell below 200 per microliter of blood or if the person had one or more of 26 specified conditions, including the new conditions of invasive cervical carcinoma, pulmonary tuberculosis, and recurrent bacterial pneumonia. The new definition reflected T-lymphocyte testing that had become increasingly common, and consequently the number of AIDS cases reported in 1993 took a significant turn upward, as Figure 4.1 illustrates. It also included more HIV-infected women since early cervical cancer often occurs concurrently with HIV infection. Moreover, the helper T-lymphocyte (CD4) count per microliter was used to classify a person's HIV infection into three categories: A count above 500 represents the least severe level of disease; between 200 and 499 reflects intermediate severity; and below 200 is the severest form.

The latest version of the case definition took effect in January 2000 when the CDC asked all states and territories to implement a program to detect persons having HIV infection (as well as those with AIDS). This expansion of the national surveillance effort to seek out those with HIV infection arose because of the impact of new therapies introduced in 1996 and the increased need for data on persons having all stages of the disease. Officials at the CDC hoped that the new data would enhance efforts to prevent HIV transmission, improve allocation of resources for treatment services, and assist evaluation of public health interventions.

The seminal element of the revised case definition is the inclusion of surveillance for HIV infection in adults and children. In issuing the guidelines, the CDC acknowledged that AIDS is the end stage of the natural history of HIV infection and that although monitoring AIDS had been valuable in the past, recent advances in therapy have slowed the progression to AIDS and reduced the ability of AIDS surveillance data to reflect trends. Thus, the need to survey HIV infection as well as AIDS.

The revision is shown in Table 4.4. It applies to infections by both HIV-1 and HIV-2, and it incorporates the previous 1993 reporting criteria for HIV infection and AIDS into a single case definition. Among the new criteria are the use of RNA or DNA tests (the "viral load" tests) to detect HIV and the isolation of HIV in viral culture. The ensuing years will show how well the new definition works.

HIV Infection

One of the primary targets of HIV is the T-lymphocyte of the immune system. More specifically, the host cells for HIV are the helper T-lymphocytes and the cytotoxic T-lymphocytes (Chapter 3). Destruction of these cells as determined by

[Handwritten at top: Know this — Definition for having AIDS]

TABLE 4.1	1983 Case Definition for Acquired Immune Deficiency Syndrome

1. Presence of a reliably diagnosed disease at least moderately indicative of cellular immunodeficiency (e.g., *Pneumocystis* pneumonia).
2. Absence of known causes of underlying reduced resistance to the disease other than due to HTLV-III/LAV infection (e.g., immunosuppressive therapy, Hodgkin's disease).*

*HTLV-III/LAV: human T-cell lymphotropic virus type III/lymphadenopathy-associated virus.

Source: Centers for Disease Control and Prevention.

TABLE 4.2	1987 Case Definition for Acquired Immune Deficiency Syndrome

Positive HIV test   *[Handwritten: look for antibodies in the bloodstream]*

Plus one or more of the following:

Cryptosporidiosis, cytomegalovirus, isosporiasis, Kaposi's sarcoma, lymphoma, lymphoid pneumonia (hyperplasia), *Pneumocystis carinii* pneumonia, progressive multifocal leukoencephalopathy, toxoplasmosis, candidiasis, coccidioidomycosis, cryptococcosis, herpes simplex virus, histoplasmosis, extrapulmonary tuberculosis, other mycobacteriosis, salmonellosis, other bacterial infections, HIV encephalopathy (dementia), HIV wasting syndrome. *[Handwritten: swelling in head]*

Source: Centers for Disease Control and Prevention.

TABLE 4.3	1993 Case Definition for Acquired Immune Deficiency Syndrome

All HIV-infected adolescents and adults with fewer than 200 T-lymphocytes per microliter

Or one or more of the following:

Cryptosporidiosis, cytomegalovirus, isosporiasis, Kaposi's sarcoma, lymphoma, lymphoid pneumonia (hyperplasia), *Pneumocystis carinii* pneumonia, progressive multifocal leukoencephalopathy, toxoplasmosis, candidiasis, coccidioidomycosis, cryptococcosis, herpes simplex virus, histoplasmosis, extrapulmonary tuberculosis, other mycobacteriosis, salmonellosis, other bacterial infections, HIV encephalopathy (dementia), HIV wasting syndrome, *pulmonary tuberculosis, recurrent pneumonia,* and *invasive cervical cancer.*

Source: Centers for Disease Control and Prevention.

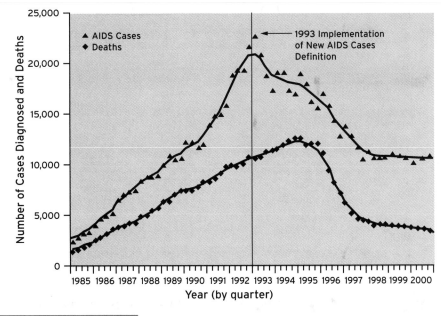

FIGURE 4.1

The estimated incidence of AIDS cases and deaths associated with AIDS in adults by quarter-years through 1998. The graph shows the increase in AIDS cases resulting from the 1993 expansion of the case definition for AIDS. Note that the revised case definition had no effect on the incidence of death, which continued to rise until 1996 when new therapies were introduced to control HIV in the body. *Source: Centers for Disease Control and Prevention.*

a T-lymphocyte count points to impending symptoms. Determining the viral load (Chapter 7) is another way of knowing that HIV infection is present.

Some of the first signs of the presence of HIV occur within weeks or months after the virus has entered the body. This is the period of acute primary HIV infection. Patients report fatigue, mild fever, sore muscles, occasional diarrhea, and the onset of swollen lymph nodes ("swollen glands"). The symptom of swollen lymph nodes is known as lymphadenopathy, and it usually reflects the fact that HIV has activated B-lymphocytes to become plasma cells and secrete HIV antibodies (Chapter 3). Apparently, HIV continues such activation for a long period of time, which accounts for the persistent swollen lymph nodes. But since HIV penetrates and resides in T-lymphocytes in the provirus form, the antibodies are ineffective against the virus.

During this stage of the disease, a test for HIV antibodies (Chapter 7) will normally give a positive result. A viral load test will also be positive. However, the count of helper T-lymphocytes does not drop to a level that compromises body defense. The count, normally about 800 cells per microliter of blood, will remain in that range. Infections by opportunistic organisms are not typically

TABLE	
4.4	**2000 Revised Surveillance Case Definition for HIV Infection**

I. In adults, adolescents, or children aged ≥18 months, a reportable case of HIV infection must meet at least one of the following criteria:

Laboratory Criteria

- Positive result on a screening test for HIV antibody (e.g., repeatedly reactive enzyme immunoassay), followed by a positive result on a confirmatory (sensitive and more specific) test for HIV antibody (e.g., Western blot or immunofluorescence antibody test)

or

- Positive result or report of a detectable quantity on any of the following HIV virologic (nonantibody) tests:

  - HIV nucleic acid (DNA or RNA) detection (e.g., DNA polymerase chain reaction [PCR] or plasma HIV-1 RNA)

  - HIV p24 antigen test, including neutralization assay

  - HIV isolation (viral culture)

OR

Clinical or Other Criteria (if the above laboratory criteria are not met)

- Diagnosis of HIV infection, based on the laboratory criteria above, that is documented in a medical record by a physician

or

- Conditions that meet criteria included in the case definition for AIDS

II. In a child aged <18 months, a reportable case of HIV infection must meet at least one of the following criteria:

Laboratory Criteria

Definitive

- Positive results on two separate specimens (excluding cord blood) using one or more of the following HIV virologic (nonantibody) tests:

  - HIV nucleic acid (DNA or RNA) detection

  - HIV p24 antigen test, including neutralization assay, in a child ≥1 month of age

  - HIV isolation (viral culture)

or

Presumptive

A child who does not meet the criteria for definitive HIV infection but who has:

- Positive results on only one specimen (excluding cord blood) using the above HIV virologic tests and no subsequent negative HIV virologic or negative HIV antibody tests

OR

Clinical or Other Criteria (if the above definitive or presumptive laboratory criteria are not met)

- Diagnosis of HIV infection, based on the laboratory criteria above, that is documented in a medical record by a physician

or

- Conditions that meet criteria included in the 1987 pediatric surveillance case definition for AIDS

Source: Centers for Disease Control and Prevention.

experienced. Some persons may experience extended headaches or brain inflammation that could indicate infection of the brain cells and AIDS dementia, as we discuss below.

An individual in the earliest stages of disease is said to be suffering from HIV infection. Symptoms of HIV infection, summarized in Table 4.5, often remain for several weeks, then disappear. However, this ensuing period of quiet should not be misinterpreted. It is only a period of "clinical latency," because HIV is multiplying rapidly in the lymph nodes and attempting to outrace the body's replacement of infected and destroyed T-lymphocytes (Chapter 3).

At this point, it is conceivable that the body could successfully clear HIV from its tissues and restore itself to a normal state of health. This possibility was pointed up in 1995 when physicians reported on a number of babies who initially tested positive for HIV and then showed up free of infection weeks or months later. The observations, described in respected scientific journals, included one case where pediatric HIV infection was confirmed by three different test methods (Chapter 7) and on three separate occasions up to 51 days of age. By the age of 1 year, however, the child was negative by every possible HIV test and no medical intervention had occurred. Four years later, the child was still HIV-negative.

It is even possible that a person may not progress beyond HIV infection for a long period of time, perhaps a decade or more. Individuals in this status are known as long-term nonprogressors, and extensive studies are currently under way to learn why they have been able to resist the progression to AIDS (Box 4.1).

AIDS-Related Complex

After the period of primary acute HIV infection, there is a quiet period that may be prolonged. For many individuals, the next consequence of infection with HIV is a set of constitutional symptoms known as AIDS-related complex (ARC). Health agencies have begun to delete "ARC" from their official vocabulary (preferring to refer to all pre-AIDS conditions as "HIV infection"), but this book uses the term because it is ingrained in the public lexicon and is part of the vernacular of AIDS. Many symptoms of ARC are similar to those of HIV infection, but usually the symptoms are exaggerated in persons with ARC.

When a person experiences ARC, lymphadenopathy once again develops in lymph nodes of the neck, armpits, and groin. Swelling can remain for three months or more. Patients also experience weight loss of up to 10 percent of baseline body weight or more than 10 pounds (Figure 4.2). Also, there is constant low-grade fever at about 37.8°C (100°F) and diarrhea extending over several weeks. In addition, the fatigue may be so overwhelming that patients cannot lift their heads from the pillow on waking in the morning.

One of the most troublesome aspects of ARC is the night sweats. Individuals perspire so heavily at night that the bed linens and nightwear become drenched with sweat. Saturation can be extensive enough to necessitate linen changes, and

TABLE 4.5 Some Symptoms of HIV Infection, ARC, and AIDS

HIV Infection

Fatigue

Mild fever

Sore muscles

Occasional diarrhea

Swollen lymph nodes (lymphadenopathy)

[handwritten: flu-like symptoms]

AIDS-Related Complex (ARC)

Extended and extensive lymphadenopathy *[handwritten: — swollen lymph nodes]*

Weight loss of as much as 10 percent of normal body weight

Constant low-grade fever (about 37.8°C, or 100°F)

Extensive diarrhea over several weeks

Overwhelming fatigue

Saturating night sweats

Thrush from *Candida albicans*

[handwritten: → could be 8-10-15 yrs. later — chronic lymphadenopathy]

[handwritten: can be A-symptomatic then sub-clinical dysfunction]

Acquired Immune Deficiency Syndrome (AIDS)

Persistent lymphadenopathy

Constant low-grade fever

Substantial nausea and fatigue

Vomiting

Severe psychological stress

Saturating night sweats

Extensive headaches

Possible wasting syndrome

Unrelenting diarrhea

Dramatic weight loss

Severe fluid imbalance

Chronic weakness and fever

Possible AIDS-dementia complex

Difficult muscle coordination

Confusion and apathy

Loss of concentration

Sudden, strong emotions

Memory loss

Difficulty in sleeping

Headache and disorientation

Possible Kaposi's sarcoma

Slow-growing tumors in blood-vessel linings

Possible opportunistic diseases

Pneumonia, esophageal diseases, blindness, brain infection, choleralike diarrhea, spinal meningitis, liver and kidney disease, tuberculosis, and many others

[handwritten: Skin + mucous membrane immune defects + systemic immune def.]

BOX
4.1

Nonprogression

Studies reported in 1995 reveal important clues as to why a small minority of HIV-infected people (about 5 percent) have remained healthy for 10 or more years without loss of immune function. The research suggests that some HIV-positive individuals can remain "frozen" in a long period of robust health. Essentially, the study gave insight into the mechanisms for delayed or arrested progression of the disease.

Researchers from the National Institutes of Health (NIH) studied fifteen HIV-infected volunteers who had not progressed beyond HIV infection, thirteen of them for over a decade. All had steady counts of helper T-lymphocytes, and seven had counts well within the normal range. The team also analyzed eighteen HIV-infected people who had progressed to AIDS, according to the CDC case definition.

To get an idea of how HIV infects long-term survivors, the researchers focused on the patients' lymph nodes. Biopsies revealed well-preserved organs in fourteen of the fifteen nonprogressors, but there was clear scarring and deterioration in the eighteen AIDS patients. In one nonprogressor, tissue samples taken nine years apart were practically identical. Although nonprogressors had various amounts of HIV in the follicular dendritic cells of their lymph nodes, the levels were consistently lower than in progressors.

There was also a discernible difference in the antibody-producing mechanisms of the two groups: Nonprogressors had a much higher level of antibodies in their plasma than progressors, indicating that both antibody-mediated and cell-mediated immunity (Chapter 3) were preserved in long-term survivors. Moreover, the blood of seven survivors had the ability to neutralize HIV, while none of the blood samples from progressors had that ability. Indeed, the scientists had great difficulty locating any HIV in the plasma or blood of the survivors, indicating a lower viral burden.

When the rate of viral multiplication was compared, researchers found that the viruses in progressors multiply four to twenty times faster than those in nonprogressors. Clearly, the rapid multiplication rate was a reflection of the aggressiveness of the virus. This observation also opened the possibility that nonprogressors were infected with a weaker form of HIV, one that the body could control. Studies with simian immunodeficiency virus (SIV) indicate that weaker strains are associated with nonprogression in monkeys; perhaps the same phenomenon is operating in humans.

The experimental results indicate that low-level, persistent HIV infection may not necessarily be associated with disease progression if efficiently controlled over time. For the almost 1 million Americans who now have HIV infection, the results give renewed hope that they can beat the virus.

sleep is fitful at best. Few other microbial diseases are accompanied by such heavy sweating.

During this stage of the disease, the number of helper T-lymphocytes has generally dropped to fewer than 400 cells per microliter, an indication of viral replication, as shown in Figure 4.3. Evidence for the declining cell numbers comes from

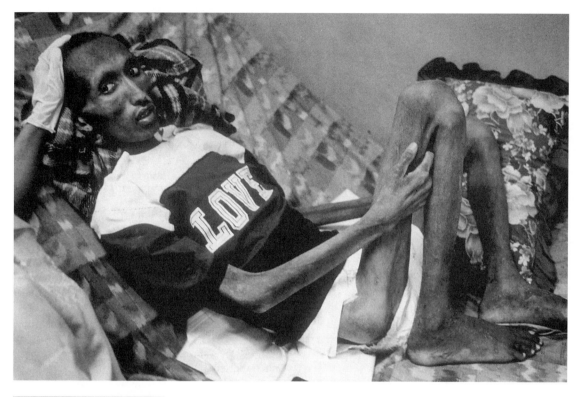

FIGURE 4.2

A photograph of an AIDS patient, displaying the severe weight loss that commonly accompanies the disease. Also visible on his legs and feet are the skin lesions of Kaposi's sarcoma, an opportunistic disease often associated with AIDS.

a number of skin tests that depend on T-lymphocyte activity. These tests, similar to the tuberculin test, elicit a response from a normal individual, but give negative results in a person with ARC because of the reduced numbers of T-lymphocytes.

Some persons with ARC also suffer an infection of the mouth known as thrush. This is a fungal disease caused by a yeastlike microorganism called *Candida albicans*. Commonly found on the skin surface and in the intestine, *C. albicans* is normally held under control by T-lymphocytes. With destruction of T-lymphocytes, however, the fungus grows on the tongue, gums, and lining of the cheeks, producing ulcers and milky, white flakes of fungal growth. Infected individuals are not inclined to eat, especially when the disease reaches the esophagus, erodes the surface tissue there, and exposes the nerve endings. Loss of appetite increases the weight loss.

For some individuals, ARC is a mild illness with limited bouts of symptoms. For others, it may be severe and may lead to physical deterioration. Moreover, the person with ARC suffers psychological stress from fear that AIDS lies ahead.

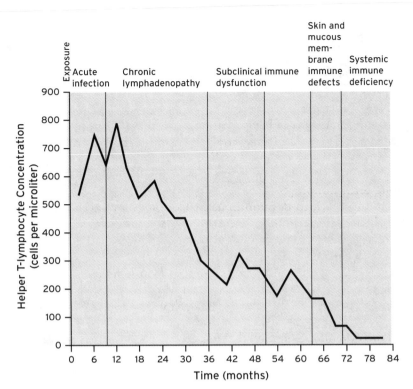

No widely accepted estimate as to how many persons with ARC will develop AIDS is available, but public health officials generally agree that a substantial number of ARC cases will progress to AIDS.

Acquired Immune Deficiency Syndrome

As HIV continues to replicate itself, the destruction of T-lymphocytes goes on methodically and inexorably. Soon the count of helper T-lymphocytes has dropped below 100 cells per microliter of blood, and crippling of the immune system is virtually complete. At any time, the symptoms of ARC can return in severe form, together with brain disease, a wasting phenomenon, and/or opportunistic infection. Then, the person has AIDS.

The average time that passes from HIV infection until AIDS (i.e., the incubation period) has been a subject of controversy for many years. At one time, the incubation period was believed to be seven years, but according to a more recent study performed at the University of California at San Francisco, the incubation period for AIDS averages about ten years. The San Francisco study was based on blood samples obtained from homosexual men in the 1970s and stored for later analysis. It also included an elaborate system of confidential blood testing in the San Francisco homosexual community. Researchers were able to track men whose blood tested positive for a period of ten years and found that it took that long, on average, for the disease to develop.

It should be noted, however, that antiretroviral therapy (Chapter 8) can lengthen the incubation period significantly. Indeed, studies show that about 5 percent of individuals infected with HIV live for 12 years or more without developing AIDS. (These individuals are the long-term nonprogressors.) At the other end of the spectrum, AIDS is known to develop in as little as six months, depending largely on the type of lifestyle the individual leads. Clinical illness cofactors such as coinfection with hepatitis B viruses or other microbes may be another determining factor.

As full-blown AIDS develops in the patient, the lymph nodes become enlarged, tender, and stiffer than normal lymph nodes. This lymphadenopathy persists for months. Also, a low-grade fever at about 37.8°C (100°F) returns. It is commonly present in the late afternoon and early evening. When another infection is present, the fever may be higher and more difficult to control. Chills and periods of sweating often accompany the fever.

Persons with AIDS suffer from substantial nausea and fatigue. The nausea is often accompanied by vomiting, and the fatigue does not seem to end. Both sap the individual's strength, making normal routines extremely difficult. Job efficiency declines, and the will to care for oneself diminishes. A headache may come and go in some individuals; in others, it remains for days. The night sweats resemble those in ARC, only they are worse (Healthline 4.2).

The diarrhea associated with AIDS can also be considerable. In its most severe form, a patient may lose a quart of water in a 24-hour period (an opportunistic disease of the intestine may make the diarrhea worse). Exhausting fatigue and considerable weight loss usually are observed. In milder cases of AIDS, two to four loose stools are passed per day, often containing blood or mucus.

The CDC Stages of Disease

It is important to understand that AIDS is the end result of HIV infection; therefore, AIDS patients represent a subgroup of the total group of HIV-infected individuals. Because patients may have HIV infection but not manifest the actual syndrome of AIDS, the CDC has classified patients with HIV infection into four stages, as Table 4.6 outlines.

Healthline 4.2

1 **Q** What is the life expectancy of persons with AIDS?

A Because the AIDS epidemic has killed so many, people are inclined to believe that the disease is always fatal. But that is not necessarily so. Such factors as quality of life, route of infection, and type of opportunistic infection influence the survival time. Drug therapies and other interventions (Chapter 8) can increase life expectancy significantly.

2 **Q** Has anyone been cured of AIDS?

A Curing AIDS would require that the immune system be returned to normal functioning. No treatment is yet available to bring this about. However, drugs are now used to extend the life of AIDS patients in hopes that a cure may one day be available. Through a combination of therapeutic drugs and a healthy lifestyle, some individuals with AIDS have lived long and fruitful lives.

3 **Q** Of those in the United States diagnosed with AIDS and fitting the case definition, how many have died of AIDS or its effects?

A Through December 2000, the majority of all individuals having AIDS have died. As of that date, 774,467 AIDS cases had been reported to the CDC, and 448,060 deaths had been recorded. It bears mention, however, that the number of deaths per year has been declining since the mid-1990s.

TABLE 4.6   CDC Classification of HIV Infections*

New Classification		Common Name
Stage I	Acute HIV infection (mononucleosislike, aseptic meningitis)	Acute infection
Stage II	Asymptomatic	Healthy carrier
Stage III	Persistent generalized lymphadenopathy	ARC
Stage IV	Other disease	
	A. Constitutional disease (fever, weight loss, diarrhea)	ARC
	B. Neurological disease (dementia, myelopathy, peripheral neuropathy)	ARC
	C. Secondary infections	
	1. CDC-defined AIDS-associated[†]	AIDS
	2. Other specified infections[‡]	ARC
	D. Secondary cancers (CDC-defined AIDS-associated)[§]	AIDS
	E. Other conditions attributed to HIV infection or immunosuppression	ARC

*CDC, Centers for Disease Control and Prevention; HIV, human immunodeficiency virus; ARC, AIDS-related complex.

[†]*Pneumocystis carinii* pneumonia, toxoplasmosis, cryptococcosis, chronic cryptospordiosis, extra-intestinal strongyloidiasis, isosporiasis, candidiasis (esophageal, bronchial or pulmonary), histoplasmosis, mycobacterial infection with *Mycobacterium avium-intracellulare* complex or *M. kansasii*, cytomegalovirus infection, chronic mucocutaneous or disseminated herpes simplex infection, and progressive multifocal leukoencephalopathy.

[‡]Multidermatomal herpes zoster, oral hairy leukoplakia, nocardiosis, tuberculosis, recurrent *Salmonella* bacteremia, oral candidiasis.

[§]Kaposi's sarcoma, non-Hodgkin's high-grade lymphoma, primary central nervous system lymphoma.

Source: Centers for Disease Control and Prevention.

The first stage of disease (Stage I) is acute HIV infection. The symptoms of HIV infection may last a few weeks or up to six months. Following acute HIV infection, Stage II disease involves few or no symptoms. Minor laboratory abnormalities may be detected, but immune-deficiency-related infections or cancers are not present. The third stage of disease, Stage III, consists of persistent generalized lymphadenopathy and is synonymous with ARC. The lymphadenopathy lasts for six months or more and occurs in two or more areas of the body, excluding the groin area. Stage IV disease is the point at which the patient begins experiencing symptoms from immunodeficiency due to the continuing loss of T-lymphocytes. This stage is further subdivided into five different sections, depending on the specific symptoms of immunodeficiency (Table 4.6). Certain sections are defined as ARC, whereas others constitute AIDS. In the paragraphs ahead, we shall explore the symptoms and conditions that distinguish AIDS.

The Walter Reed Classification System

Many physicians favor a classification system that incorporates stages of illness defined by specific immunologic markers. Such a system has been proposed by physicians at Walter Reed Hospital in Washington, D.C. The Walter Reed classification system charts the course of patients from exposure to HIV (WR0 for "Walter Reed zero") and onset of infection (WRI) through stages of continuing immune system destruction. The essential criteria by which patients are assigned to each stage always include laboratory evidence of HIV infection, as Table 4.7 indicates.

According to the Walter Reed classification system, lymphadenopathy appears at WR2, and WR3 is reached when the helper T-lymphocyte count drops below 400 cells per microliter of blood. The fourth stage (WR4) occurs when a person is unable to effectively mount the delayed hypersensitivity reactions associated with T-lymphocytes (a skin test for tuberculosis, for example). The next stage (WR5) is present when the patient cannot respond to skin tests at all or when thrush develops. By this time, the T-lymphocyte count has remained abnormal for at least three months, and lymphadenopathy has been consistent. When patients enter WR6, they are said to have AIDS. In this stage, the HIV wasting syndrome may ensue or AIDS-dementia complex may be observed. In addition, cancers or opportunistic diseases may be present. We shall now examine each of these conditions.

[handwritten: goes from 0-6 + have to have antibody]

TABLE 4.7	The Walter Reed Classification System*					
Stage	HIV Antibody and/or Virus	Chronic Lymphadenopathy	Helper T-Lymphocytes per cu mm	Delayed Hyper-sensitivity	Thrush	Opportunistic Diseases
WR0	–	–	>400	NORMAL	–	–
WR1	+	–	>400	NORMAL	–	–
WR2	+	+	>400	NORMAL	–	–
WR3	+	+/–	<400	NORMAL	–	–
WR4	+	+/–	<400	P	–	–
WR5	+	+/–	<400	P/C	+/–	–
WR6	+	+/–	<400	P/C	+/–	+

*P, partial reaction; P/C, partial or complete reaction; +/-, may or may not occur.

Source: Data from R. R. Redfield, et al., "The Walter Reed Staging Classification for HTLV-III/LAV Infection," in New England Journal of Medicine, 314: 131-139, 1986.

HIV Wasting Syndrome

For some patients, the diarrhea associated with AIDS can be so profound that a condition called HIV wasting syndrome ensues. This condition is accompanied by a dramatic weight loss of more than 10 percent of a person's baseline body weight plus either chronic diarrhea lasting at least 30 days or chronic weakness and fever lasting 30 days. For the definition of AIDS to apply, no other illness, such as opportunistic disease, or any condition other than HIV infection need be present. In such an instance, the diagnostic criteria for HIV wasting syndrome, shown in Table 4.8, have been fulfilled.

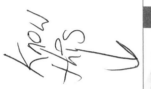

TABLE
4.8   Diagnostic Criteria for HIV Wasting Syndrome
Findings of involuntary loss of more than 10% of baseline body weight plus either chronic diarrhea (two or more loose stools per day for 30 or more days) or chronic weakness and documented fever (for 30 days or longer, intermittent or constant) in the absence of a concurrent illness or condition other than HIV infection that could explain the findings (e.g., cancer, tuberculosis, cryptosporidiosis, or other specific enteritis).

HIV wasting syndrome is a major cause of morbidity and mortality in patients with AIDS. In addition to decreased quality of life, the syndrome has been associated with a lower survival rate independent of the count of T-lymphocytes. Although the precise cause remains unknown, various researchers have related the syndrome to altered energy intake, secondary infections, altered body metabolism, and abnormalities in the body's hormone balance. The appetite loss is due to such things as mouth soreness, vomiting, lethargy, and depression.

The most common hormone abnormality associated with the wasting syndrome is hypogonadism, or low level of the sex hormone testosterone. Low testosterone levels may manifest themselves as poor tissue preservation, and researchers are investigating whether treating patients with anabolic steroids is beneficial. Over 50 percent of men with advanced HIV disease display low testosterone levels.

Another approach to forestalling HIV wasting syndrome is to strengthen the muscles with exercise. Many AIDS sufferers are reluctant to work with weights for fear of stimulating further muscle loss, but research reported in 1998 indicates that HIV levels do not rise as a result of strenuous workouts.

AIDS-Dementia Complex

There is much accumulated evidence that HIV can also replicate in the brain cells of infected individuals and cause AIDS-dementia complex. This condition may account for the periods of depression occurring as an early symptom of HIV infection. Persons with AIDS also display signs of confusion and have trouble coordinating their muscular activities. Apathy, along with fatigue, nausea, and loss of concentration, is another signal that the nervous system is involved. AIDS patients often experience a sudden, strong emotion unprecipitated by anything they can recall.

Public health officials estimate that roughly one-third of persons with AIDS develop AIDS-dementia complex. Such individuals display mental and physical deterioration traced to brain infection. They suffer memory loss, concentration lapses, minor disturbances in thought processes, and difficulty in sleeping. Headache, disorientation, and a general feeling of the "blues" are often experienced. Unsteady gait, slurred speech, and tremors may be other signs that the AIDS-dementia complex has developed. The patient often experiences absence of feeling in the arms and legs, leading to loss of such basic functions as walking.

Mounting evidence indicates that AIDS-dementia complex is a true viral infection of the brain. For example, HIV has been isolated from brain cells called astrocytes, shown in Figure 4.4, and from their surrounding fluid. Moreover, infection of the brain can be induced by inoculating animals with brain tissue obtained at autopsy from deceased individuals. The actual mechanism of HIV involvement with the brain cells is unclear, but one possibility is that the gp120 protein of HIV (Chapter 2) may be released in brain tissue and act as a neurotoxin that interferes with normal maintenance processes in the brain. Most researchers agree that the virus does not destroy brain cells simply by multiplying within them, but by mechanisms not yet understood. One possibility is apoptosis, a form of cell suicide discussed in Chapter 3.

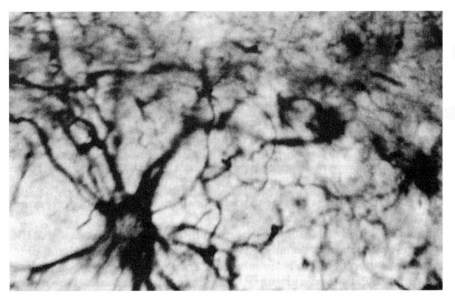

FIGURE 4.4
A photomicrograph of human brain tissue showing astrocytes, the star-shaped cells with multiple long extensions. The astrocytes may be targets of HIV, and the result of the infection may be AIDS-related dementia.

For HIV to infect human brain tissue, the virus would have to interact with brain cells much as it interacts with T-lymphocytes. Such an interaction would require receptor molecules on brain cells similar to the CD4 molecules on T-lymphocytes (Chapter 2). As early as 1986, scientists from New York's Columbia University located protein molecules at the surface of brain cells and provided the clue to how HIV and brain cells interact.

How HIV enters the brain tissue was another problem requiring resolution. Normally the brain is shielded from the blood and its constituents by the so-called blood-brain barrier. This barrier of membranes and substances allows only selected materials and cells to pass from blood to brain tissue. In 1987, scientists learned how HIV passes this barrier. Apparently the virus remains sequestered inside a macrophage (Chapter 3) while the latter squeezes through the barrier (macrophages are one of the few types of cells that can pass the barrier). Thus, the macrophage appears to be the key to HIV delivery into the brain. Indeed, the emerging consensus is that the central nervous system is a reservoir for HIV, probably in the macrophages of the brain tissue.

The ability of HIV to attack brain cells as well as T-lymphocytes has changed the outlook on AIDS significantly. No longer is AIDS considered solely a disease of the immune system. Rather, the substantial effects of HIV on the nervous system indicate that AIDS affects at least a second system of the body and pushes concerns about the disease another notch higher. Moreover, the infection of brain tissue implies further demands on already overburdened public health facilities. People with mild dementia, for example, cannot perform routine day-to-day activities, and those with severe dementia resemble senile patients—they cannot get around on their own or find their way in their own homes. The irrational and unpredictable behavior they sometimes display adds a mental component to the loss of immune function.

Another disquieting note was sounded in 2000 when researchers noted the inability of protease inhibitor drugs to cross the blood-brain barrier and penetrate the brain tissue. This observation raised concerns that although infected patients may live longer as a result of the drug therapy, they may face an increased risk of developing AIDS-dementia complex. Opponents of this conclusion point out that the incidence of the complex has declined since the drugs were introduced.

AIDS-dementia complex necessitated modification of the definition for AIDS. As previously mentioned, the original definition of AIDS specified that some other infectious disease involving immunodeficiency be present; as we shall discuss presently, that requirement still holds for the majority of cases. However, the case definition was expanded in 1987 to include neurological disease (technically called HIV encephalopathy), even though some other microbial disease is not present (Table 4.9 provides the diagnostic criteria for HIV encephalopathy). Thus, a person may fulfill the case definition for AIDS if they have AIDS-dementia complex.

Kaposi's Sarcoma

One of the conditions associated with AIDS is a type of cancer known as Kaposi's sarcoma, named for Moritz Kaposi, who first described it in 1924. The original

TABLE	
4.9	**Diagnostic Criteria for HIV Encephalopathy**

Clinical findings of disabling cognitive and/or motor dysfunction interfering with occupation or activities of daily living, or loss of behavioral developmental milestones in a child, progressing over weeks to months, in the absence of a concurrent illness or condition other than HIV infection that could explain the findings. Methods to rule out such concurrent illness must include cerebrospinal fluid examination and either brain imaging (computed tomography or magnetic resonance imaging) or autopsy.

case definition of AIDS included Kaposi's sarcoma because it was frequently present in homosexual men who displayed immune deficiency. As of 1990, almost one-quarter of all persons with AIDS suffered from Kaposi's sarcoma, and the condition remains one of the most common diseases associated with AIDS. The case definition for AIDS, set down in 1987 and revised in 1993, continues to include the presence of Kaposi's sarcoma as a basis for AIDS.

Before the AIDS epidemic, Kaposi's sarcoma was a rare form of cancer found primarily in older men of Mediterranean descent. In this population, Kaposi's sarcoma is characterized by slow-growing tumors in the blood-vessel linings, with patches of red to violet-red on the lower extremities (Figure 4.5). Eventually, the patches become darkened purplish-brown nodules. Kaposi's sarcoma by itself is rarely fatal; patients live for many years and often die of an unrelated disease.

When associated with AIDS, Kaposi's sarcoma is a much more serious disease. Nodules appear on the lower extremities as well as in scattered patches all over the body. The upper body and face are often the site of the purplish-brown patches, and the oral cavity may be involved. Internal organs such as the lymph nodes, gastrointestinal tract, liver, and spleen are possible nodule sites, and any soft tissue appears to be susceptible. Kaposi's sarcoma is often accompanied by diarrhea, weight loss, fever, and intense sweating at night. The disease is so aggressive that affected individuals survive an average of less than two years. This span may be even shorter if a microbial infection occurs concurrently.

Evidence is lacking on why Kaposi's sarcoma is so prevalent in persons with AIDS and why it is so aggressive. However, research results indicate that HIV itself may promote the disease. Scientists at the National Cancer Institute transplanted genes from HIV into unborn mice. They then noted that a significant percentage of mice born with certain of the transplanted genes had abnormal skin growths similar to those in Kaposi's sarcoma. The HIV genes were located in cells distant from the growths, suggesting that a protein encoded by the genes was responsible for the cancer-promoting effect. Scientists have reported that the *tat* gene of HIV (Chapter 2) was the critical protein-encoding gene.

Observations of a different sort indicate that Kaposi's sarcoma may be caused by a separate viral agent transmitted coincidentally with HIV. In 1990, a promi-

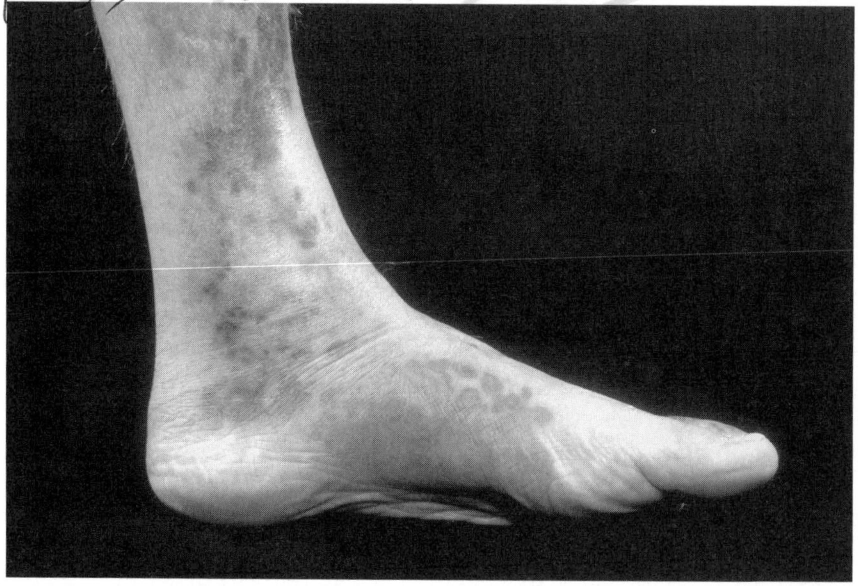

Kaposi Sarcoma(tumor) leisions - spreads out on skin

FIGURE 4.5

The foot of a patient with AIDS, displaying the patches of Kaposi's sarcoma that commonly develop on the lower extremities.

nent New York physician reported 12 cases of Kaposi's sarcoma in homosexual men testing negative for HIV. The suggestion was made that a Kaposi's sarcoma agent may have entered the human population at approximately the same time as HIV but was becoming uncoupled from AIDS. This speculation was fueled by a 1998 report that the number of cases of Kaposi's sarcoma in homosexual men with AIDS had dropped to 21 percent (compared with nearly 50 percent in the early years of the AIDS epidemic).

Further insight was provided in 1995 when Patrick S. Moore and Yuan Chang of Columbia University identified human herpesvirus type 8 (HHV-8) as the cause of Kaposi's sarcoma. The investigators determined the DNA sequence of the virus and identified the sequence in lesions associated with Kaposi's sarcoma, including lesions from patients living in widely separated areas of the United States. Many physicians believe that HIV infection promotes HHV-8 replication by impairing the immune system of the host. However, in 1997, Robert Gallo and his coworkers postulated that the *tat* protein encoded by HIV acts as a toxin and attracts HHV-8 into the cellular area that becomes a Kaposi's sarcoma lesion. This work suggests that HHV-8 may be a mere "visitor" to the site, a virus that takes advantage of the conditions altered by HIV. Thus, HHV-8 may be necessary to establish Kaposi's sarcoma, although it does not act alone. In some reports, the virus is called KS-associated herpesvirus, or KSHV. Its isolation from salivary secretions in 1997 may give a glimpse of how it is transmitted. The virus lives in the back of the mouth and throat, and kissing is thought to be one route of transmission.

Opportunistic Diseases

Another hallmark of AIDS is the presence of disease caused by an opportunistic organism. Opportunistic organisms are organisms that often exist in the body but cause no harm because the body's immune system and other natural defenses keep them under control. When the natural defenses are compromised, however, the organisms seize the "opportunity" to invade the tissues and cause disease. The occurrence of diseases caused by opportunistic organisms illustrates the delicate balance that exists between infectious organisms and natural defenses. Once the defenses break down, the opportunists invade.

The majority of persons with AIDS suffer from one or several diseases caused by opportunistic organisms. These diseases have euphemistically been called opportunistic diseases. Though technically incorrect (because the organisms are opportunistic, not the diseases), the term "opportunistic disease" has become part of AIDS terminology, and so we shall use it here.

When the original definition of AIDS was promulgated in 1981, the CDC specified that an opportunistic disease or Kaposi's sarcoma had to be present before doctors could report a case as AIDS. With the realization that dementia and wasting could be key factors, the 1987 definition of AIDS incorporated neurological disease (HIV encephalopathy) and HIV wasting syndrome as other bases for identifying a case of AIDS. Then, the 1993 case definition specified a count of helper T-lymphocytes (CD4 cells). Nevertheless, the presence of an opportunistic disease remains a prime criterion in the case definition of AIDS, and a majority of persons with AIDS suffer from at least one opportunistic disease.

The opportunistic disease most prevalent among persons with AIDS is *Pneumocystis carinii* pneumonia, commonly referred to as *Pneumocystis* pneumonia or sometimes as PCP. The disease is due to *Pneumocystis carinii*, a protozoan first described by John Carini in 1910 and depicted in Figure 4.6a. We should note that biochemical studies have encouraged some researchers to consider *Pneumocystis carinii* a fungus, but the prevailing opinion is that the organism is a protozoan. The protozoan is a benign inhabitant of the lungs in many people. Disease occurs when the *Pneumocystis* organisms multiply furiously and take up all the lung's air spaces (Figure 4.6b). The patient experiences rapid, labored breathing, a nonproductive (no mucus) cough, and extreme anxiety because enough oxygen cannot be drawn from the air into the bloodstream. Symptoms may be relieved by administering high concentrations of oxygen through a face mask or, when symptoms are extreme, by using a respirator machine connected to a tube placed in the windpipe. The respirator reduces the effort to breathe, but the procedure can be frightening and cause some physical discomfort.

Patients with *Pneumocystis carinii* pneumonia can be treated with a drug called pentamidine isethionate (Chapter 8). Although this drug kills the protozoa, the damage to the lungs may be irreversible, and the drug may impair kidney and liver function and cause painful abscesses at the injection site. As

FIGURE 4.6

Pneumocystis carinii, an opportunistic protozoan associated with AIDS. (a) The protozoan is seen in the throat washings of an AIDS patient. The parasite appears as dark spheres in this specimen as it might be viewed by a pathologist (×250). (b) An X ray of the lungs of an AIDS patient infected with P. carinii. The dark areas reflect regions of protozoal involvement and demonstrate the extensive nature of the infection. The organisms occupy the spaces normally used for the transfer of gases and make breathing very difficult.

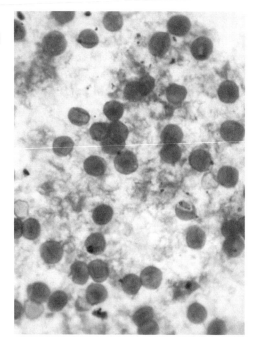

(a)

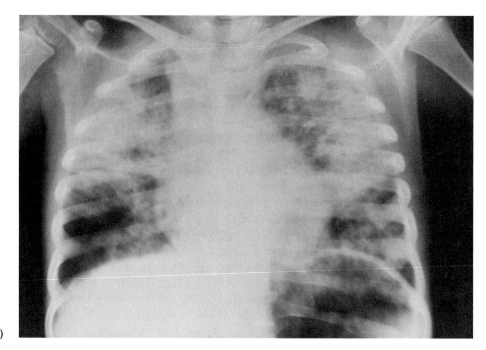

(b)

of 1996, more than 50 percent of individuals who died from complications of AIDS died from *Pneumocystis* pneumonia. Because the disease is rarely seen elsewhere, a diagnosis of *Pneumocystis* pneumonia is a reliable indicator that HIV is present.

Another opportunistic disease often associated with AIDS is toxoplasmosis. The agent of this disease *is Toxoplasma gondii,* a protozoan shown in Figure 4.7a. Normally, toxoplasmosis is a mild, mononucleosislike disease, but in persons with AIDS, the protozoan attacks the brain tissue, causing lesions, cerebral swelling, and seizures. Severe headaches, sensitivity to light, neck stiffness, and loss of some motor or sensory functions may also occur. Several drugs are available to control toxoplasmosis, but since the person is usually quite weak, these are of limited value. Domestic housecats often harbor *T. gondii,* so persons with HIV infection are advised to avoid cats.

Another protozoal opportunist is *Cryptosporidium coccidi* (Figure 4.7b). This organism infects the intestine in AIDS patients and induces unrelenting, voluminous, watery diarrhea, progressing to dehydration, loss of important body salts, and malnutrition. The results are extreme weight loss, wasting of muscle tissue, and loss of skin tone, as well as poor tissue healing and repair. In its severest form, cryptosporidiosis may result in loss of up to a gallon of fluid per day. Dehydration and emaciation accompany this disease, and intravenous fluid replacement is required to maintain the body's water balance.

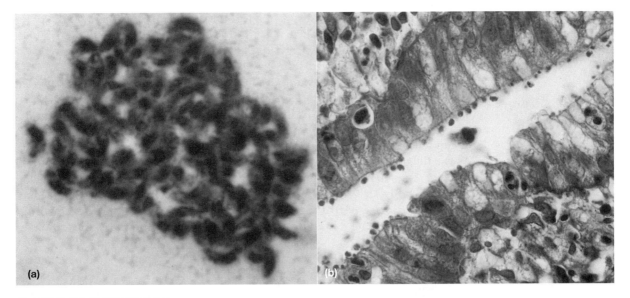

FIGURE 4.7

Two opportunistic protozoa associated with AIDS. (a) *Toxoplasma gondii,* the cause of toxoplasmosis. In this scanning electron micrograph, the protozoan appears in its crescent form (×31,000). (b) A light micrograph of *Cryptosporidium coccidi,* the cause of cryptosporidiosis. The 4–5 micron protozoans are seen here lining the lumen of the colon in a 29-year-old man with AIDS.

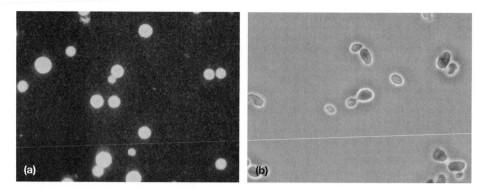

FIGURE 4.8

Two opportunistic fungi associated with AIDS. (a) A light microscope view of *Cryptococcus neoformans*, the agent of cryptococcosis. Each cell is round to oval and is surrounded by a distinctive capsule. The capsule provides resistance to phagocytosis and enhances the pathogenicity of the fungus. (b) *Candida albicans*, the cause of thrush. In this light micrograph, the fungus appears as oval cells with a tendency to cling together in long filamentlike strands.

One fungus that causes an opportunistic disease is *Cryptococcus neoformans* (Figure 4.8a). This organism, a common resident of the lungs, is usually inhaled from the air. It grows actively in the droppings of pigeons and enters the air in windborne particles. The fungus is generally noninfectious, but in persons with AIDS, it multiplies in the lungs, spreads to the blood, and localizes on the brain and its coverings. Piercing headaches, stiff neck, paralysis, and mental dysfunction accompany the infection. Changes in behavioral patterns and mental confusion may also be observed. The disease is termed cryptococcosis.

Another fungus of substantial consequence for AIDS patients is *Candida albicans*, the yeastlike microorganism mentioned earlier in the discussion on ARC and portrayed in Figure 4.8b. In a person with AIDS, *C. albicans* grows in the mouth as patches of white, curdlike material, producing a condition called thrush or candidiasis. When scraped off, the patches reveal a painful, red, inflamed base. As the fungus spreads to the esophagus, tissue erosion occurs, and the exposed nerve endings make eating an excruciating experience. The appetite is quickly lost, and body deterioration ensues, sometimes necessitating liquid feeding through a tube inserted through the nose into the stomach. Though several drugs are available to control candidiasis, repairing the damage to the esophagus takes considerable time.

One virus that can cause an opportunistic disease is the cytomegalovirus (CMV). This virus is so named because in the laboratory it causes cells to assume an enlarged size (*cyto* means "cell"; *megalo* refers to "giant" size). Normally, CMV is present without consequence in many body tissues, but when the immune system is compromised, the virus multiplies aggressively in lung tissues, where it induces pneumonia. The virus also multiplies in other tissues: in the liver and kidney tissues, where it causes tissue death; in salivary gland tissues, where it brings on swollen glands; and on the retina (CMV retinitis), where it leads to partial or complete blindness (Healthline 4.3). Indeed, over 30 percent of AIDS patients develop eye disease due to CMV and experience "floaters," flashes of light, blind spots, or blurred vision.

In addition, the cytomegalovirus appears to invade helper T-lymphocytes, thus accelerating the destruction of those cells begun by HIV. An interesting corollary to this observation was made in 1997 when French investigators reported that cells invaded by CMV produce proteins that act as receptors identical to CCR5. The implication is that cells infected with CMV become unusually receptive to HIV. Although the evidence is controversial and somewhat contradictory, if proved true, it would imply a tight relationship between HIV and its accomplice CMV. Skeptics of the findings point out, however, that although CMV is known to infect brain cells (as well as cells of the retina), there is little evidence that coinfection of helper T-lymphocytes with both HIV and CMV is a common event. Figure 4.9a shows the cytomegalovirus.

Opportunistic diseases of bacterial origin have also been observed. One example, tuberculosis, has always been a significant cause of death worldwide. In the United States, for example, tuberculosis was responsible for one death in seven (from all causes) in the early 1900s. Today's statistics, though improved, are still alarming: Over 25,000 cases of the disease are reported each year in the United States. The cause of tuberculosis is a small bacterial rod called *Mycobacterium tuberculosis* (Figure 4.9b). A generally good quality of life together with natural controls centered in T-lymphocytes prevent the disease from proliferating in most individuals. For those with AIDS, however, the controls break down and tuberculosis develops. Progressive deterioration of the lung tissue leads to labored breathing and a cough that brings up a mucousy pus and, sometimes, blood. Chest pain is substantial, shortness of breath is obvious, and the disease may spread to other organs. Without treatment, the patient often becomes emaciated and dies. It is not coincidental that the spread of HIV in recent years has paralleled an increase in the incidence of tuberculosis.

Another species of *Mycobacterium* can also be a serious threat to those with HIV. This bacterium is called *Mycobacterium avium-intracellulare* (or MAI). Like *M. tuberculosis*, the organism invades lung tissue as the T-lymphocyte count drops and causes a progressive destruction of tissue that can be fatal. Drugs are available for treating both MAI infection (also called mycobacteriosis) and tuberculosis, but drug therapy must be aggressive and must extend over a period of many months.

Healthline 4.3

1 Q Can persons with HIV infection minimize the risk of acquiring opportunistic diseases?

A Unfortunately, most opportunistic diseases are caused by organisms already in the body. However, there are some precautions that can be taken to minimize exposure to organisms not already present. Cats, for example, are often infected with *Toxoplasma*, so it makes sense for individuals with HIV infection to avoid contact with cats and their waste products. Also, poorly cooked meat and fish may contain infectious microbes that can be avoided. In addition, the pentamidine isethionate and other drugs are available in an aerosolized form to help prevent development of *Pneumocystis carinii* pneumonia.

2 Q Is any one opportunistic disease more common than the others?

A Very definitely. Among patients with AIDS, more than 50 percent have died from *Pneumocystis carinii* pneumonia. While this protozoal disease can be treated with drugs, the therapy is less successful in AIDS patients than in patients who do not have AIDS or HIV infection.

3 Q Must a person have an opportunistic disease to fit the case definition for AIDS?

A No, a person need not have an opportunistic disease to have AIDS. The case definition for AIDS can be fulfilled if a person has AIDS-dementia complex or HIV wasting syndrome, neither of which is accompanied by opportunistic microorganisms.

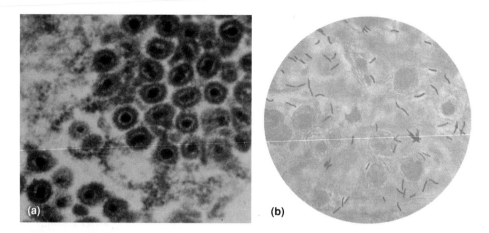

FIGURE 4.9

Viral and bacterial opportunists associated with AIDS. (a) An electron micrograph of the cytomegalovirus cultivated in tissue cells. Some viral particles are within the nucleus of the cell, but others have budded through the nuclear membrane and are now in the cellular cytoplasm. The thicker covering of these viruses reflects the envelope they have acquired during budding. Note the very small size of the viruses relative to the host cell (×45,000). (b) A photomicrograph of *Mycobacterium tuberculosis,* the agent of tuberculosis. This rod-shaped bacillus has been cultivated outside of living tissue in laboratory medium (×1000).

The list of opportunistic organisms is not exhausted by those we have considered. Also included on the list are the fungus *Histoplasma capsulatum,* the protozoan *Isospora belli,* and the herpes simplex virus (Table 4.10 summarizes the list). Like the others, each of these organisms attacks body tissues when the immune system is depressed, and each may be a cause of death in AIDS patients. It is apparent that opportunistic disease is a key element in the definition of AIDS. Except for deaths caused by AIDS-dementia complex and HIV wasting syndrome, it is not technically correct to say that a person has died of AIDS. Rather, the person has succumbed to one of the opportunistic diseases.

It is equally clear that the person with HIV infection or AIDS-related complex does not have AIDS. In the great majority of cases (the exceptions being patients with AIDS-dementia complex or HIV wasting syndrome), an opportunistic disease must be present for the case definition to be fulfilled. Such a requirement was established in the original case definition (1981) and continued in the modified definition (1987), but was made optional in the latest definition (1993).

Pediatric AIDS

In 1982, when a prominent researcher wrote that babies were contracting AIDS, few colleagues believed him. Today, there is little doubt that HIV can be passed from a pregnant woman to her offspring. Indeed, as of June 2000, a total of 8804 cases of pediatric AIDS were reported to the CDC.

| TABLE 4.10 | A Summary of Opportunistic Diseases Associated with AIDS |

Microbial Agent	Type of Microorganism	Disease	Manifestations
Pneumocystis carinii	Protozoan	Pneumocystis carinii pneumonia	Pneumonia, difficult breathing, suffocation
Toxoplasma gondii	Protozoan	Toxoplasmosis	Fatigue, brain lesions, seizures, cerebral swelling
Cryptosporidium coccidi	Protozoan	Cryptosporidiosis	Extreme diarrhea, dehydration, shock, emaciation
Isospora belli	Protozoan	Isosporiasis	Diarrhea, nausea, abdominal pain
Cryptococcus neoformans	Fungus	Cryptococcosis	Pneumonia, piercing headaches, paralysis (meningitis) — _spinal column & fluid_
Candida albicans	Fungus	Candidiasis	Oral patches of white fungus, erosion of esophagus
Histoplasma capsulatum	Fungus	Histoplasmosis	Pneumonia, lesions of visceral organs, paralysis
Cytomegalovirus	Virus	Cytomegalovirus disease	Pneumonia, liver and kidney disease, impaired vision
Herpes simplex virus	Virus	Herpes simplex	Body sores and blisters
Mycobacterium tuberculosis	Bacterium	Tuberculosis	Lesions of lungs, difficult breathing, lesions of visceral organs
Mycobacterium avium-intracellulare	Bacterium	Mycobacteriosis (MAI infection)	Lesions of lungs and visceral organs

The prevailing theory is that HIV is transferred from mother to child by crossing the placenta from the woman's blood to the child's blood, as we discuss in Chapter 5. There is also evidence that transmission may take place during the birth process or during breast-feeding (since HIV has been isolated from breast milk). In addition, a small percentage of cases have been traced to contaminated blood used in a transfusion.

Children with AIDS fail to thrive (Figure 4.10). They do not demonstrate the expected growth patterns after birth, nor do they respond to aggressive nutritional therapy. Many children achieve their normal height for a particular age,

FIGURE 4.10

A child dying of AIDS in Nigeria.

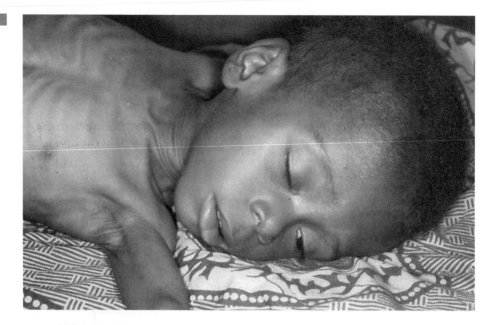

but they experience weight loss that does not reverse itself. Persistent diarrhea may contribute to the weight loss.

Another symptom of pediatric AIDS is decreased cognitive skills, most likely due to HIV infection in the brain. Researchers have discovered that brain disease in the fetus can begin during the first stages of pregnancy and can lead to dementia. Expected intelligence milestones are not reached, and on tests of cognitive skills, children with AIDS consistently score in the lowest 2 percent of their age group. In some cases, children lose the use of their arms and legs and become blind and deaf by the age of 2.

Children with AIDS suffer from opportunistic diseases, but the sources are generally bacteria; in contrast, in adults, protozoa, fungi, and viruses are important. In newborns and children with AIDS, the common opportunistic diseases are due to *Salmonella* species (intestinal infections), streptococci (respiratory infections), and staphylococci (skin and blood infections). It is conceivable that susceptibility to these bacterial diseases may reflect the inability of infected children to develop the antibody-producing B-lymphocytes necessary for protection against them. Candidiasis is also a significant symptom in children with AIDS, as are lymphadenopathy and swollen salivary glands. The latter symptom usually does not occur in adults.

Probably the only common denominator among children with AIDS is that their immune systems have been compromised. No two cases are identical. Indeed, no two cases in adults are alike, because the symptoms of AIDS vary within very broad parameters. In the final analysis, there is no one single entity called AIDS, but instead, myriad conditions and diseases. For this reason, defining and recognizing AIDS can be a formidable task.

Defining acquired immune deficiency syndrome (AIDS) is a complex matter because there are many phases to the disease. It is important that the disease be defined, however, because diagnosis, treatment, and public health record-keeping are based on a clear understanding of it. The earliest definition, promulgated by the CDC in 1981, spelled out AIDS as a condition in which certain diseases exist in the patient and reflect an impaired immune system. The revised definition, issued in 1987, included in the case definition evidence of the presence of human immunodeficiency virus (HIV) and three distinctive conditions that can accompany HIV infection: HIV wasting syndrome, AIDS-dementia complex, and opportunistic diseases. The 1993 case definition includes a helper T-lymphocyte (or CD4 cell) count below 200 cells per microliter of blood or pulmonary tuberculosis, recurrent pneumonia, or invasive cervical cancer; and the 2000 expansion of the case definition includes reporting of individuals with HIV infection.

Infection with HIV is the first phase of a multiphase disease that may progress to AIDS. Among its signs are swollen lymph nodes, headaches, and a positive viral load test and test for HIV antibodies. For many individuals, AIDS-related complex (ARC) follows. Extensive and persistent lymphadenopathy, night sweats, diarrhea, and thrush are signals of ARC. AIDS is actually the final phase of the progression, when wasting of the body is substantial, when brain involvement is severe, or when opportunistic diseases develop. Kaposi's sarcoma, now known to be caused by a separate virus, is accompanied by slow-growing tumors in the blood vessels and splotches on the skin.

Opportunistic diseases are caused by microorganisms normally present in the body and controlled by a healthy immune system. When the system is weakened, the microorganisms seize the "opportunity" to infect. The most prevalent opportunistic disease is *Pneumocystis carinii* pneumonia, a severe lung disease accompanied by lung consolidation and difficult breathing. Toxoplasmosis of the brain, *Cryptosporidium* infection of the intestine, and *Cryptococcus* infection of the nervous system are other opportunistic diseases. In many cases, an opportunistic disease is fatal to the patient who has AIDS.

Pediatric AIDS is acquired by a newborn from its mother, in most cases by transfer of HIV across the placenta. Children with AIDS fail to thrive. They display reduced cognitive skills, loss of use of their motor organs, and opportunistic diseases, often due to bacteria. Although antiretroviral therapy in pregnant women has successfully reduced the number of cases of pediatric AIDS, the number of cases remains substantial, as we explore in Chapter 5.

Having studied the pathology of AIDS, you should be familiar with the signs, symptoms, and progress of the stages of the disease. To test your knowledge, enter at the left the word or words that best complete each thought. The correct answers are listed in Appendix A.

1. *AIDS- Dimensia Complex* is the name of the brain disorder occurring in roughly one-third of persons with AIDS.

2. *Walter Reed* is the hospital whose physicians devised a six-stage classification system of the stages leading to AIDS.

3. *Kaposi's Sarcoma* is the cancer of the skin often observed in persons with AIDS.

4. *Cytomegalovirus* is the virus that forms giant cells in the laboratory and that invades many cells of many organs as an opportunist.

5. *Pneumocystis Carinii* is the name of the protozoan that causes lung disease as an opportunistic disease accompanying AIDS.

6. *10 yrs.* is the approximate incubation period for AIDS.

7. *HIV Infection* is the name assigned to the condition where a patient harbors HIV but shows no symptoms of disease.

8. *lymphadenopathy* is the term given to the swollen lymph nodes commonly associated with HIV infection, ARC, and AIDS.

9. *6000* is the approximate number of cases of pediatric AIDS reported through 2000.

10. *800* is the normal count of T-lymphocytes per microliter of blood.

11. *Candida albicans* is the yeastlike fungus that causes the infection of the mouth called thrush, an early sign of impending AIDS.

12. *gastrointestinal sys.* is the system of the body attacked by the opportunistic microorganism *Cryptosporidium*.

13. *HIV Wasting Syndrome* is the name given to the chronic diarrhea and dramatic weight loss that can fulfill the definition for AIDS.

14. *Pentamidine isethionate* is the drug used to treat patients who experience *Pneumocystis carinii* pneumonia.

15. *Cats* are the animals that harbor *Toxoplasma* and that should be avoided by a person infected by HIV.

Altman, L. K. 1990. "Unlocking the secrets of a microbe." *New York Times,* September 4.

Caldwell, M. 1994. "Blessed with resistance." *Discover,* January.

Cockerell, C. J. 1995. "Cutaneous fungal infections in HIV/AIDS." *J. Intl. Assn. Phys. AIDS Care,* February.

Fackelmann, K. 1995. "Staying alive: scientists study people who outwit the AIDS virus." *Science News* 147: 172–175.

Gallo, R. C. 1998. "The enigmas of Kaposi's sarcoma." *Science* 282: 1837–1839.

Gartner, S. 2000. "HIV infection and dementia." *Science* 287: 602–605.

Gorman, C. 1993. "Are some people immune to AIDS?" *Time,* March 22.

Hughes, W. 1987. "*Pneumocystis carinii* pneumonitis." *New Engl. J. Med.* 317: 1021–1023.

Kerr, R. A. 1997. "Does a common virus give HIV a helping hand?" *Science* 276: 1794.

Montgomery, G. 1989. "The infant brain." *Discover,* August.

Navin, T. R., and A. M. Hardy. 1987. "Cryptosporidiosis in patients with AIDS." *J. Infect. Dis.* 155: 150–157.

Price, R. W., et al. 1988. "The brain in AIDS: central nervous system HIV-1 infection and AIDS dementia complex." *Science* 239: 586–592.

Redfield, R. R., and D. S. Burke. 1988. "HIV infection: the clinical picture." *Scientific American* 259(4): 91–98.

Whitcup, S. M. 1996. "Ocular manifestations of AIDS." *JAMA* 275: 142–144.

The Epidemiology of AIDS

LOOKING AHEAD

Scientists have identified several methods by which AIDS spreads among individuals. This chapter explores those methods and discusses the principles that underlie them. On completing the chapter, you should be able to . . .

- Describe the work of epidemiologists during the AIDS epidemic and appreciate their contributions to public health care.
- Summarize current statistics on reported cases and groups affected by the AIDS epidemic.
- Understand the methods by which the human immunodeficiency virus (HIV) spreads among sexually active homosexual men, injection drug users, and heterosexual couples, and how HIV can pass to newborns.
- Compare the patterns by which the AIDS epidemic is spreading in the United States, Africa, and the rest of the world.
- Make some generalizations about the spread of AIDS in society, schools and colleges, and health care settings.

INTRODUCTION

During July 1976, the Bellevue-Stratford Hotel in Philadelphia was the site of the 58th annual convention of the Pennsylvania contingent of the American Legion. Toward the end of the convention, 149 Legionnaires and 72 others in or near the hotel experienced fever, coughing, and pneumonia. Within days, 34 had died. Microbiologists began an intensive search for a causative agent, but no pathogenic microorganisms could be found within the tissues of victims.

As the weeks wore on, the illness came to be known as Legionnaires' disease, and its enigma deepened. There were hints that a cause might never be identified. There were even some allegations of foul play, including a charge that the disease was caused by genetically engineered microorganisms stolen from U.S. Army laboratories.

Then, on January 6, 1977, less than six months after the outbreak, the mystery was resolved. Scientists from the Centers for Disease Control and Prevention (CDC) identified the responsible bacterium and named it *Legionella pneumophila*. Two things about *L. pneumophila* were significant: First, the organism was a species of bacterium never before encountered; second, the organism existed where water collected and was blown into the air by wind currents. Public health officials now had two important facts to help them interrupt the epidemic: They knew what was causing it, and they understood the source of the causative agent. They soon brought the outbreak of Legionnaires' disease under control by identifying the bacterium in infected water supplies and treating the water with disinfectants.

A somewhat similar situation has existed during the AIDS epidemic. Since the spring of 1984, scientists have known that HIV is the responsible agent, and as early as 1982, they were fairly certain how the agent is transmitted. Armed with this information, public health officials could predict which groups the epidemic would affect the most and how it was likely to spread in the future. Their predictions were largely correct. Then came the task of educating those at risk and showing individuals how to protect themselves from infection. As we shall see in this chapter, that goal has been difficult to accomplish since protection often involves changes in lifestyle and behavior. Interrupting the epidemic of Legionnaires' disease, by comparison, was relatively easy, because it involved disinfecting the water where bacteria collect. In addition, Legionnaires' disease can be successfully treated with antibiotics and the patient will return to good health. No such option is yet available for AIDS.

AIDS and the Epidemiologist

Epidemiology is the study of relationships that influence the frequency and distribution of diseases in a community. Discovering that an epidemic is in progress and defining the circumstances under which it spreads are two tasks of the epidemiologist. In the public health system, the epidemiologist also studies a disease's pattern of distribution and makes recommendations on controlling it in a population. Controlling an epidemic can be a substantial challenge because the epidemiologist must often work in a situation where no drugs or vaccines are available.

The best epidemiologists were put to the test in June 1981, when doctors at the CDC described five cases of *Pneumocystis carinii* pneumonia in homosexual men living in the Los Angeles area (Figure 5.1 shows the original report). At about the same time, the CDC received several requests for pentamidine isethionate, a drug used to treat *Pneumocystis carinii* pneumonia (only two requests had been received in the previous ten years). They also received reports of an unusual number of cases of Kaposi's sarcoma and suppressed immune systems in patients. A microbiology textbook author, writing in 1982, reflected the

FIGURE 5.1

The issue of *Morbidity and Mortality Weekly Report* in which CDC epidemiologists summarized five cases of *Pneumocystis carinii* pneumonia. This issue of June 5, 1981 is considered to be one of the beginning points of the AIDS epidemic. *Source: Centers for Disease Control and Prevention, Morbidity and Mortality Weekly Report, June 5, 1981.*

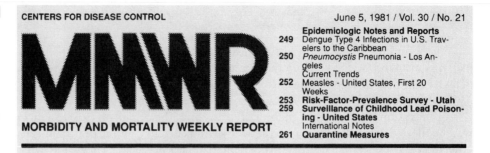

CENTERS FOR DISEASE CONTROL

June 5, 1981 / Vol. 30 / No. 21

MORBIDITY AND MORTALITY WEEKLY REPORT

Epidemiologic Notes and Reports
249 Dengue Type 4 Infections in U.S. Travelers to the Caribbean
250 *Pneumocystis* Pneumonia - Los Angeles
Current Trends
252 Measles - United States, First 20 Weeks
253 **Risk-Factor-Prevalence Survey - Utah**
259 **Surveillance of Childhood Lead Poisoning - United States**
International Notes
261 **Quarantine Measures**

Pneumocystis Pneumonia — Los Angeles

In the period October 1980-May 1981, 5 young men, all active homosexuals, were treated for biopsy-confirmed *Pneumocystis carinii* pneumonia at 3 different hospitals in Los Angeles, California. Two of the patients died. All 5 patients had laboratory-confirmed previous or current cytomegalovirus (CMV) infection and candidal mucosal infection. Case reports of these patients follow.

Patient 1: A previously healthy 33-year-old man developed *P. carinii* pneumonia and oral mucosal candidiasis in March 1981 after a 2-month history of fever associated with elevated liver enzymes, leukopenia, and CMV viruria. The serum complement-fixation CMV titer in October 1980 was 256; in May 1981 it was 32.* The patient's condition deteriorated despite courses of treatment with trimethoprim-sulfamethoxazole (TMP/SMX), pentamidine, and acyclovir. He died May 3, and postmortem examination showed residual *P. carinii* and CMV pneumonia, but no evidence of neoplasia.

Patient 2: A previously healthy 30-year-old man developed *P. carinii* pneumonia in April 1981 after a 5-month history of fever each day and of elevated liver-function tests, CMV viruria, and documented seroconversion to CMV, i.e., an acute-phase titer of 16 and a convalescent-phase titer of 28* in anticomplement immunofluorescence tests. Other features of his illness included leukopenia and mucosal candidiasis. His pneumonia responded to a course of intravenous TMP/SMX, but, as of the latest reports, he continues to have a fever each day.

Patient 3: A 30-year-old man was well until January 1981 when he developed esophageal and oral candidiasis that responded to Amphotericin B treatment. He was hospitalized in February 1981 for *P. carinii* pneumonia that responded to oral TMP/SMX. His esophageal candidiasis recurred after the pneumonia was diagnosed, and he was again given Amphotericin B. The CMV complement-fixation titer in March 1981 was 8. Material from an esophageal biopsy was positive for CMV.

Patient 4: A 29-year-old man developed *P. carinii* pneumonia in February 1981. He had had Hodgkins disease 3 years earlier, but had been successfully treated with radiation therapy alone. He did not improve after being given intravenous TMP/SMX and corticosteroids and died in March. Postmortem examination showed no evidence of Hodgkins disease, but *P. carinii* and CMV were found in lung tissue.

Patient 5: A previously healthy 36-year-old man with a clinically diagnosed CMV infection in September 1980 was seen in April 1981 because of a 4-month history of fever, dyspnea, and cough. On admission he was found to have *P. carinii* pneumonia, oral candidiasis, and CMV retinitis. A complement-fixation CMV titer in April 1981 was 128. The patient has been treated with 2 short courses of TMP/SMX that have been limited because of a sulfa-induced neutropenia. He is being treated for candidiasis with topical nystatin.

*Paired specimens not run in parallel.

uncertainty of the times by suggesting that "[the relationship of Kaposi's sarcoma] to pneumocystosis and the suppressed condition of the patient's immune system is unclear as of this writing."

By the end of 1982, epidemiologists had given the name *acquired immune deficiency syndrome (AIDS)* to the disease and were collecting data on its symptoms. Because the cities involved were far apart (New York, San Francisco, Miami, Los Angeles), epidemiologists surmised that there was a common denominator within the separate populations. And as data on the long incubation period became apparent, they guessed that a larger pool of individuals was infected and would be manifesting the disease in the future.

To gather additional data, epidemiologists used case-control studies. In such a study, people having the disease ("cases") are compared with people from a population whose members are not ill ("controls"). One of the first case-control studies was performed in 1981. This study led scientists to believe that among homosexual men, the number and frequency of a person's sexual contacts were factors affecting the incidence of AIDS. Results of another study conducted in 1982 indicated that the sexual partners of homosexual and bisexual men were at risk and that more than 20 percent of all known cases were occurring in men who had had a sexual relationship with an infected person. It was becoming clear that a transmissible agent was involved.

By 1983, epidemiologists had accumulated enough data to develop a case definition for AIDS (Chapter 4). Then they developed a set of recommendations for avoiding the disease (even though they did not know what was causing it). As physicians continued to report cases, the data made it apparent that blood and semen were the two principal sources of the disease agent. Hemophiliacs were contracting the disease from blood products; transfusion recipients were being infected by contaminated blood, the number of cases was rising among sexually active homosexual men; and heterosexuals were contracting the disease.

The identification of the human immunodeficiency virus (HIV) in the spring of 1984 and the development of the AIDS antibody test in 1985 gave public health officials the ability to track the epidemic with more confidence. It was assumed that if a person's blood had HIV antibodies, exposure to HIV had taken place (Chapter 7). Now epidemiologists could confirm a diagnosis, measure the extent of the epidemic, and screen the blood supply. They could also make more specific recommendations on halting the spread of AIDS. They targeted certain groups for prevention and control campaigns, and devised a more complete case definition (Chapter 4). Some of the major goals of epidemiology were thereby fulfilled.

The Spreading Epidemic

In the early 1980s, public health officials hoped that the number of AIDS cases would be small and that researchers would quickly develop an effective drug or vaccine. Their hopes, unfortunately, would not be fulfilled. As of December 2000, almost 775,000 Americans had been diagnosed with AIDS, most from metropolitan areas (Table 5.1), and over 448,000 had died. The good news was

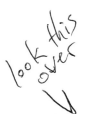

	Cumulative Totals		
	TABLE 5.1 AIDS Cases by Area of Residence and Age Group, through June 2001		

TABLE

5.1 AIDS Cases by Area of Residence and Age Group, through June 2001

Area of Residence	Adults/ Adolescents	Children <13 Years Old	Total
Metropolitan areas with 500,000 or more population	656,916	7,626	664,542
Central counties	*643,669*	*7,488*	*651,157*
Outlying counties	*13,247*	*138*	*13,385*
Metropolitan areas with 50,000 to 499,999 population	76,017	834	76,851
Central counties	*70,982*	*760*	*71,742*
Outlying counties	*5,035*	*74*	*5,109*
Nonmetropolitan areas	47,081	504	47,585
Total[1]	**784,032**	**8,994**	**793,026**

[1] Totals include 4,048 persons whose area of residence is unknown.

Source: Courtesy of CDC, HIV/AIDS Surveillance Report, 13(1), June, 2001.

that AIDS deaths began to decline in 1996 (primarily as a result of new anti-HIV therapies). Moreover, since the mid-1990s, the incidence of new AIDS cases has been declining. For example, between July 1996 and June 1997, 64,597 new AIDS cases were reported, but between 1997 and 1998 that number was down to 54,140 cases. Between 1998 and 1999, it was 47,083, and for 1999 to 2000, it was 42,156. Unfortunately, CDC officials estimate that up to 1 million Americans continue to live with HIV infection and that at least a third do not know that they are infected. Moreover, 4 to 5 million Americans continue to engage in behaviors putting them at high risk for contracting HIV infection (as we shall discuss presently). It is clear that AIDS will not fade from memory until well into the twenty-first century.

The CDC has also tracked the AIDS epidemic in various groups. Reports accumulated by the CDC since 1981 indicate that through June 2000, 47 percent of all reported cases of AIDS occurred in homosexual or bisexual men who had no history of injection drug abuse. Injection drug users accounted for 25 percent of cases. Another 6 percent of cases were homosexual or bisexual men who used injection drugs; 10 percent were individuals in a heterosexual relationship; 1 percent were individuals who received a blood transfusion, primarily before 1985, when blood screening was instituted; and about 1 percent were hemophiliacs. The final 9 percent of adults with AIDS fell into an undetermined category, where the source of infection may have included several risk factors (Figure 5.2). It is worth repeating that these figures represent all cases reported since 1981.

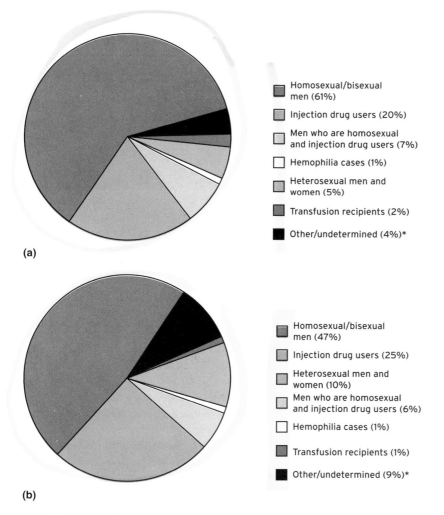

(a)

Homosexual/bisexual men (61%)

Injection drug users (20%)

Men who are homosexual and injection drug users (7%)

Hemophilia cases (1%)

Heterosexual men and women (5%)

Transfusion recipients (2%)

Other/undetermined (4%)*

(b)

Homosexual/bisexual men (47%)

Injection drug users (25%)

Heterosexual men and women (10%)

Men who are homosexual and injection drug users (6%)

Hemophilia cases (1%)

Transfusion recipients (1%)

Other/undetermined (9%)*

FIGURE 5.2

An analysis of cases of AIDS among different groups as reported to the CDC (a) through September 30, 1990 and (b) through June 30, 2001. The greatest percentage of cases has occurred among homosexual men, and the second greatest percentage among intravenous drug users. In recent years, the percentage among heterosexuals has been increasing, while the percentage among homosexual men has been decreasing. Percentages do not add to 100 percent because of rounding.

As Figure 5.2 shows, the percentages have changed over the years, reflecting the changing incidence of AIDS in various groups. For example, the percentage of cases involving homosexual men has declined since the 1990s, whereas the percentage in injection drug users has increased concurrently. The percentage in heterosexual men and women has also risen during this period.

Additional figures reported at the beginning of 2000 show the current distribution of the AIDS epidemic in various groups in the United States. According to the CDC, 82 percent of all cases through 2000 occurred in men, 18 percent in women, and 1 percent in children under age 13. Forty-three percent of cases occurred in whites, 37 percent in blacks, 18 percent in Hispanics, and less than one percent in Asians, Pacific Islanders, American Indians, and Alaskan Natives. The 1990s saw a gradual shift of the epidemic away from sexually active homosexual men and toward blacks, Hispanics, and women. Of note is the fact that the proportion of women among AIDS patients in the United States (annual statistics) has increased steadily each year since the beginning of the epidemic, reaching 30 percent in 2000. We shall explore the implications of this increase later in this chapter.

In the world, the statistics are somewhat different. As of 2002, AIDS was the leading global cause of death from an infectious disease and the fourth ranked cause of death overall. AIDS was outranked on the international list of killers only by ischemic heart disease, cerebrovascular disease, and lower respiratory diseases. As we shall see later in this chapter, AIDS is the number one killer in Africa (surpassing malaria), and the UNAIDS estimates that worldwide new infections are increasing by 6 million per year. Of particular concern is the growing epidemic in the countries of the former Soviet Union, where injection drug use is a prime mode of transmission. The epidemic is more recent but no less important in Asia because half the world's population resides on that continent.

The Fragility of HIV

AIDS is a bloodborne disease caused by a fragile virus (Figure 5.3). Outside the body, HIV quickly disintegrates because its molecular structure cannot resist environmental pressures such as drying, heat, and various chemical substances. In a loose sense, the virus "dies." Certain other viruses, by contrast, are more resistant to environmental agents. The virus of hepatitis A, for example, can remain active ("alive") outside the body and, therefore, can be transmitted by contaminated food such as raw shellfish or by water contaminated with intestinal matter.

Because of its fragile nature, HIV must pass directly from person to person in such fluids as blood and semen. In addition, a large number of the viral particles must be passed during transmission, because many of them will be unable to survive the transfer to the recipient host and remain active in the new environment. Although HIV has been found in saliva, tears, and sweat, the number of viral particles in these fluids is extraordinarily low, too low, public health officials maintain, to effect HIV transmission. Infected semen and blood remain the major transferring substances, and for this reason, individuals coming in contact with infected semen and/or blood are at risk. A 2000 report from the CDC indicates that 4 to 5 million Americans (about 4 percent of the population) engage in behaviors putting them in danger of contacting these fluids.

Other factors that contribute to risk of infection are the volume of fluid introduced into the recipient (higher volume, higher risk), the general state of health of the recipient (better health, lower risk), and the inoculation site of the fluid (blood or semen must enter the recipient's blood system). As we shall see presently, maternal-fetal transfer is also possible because the virus can cross the placenta. Still other factors shall become apparent as we proceed.

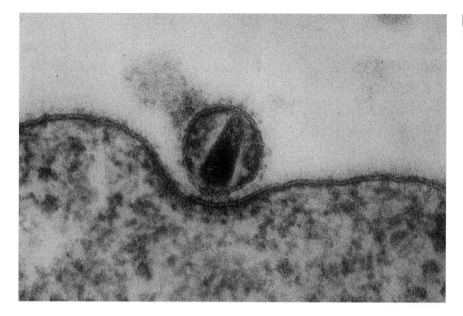

FIGURE 5.3
Electron micrograph of HIV.

AIDS in Homosexual Men

When the AIDS epidemic was revealed in 1981, the first cases were reported among sexually active men living a homosexual lifestyle (Healthline 5.1). Epidemiologists were uncertain whether the frequent use of certain drugs was to blame or whether a series of sexually transmitted diseases might be depressing the immune system's function in these individuals. When it became apparent that a transmissible agent was involved, epidemiologists focused on the type and frequency of sexual activities among homosexual men. Those men having few sex partners were less likely to have AIDS; men having unusually high rates of sexual activity had a correspondingly high chance of acquiring AIDS.

For homosexual men, the primary mechanism of HIV transfer is anal intercourse. In this practice, the penis of one male (the insertive partner) is placed into the rectum of the second male (the receptive partner) and semen is ejaculated. During the process, the delicate lining of the rectum may tear and bleed, because the rectal tissue is composed of columnar epithelial cells, which are easily damaged. Also, the rectum is highly susceptible to abrasions and bleeding because, like the rest of the digestive tract, it is rich in blood capillaries for absorbing nutrients. Thus, if the insertive partner is infected with HIV and if the virus is present in the semen, the viruses can easily penetrate the rectal lining and enter the blood of the receptive partner. T-lymphocytes

Healthline 5.1

1 **Q** Why are sexually active homosexual men at risk for AIDS?

A Cases of AIDS among homosexual men are associated with the practice of anal intercourse. When the penis enters the rectum, the surface tissue often tears and bleeds, thereby allowing HIV-infected semen to enter the blood of the sexual partner.

2 **Q** Can infected heterosexuals spread AIDS if they practice anal intercourse?

A Yes. If the man's penis causes abrasions or bleeding in the lining of the woman's rectum, then semen-to-blood contact can take place. Should the semen contain free HIV or HIV-infected T-lymphocytes, the possibility of viral transmission is substantial.

3 **Q** Can lesbians (female homosexuals) spread AIDS from one to another?

A A lesbian relationship does not involve anal intercourse or blood-to-blood contact. Because these behaviors are excluded, transmission of HIV is not likely.

infected with HIV may also be present in the semen and may carry HIV in its provirus form into the receptive partner.

Anal intercourse also poses a risk for the insertive partner. It has been found, for example, that HIV-infected T-lymphocytes accumulate within the rectum (T-lymphocytes are normally found in this organ). It is possible that during anal intercourse, infected T-lymphocytes from the receptive partner can enter the urethra (the tube within the penis) of the insertive partner. If the cells make their way through an eroded urethral lining into the circulation, the insertive partner is infected. Moreover, the insertive partner may have external lesions of the penis due to such diseases as syphilis and genital herpes. When the penis enters the rectum, free viruses or infected T-lymphocytes can pass from the rectal fluid through the open lesion into the insertive partner's blood.

Public health epidemiologists point out that those who engage in anal intercourse are at extraordinarily high risk for AIDS. Practicing a homosexual lifestyle is immaterial, they note, but engaging in anal intercourse is of great consequence ("It's not who you are. It's what you do"). For that reason, this book specifies "sexually active" homosexual men (Figure 5.4). To minimize the risk of transfer via semen, epidemiologists recommend using condoms (Chapter 6). To further reduce the risk, they suggest reducing the number of sexual partners, thereby reducing the possibility of coming in contact with an HIV carrier.

As of 2000, over 50 percent of all reported cases of AIDS in the United States since the beginning of the epidemic occurred in sexually active homosexual men.

FIGURE 5.4

The greatest number of AIDS cases in the United States have occurred among homosexual men, but the homosexual lifestyle has little to do with the transmission of AIDS. Rather, engaging in anal intercourse is of great consequence, whether it is performed by homosexual men or by a heterosexual couple. AIDS education groups point out, "It's not who you are. It's what you do."

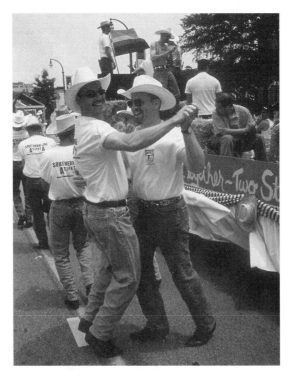

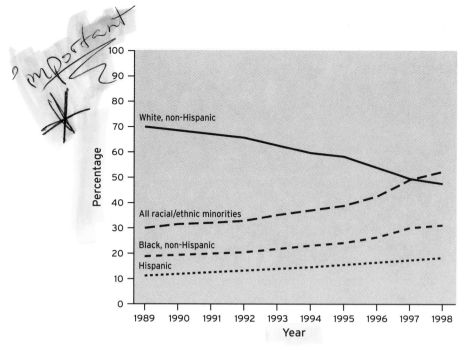

FIGURE 5.5

Percentage of AIDS cases among sexually active homosexual men by race/ethnicity and year of diagnosis. *Source: Centers for Disease Control and Prevention, MMWR, 49(1), January 14, 2000.*

Within this group, the percentages were changing. In 2000, the CDC reported that among sexually active homosexual men, racial/ethnic minority populations are accounting for an increasing proportion of AIDS cases. Epidemiologists at the CDC learned that in the period between 1989 and 1998, the proportion of AIDS cases declined significantly among white, non-Hispanic males, but increased among black, non-Hispanic males, while remaining constant among Hispanic males (Figure 5.5).

Although epidemiologists are not certain why these shifts have occurred, they point to studies indicating that black and Hispanic males are less likely than white males to identify themselves as homosexuals or to seek AIDS prevention and treatment services. Minority groups see AIDS as more of a stigma than white do, which may explain the reluctance to seek services. The report also found that 85 percent of the infected black and Hispanic homosexual males live in metropolitan areas with populations of 500,000 or more. Public health officials in New York City pointed out that 18 percent of the infected whites had spent at least one night in jail or prison, while the figure was 47 percent for blacks and 39 percent for Hispanics. The implication was that HIV was acquired while the men were incarcerated, a factor that should encourage prisons to give serious consideration to distributing condoms to inmates (a practice now banned in several states).

Another reporting category is sexually active homosexual males who are also injection drug users. These individuals pose unique challenges to the public health system because the men have multiple risks for acquiring HIV and transmitting it to heterosexual women, as well as other injection drug users and homosexual men. In a report filed in 2000, epidemiologists found that between 1990 and 1998,

FIGURE 5.6

Estimated incidence of AIDS among a cross-section of selected homosexual men who also inject drugs. *Source: Centers for Disease Control and Prevention, MMWR, 49(21), June 2, 2000.*

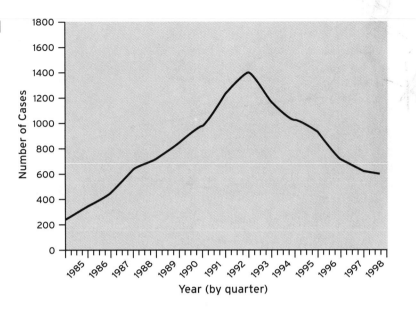

the proportion of all AIDS cases dropped from 8 percent to 5 percent among these men (after increasing in the previous period studied). Figure 5.6 shows the numbers reported. Possible reasons for the decline include increased use of antiretroviral drug therapies as well as vigorous testing and counseling programs. The decline was viewed as encouraging because it could result in interruption of HIV spread to several groups, including injections drug users, as we discuss next.

AIDS in Injection Drug Users

HIV is more prevalent among injection drug users because these individuals often share contaminated syringes and needles (Healthline 5.2). Sharing one's "works" is a common practice among groups of heroin addicts and other drug users. A syringe and needle become bloodstained when they are used to inject the drug into the veins (i.e., intravenously). Then the syringe and needle are passed to the next person, who uses them without the benefit of disinfection and is exposed to the first person's blood. Thus, the virus passes easily between the two individuals. Rinsing the syringe and needle in a bleach solution can eliminate the virus and interrupt transmission (Chapter 6).

Another practice often followed by injection drug users in a group is basically the same as a blood transfusion: One addict fills the syringe with the drug, inserts the needle, pulls back on the plunger, and draws blood into the syringe. Then he or she pushes some but not all of the drug-blood mixture back into the vein. The needle is then passed to the second individual who also draws blood back into the syringe to mix with the first person's blood. Now some of the drug-blood mixture is injected into the vein, and the syringe is passed to the third individual, who continues the pattern. The possibilities for HIV transmission during this practice are multifold.

For many years, the overall percentage of AIDS cases represented by injection drug users hovered in the range of 16 to 17 percent. As of 2000, however, it had risen to 25 percent overall, with 41 percent of that total being women, as Table 5.2 indicates, and public health officials were predicting that the percentage would rise higher.

Since injection drug users and their sex partners are concentrated in the nation's inner cities, the problems created by the AIDS epidemic have been linked directly to problems of urban decay, drug traffic, and homelessness (Figure 5.7). Thus, the AIDS epidemic is gradually undergoing a face change and is taking on sociological, political, and economic overtones that differ from those of the past (Chapter 10). In past years, for example, homosexual men were able to exert political pressure to have funds appropriated for AIDS research; no such political pressure can be expected from injection drug users.

AIDS in Heterosexuals

For individuals in a heterosexual relationship, the risk of contracting AIDS can be substantial, depending on circumstances. Heterosexuals generally practice vaginal intercourse. Normally, the lining of the vaginal tract will not erode or tear during intercourse. If, however, there are wounds, lesions, or abrasions along the lining, then viruses can enter a woman's bloodstream through the opening (Healthline 5.3). An infection such as gonorrhea, syphilis, or genital herpes can be the source of such lesions or abrasions. Moreover, should vaginal intercourse take place at the beginning of or during a woman's menstrual period, the viruses could pass through the lining of the uterus, which is then more fragile because the blood vessels are breaking down and rebuilding at this time. Researchers have also suggested that macrophages infected with HIV can pass through the tissue of the cervix at the opening to the uterus. Additional information on AIDS in women is presented in the next section.

In a heterosexual relationship, the male may also be at risk. It may happen, for instance, that the male has lesions on the outside surface of the penis, perhaps due to a herpes simplex infection. If the female is infected, her vaginal fluid may contain free viruses and/or HIV-infected T-lymphocytes, and these could pass through the lesions on the penis into the circulation. It is also possible that viruses or infected T-lymphocytes could enter the urethra of the penis at the conclusion of ejaculation and penetrate an internal lining eroded by a sexually transmitted disease such as gonorrhea.

From the foregoing, it follows that abstinence from sexual intercourse with individuals of unknown health status is the most sensible and efficient way of

Healthline 5.2

1 **Q** Why does injecting drugs put one at risk for AIDS?

A Injecting drugs does not in itself put one at risk for AIDS, but sharing blood-contaminated syringes and needles is very risky. If a person has AIDS, the virus is in the blood or in infected T-lymphocytes, and a blood-contaminated syringe may therefore carry the virus. If the syringe is shared, the next person's blood will come in contact with the infected blood, and the virus will be transmitted.

2 **Q** Can anything be done to reduce the risk of HIV transmission among injection drug users?

A The most obvious way of reducing exposure to HIV is to avoid drugs that require injection. If this is not possible, then the risk of acquiring AIDS can be reduced by using clean needles or syringes. The risk can be reduced even further by rinsing the needle and syringe with a disinfectant, such as a solution of household bleach.

3 **Q** What is the connection between AIDS in newborns and injection drug users?

A To date, most cases of AIDS in newborns have been transferred by mothers who were injection drug users or who had sexual intercourse with injection drug users. After acquiring HIV in either of these ways, the mothers passed the virus to their offspring across the placenta during fetal development or shortly after birth, probably by breast-feeding.

TABLE

5.2 AIDS Cases in Adults By Exposure Category and Sex, through June 2001

Adult/Adolescent Exposure Category	Males		Females		Totals	
	Number	(Percentage)	Number	(Percentage)	Number	(Percentage)
Sexually active homosexual men	361,867	(56)	–	–	361,867	(46)
Injection drug use	142,888	(22)	54,203	(40)	197,091	(25)
Sexually active homosexual men who inject drugs	50,066	(8)	–	–	50,066	(6)
Hemophilia/coagulation disorder	4,949	(1)	285	(0)	5,234	(1)
Heterosexual contact:	30,956	(5)	54,782	(41)	85,738	(11)
Sex with injecting drug user	9,496		21,111		30,607	
Sex with bisexual male	–		3,672		3,672	
Sex with person with hemophilia	67		422		489	
Sex with transfusion recipient with HIV infection	436		614		1,050	
Sex with HIV-infected person, risk not specified	20,957		28,963		49,920	
Receipt of blood transfusion or blood components	5,031	(1)	3,863	(3)	8,894	(1)
Other/risk not reported or identified	53,429	(8)	21,712	(16)	75,142	(10)
Total	649,186	(100)	134,845	(100)	784,032	(100)

Source: Courtesy of CDC, HIV/AIDS Surveillance Report, 13(1), June, 2001

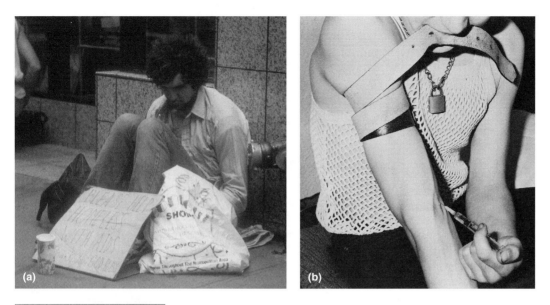

FIGURE 5.7

The percentage of total cases of AIDS reported since 1981 continues to rise among intravenous drug users and is expected to remain on that path well into the twenty-first century. (a) A homeless intravenous drug user. (b) Heroin addict shooting up.

minimizing the risk of transmitting AIDS. For those who are sexually active, public health officials advise using condoms to reduce the possible passage of semen and viruses (Chapter 6). They also recommend limiting the number of sexual partners. As we have noted, more than a million Americans may currently be carrying the virus. Having multiple sex partners dramatically increases the odds of coming in contact with HIV.

The truth of this last statement was demonstrated among young people living in a small town in rural Mississippi. During 2000, public health investigators studied a group of individuals who had shared sex partners and identified seven who had become HIV-infected. Forty-four other adolescents and young adults were pinpointed in the network, and their HIV status was either negative or unknown at the time of the study (Figure 5.8). Antiretroviral therapy was recommended for all those found to be infected. The study underscores the importance of HIV counseling and testing services in rural areas.

In 1999, the CDC reported that 15 percent of all cases reported that year could be traced to vaginal intercourse among heterosexuals who had no other risk factors (such as injection drug use). Two years previously, the percentage was 14 percent. This figure has changed appreciably since the 1980s, when the percentage was closer to 5 percent. Indeed, of the 793,026 AIDS cases reported to the CDC from the epidemic's beginning up to June 2001 almost 11 percent (85,738 cases) were transmitted by heterosexual contact, with no other risk factor involved. Moreover, some cases related to injection drug use may, in fact,

1 **Q** Why is AIDS more likely to be transmitted from men to women than from women to men during vaginal intercourse?

A Most studies indicate that a woman is more likely to contract AIDS from a male than the reverse. The reason is probably linked to the fact that the concentration of HIV is higher in the semen than in the vaginal secretions. Thus, an uninfected woman is exposed to more viruses than an uninfected man. In addition, the semen can remain for a long time in the vagina, thereby increasing the length of exposure to HIV.

2 **Q** Can you get AIDS by kissing?

A Social kissing is not considered a risky behavior, but deep, or "French," kissing can present a slight risk. In some cases, small amounts of HIV have been found in the saliva of infected individuals, and a substantial transfer of saliva coupled with lesions in the mouth of the recipient could permit viral transmission.

3 **Q** Is it possible to acquire HIV by oral sex?

A Acquiring HIV may be possible by engaging in oral sex. Although public health officials cannot be certain of the degree of risk because few couples engage in this sexual practice exclusively, it seems reasonable to assume that an exposure to infected semen can put one at risk for AIDS. The risk is increased if lesions exist in the mouth or if microscopic tears or abrasions are present in the tissues lining the mouth.

have occurred by heterosexual transmission, and some of the apparently homosexual men may have been bisexual and may have acquired HIV during vaginal intercourse with women.

Epidemiologists also point out that the characteristics of the heterosexual transmission group are changing. Before 1985, most cases linked to heterosexual contact occurred in people born in other countries (hence, HIV was "imported"). Since 1985, most such cases have occurred in persons in a sexual relationship with an infected person or with a person at high risk for AIDS (for example, an injection drug user). The HIV was, therefore, "domestic."

Elderly individuals (55 and older) represent a special subgroup among the heterosexual population. Researchers point out that the elderly are far less likely to practice "safer sex" methods (such as using condoms); moreover, they have weaker immune systems with which to battle HIV than younger people do; and their HIV infection is less likely to be diagnosed by doctors, especially since fatigue, pneumonia, dementia, weight loss, and other AIDS symptoms are often related to advanced age or illnesses associated with aging. Nevertheless, elderly Americans, especially males, represent a significant number of the total AIDS cases in the United States.

During the 1980s, most older Americans with AIDS contracted HIV as a result of receiving a transfusion of contaminated blood, but currently, the vast majority have become infected as a result of heterosexual contact. Public health epidemiologists point out that the number of cases and deaths in this group is expected to increase further because of the new treatments that prolong life. Good nutrition, exercise, and an upbeat attitude also contribute to extending one's life. For many elderly patients, overcoming the denial that AIDS can strike them is a major obstacle in treatment.

AIDS in Women

AIDS transmitted by heterosexual contact has raised special concerns among women. In 1994, for example, 18 percent of all U.S. cases of AIDS since the epidemic's beginning were reported in women, but by June 2001 the number was 17 percent. (These figures stand in stark contrast to 1985 statistics; only 7 percent of all AIDS cases to that time had occurred in women.) Two modes of transmission are primarily associated with HIV infection in women: use of injection drugs and heterosexual contact with a partner at risk.

To deal with their special needs, women's groups have started preventive counseling programs and care centers for the children of infected women to supplement publicly sponsored programs. Educational campaigns have also been directed at women, including

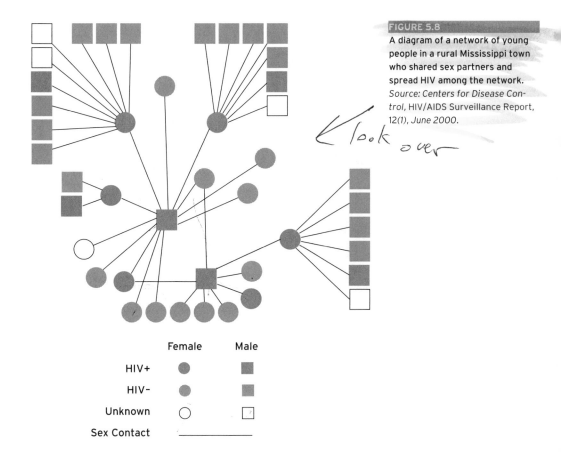

FIGURE 5.8
A diagram of a network of young
people in a rural Mississippi town
who shared sex partners and
spread HIV among the network.
*Source: Centers for Disease Con-
trol,* HIV/AIDS Surveillance Report,
12(1), June 2000.

	Female	Male
HIV+	●	■
HIV–	●	■
Unknown	○	□
Sex Contact	————	

suggestions that women carry condoms (Figure 5.9), and researchers have developed vaginal condoms. The basic theme of these campaigns is that AIDS is not solely a disease of homosexual men. Among women, the fear of HIV transmission has added to the trauma of rape and has exacerbated the torture of its aftermath.

In women, vaginal infections represent a unique problem that contributes to the risk of acquiring HIV infection. In addition to the well-known sexually transmitted diseases (STDs), a microbial infection called bacterial vaginosis increases a woman's susceptibility to HIV infection because the disease interferes with the normal metabolism of cells lining the vaginal cavity. The bacteria produce offensive odors and cause internal pruritis (itching) and excessive vaginal discharge. Although there is little of the ulceration and inflammation associated with STDs such as gonorrhea or syphilis, bacterial vaginosis has a higher incidence rate and thus may be equally important to the spread of HIV. For example, researchers studied 1196 pregnant women in Malawi and found that those with bacterial vaginosis were 3.7 times more likely to acquire HIV than those without vaginosis. Furthermore, the study showed that a man's risk of acquiring HIV rises when he has intercourse with an HIV-infected woman who has vaginosis. In the United States, vaginosis is more common among African-American and Hispanic American women.

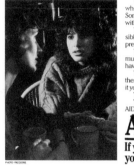

Talk about AIDS before it hits home.

"I really don't have to tell Linda about AIDS. They're teaching about it in school."
"Why discuss AIDS with my Johnny? He isn't gay."
"If I talk to them about AIDS, they'll think it's okay to have sex."

If you're thinking any of these thoughts, you're not doing all you should to protect your teenager from AIDS.

So put your embarrassment and your fear of encouraging sex aside.

Just sit down and tell them the facts.

Tell them that you just can't be sure who's infected with the AIDS virus. Sometimes it can be carried for years without any symptoms.

Tell them that since they can't possibly know who's infected they must use precautions to protect themselves.

Tell them if they're having sex, they must always use a condom. And not having sex is still the best protection.

Tell them that AIDS is incurable, there's no vaccine, and once you get it you'll likely die.

Then tell them it's preventable.

Tell them everything you can about AIDS. But make sure you tell them now.

AIDS Because by the time you think they're old enough to know, it might be too late.

If you think you can't get it, you're dead wrong.

NEW YORK CITY DEPARTMENT OF HEALTH. FOR MORE INFORMATION CALL: 1 (718) 485-8111

Researchers have also found that opportunistic diseases are equally prevalent in HIV-infected women and men, with the exception of cervical cancer and Kaposi's sarcoma. Erosion of the esophagus with *Candida albicans* and infections due to herpes simplex virus and cytomegalovirus appear to occur in higher incidence in HIV-positive women who inject drugs (although the reason is not clear). Gynecological complications associated with STDs, including abscesses of the ovaries and oviducts, also require special attention. Abnormalities of cells of the cervix can occur at any stage of HIV infection, but it is more frequent as the number of T-lymphocytes declines. Human papilloma viruses may cause the abnormalities and induce a progression to cervical cancer, but Pap smears detect early signs of infection, and antiviral therapy for papilloma viruses is helpful. Antiretroviral therapy against HIV has also been shown effective for reducing papilloma infection.

In women who are pregnant, determining HIV status (Box 5.1) is particularly important because intervention with AZT can interrupt viral passage to the fetus (as we discuss in the next section). Moreover, during delivery, an obstetrician will postpone rupture of the amnionic membranes or other potentially invasive procedures that might encourage HIV transmission.

AIDS in Newborns

Among the more tragic cases of AIDS are those in infants born to women infected with HIV. As Table 5.3 indicates, up through June 2001, the CDC had reports of

BOX
5.1

Head, Tails, and the Truth

Studies linking disease to sexual behavior are difficult to perform because people are reluctant to reveal details of their private lives. For example, asking a man whether he has had a sexual encounter with anyone other than his wife often elicits a look of skepticism and an unreliable answer. Try as they might, researchers can rarely be certain they are getting the truth when they ask such questions.

In 1987, Joel E. Cohen, a mathematical biologist from Rockefeller University, suggested a statistical tool that could add reliability to the answer. The technique was invented in 1965 by Stanley Warner of Ontario's York University. It has been used periodically since then. Its basic premise is that people will reveal the truth if they believe their answers are secret.

The method involves a question and a coin flip. For example, a questioner asks a man, "Have you ever had a sexual encounter with anyone other than your wife?" The man then flips the coin in privacy. He answers no if he has not had an encounter *and* if the coin comes up tails. Otherwise, he must answer yes.

Using this method, a man can answer no because the flip resulted in tails, and he can answer yes, also because of the coin. A yes does not necessarily incriminate him; a no does not necessarily mean he is lying.

Totaling the results, the researcher simply doubles the number of no answers to get an almost correct number of nos. The theory is simple: Given enough flips, the coin should come up tails half the time; this means that only half of the total number of men who actually had encounters said no. Therefore, doubling the number of nos gives a fairly accurate picture of the true number of nos. Subtracting the number of nos from the total number of men questioned reveals the number of yes answers.

more than 8994 confirmed cases of so-called pediatric AIDS in the United States and over 5000 deaths (worldwide cases in children numbered over a million). The tragedy is compounded by the fact that thousands of other babies have probably been born infected but do not yet have symptoms. In the great majority of cases, the mother had AIDS or was at risk for AIDS, meaning that she was an injection drug user, the sexual partner of an injection drug user, or engaged in prostitution and thus had sexual relations with multiple partners. Table 5.4 shows the breakdown of exposure routes by which newborns acquired HIV. Note that 91 percent were born to mothers at risk for HIV infection and that more than a third of the mothers were injection drug users.

Research studies indicate that HIV is able to pass the placental barrier and infect the fetus while it is still developing in the uterus. (A 1999 study concluded that the amount of HIV in a woman's bloodstream is a critical factor in whether transmission can occur.) Infection can therefore take place within the woman's body. In addition, public health officials have received reports of women who contracted HIV infection after giving birth, then infected their infants. Because

TABLE		
5.3 AIDS Cases By Sex and Age At Diagnosis, through June 2001		

Male Age at diagnosis (years)	Total	
	Number	**(Percentage)**
Under 5	3,492	(1)
5–12	1,130	(0)
13–19	2,450	(0)
20–24	19,886	(3)
25–29	82,465	(13)
30–34	144,890	(22)
35–39	148,315	(23)
40–44	111,260	(17)
45–49	66,296	(10)
50–54	35,312	(5)
55–59	19,122	(3)
60–64	10,483	(2)
65 or older	8,707	(1)
Male subtotal	653,808	(100)

Female Age at diagnosis (years)		
Under 5	3,436	(2)
5–12	936	(1)
13–19	1,769	(1)
20–24	7,994	(6)
25–29	20,620	(15)
30–34	30,453	(22)
35–39	29,444	(21)
40–44	20,458	(15)
45–49	10,856	(8)
50–54	5,660	(4)
55–59	3,301	(2)
60–64	1,932	(1)
65 or older	2,358	(2)
Female subtotal	139,217	(100)
Total	793,026	

Source: Courtesy of CDC, HIV/AIDS Surveillance Report, 13(1), June 2001.

5.4 Pediatric AIDS Cases By Exposure Category and Sex, through June 2001

Pediatric (<13 Years Old) Exposure Category	Males		Females		Totals	
	Number	(Percentage)	Number	(Percentage)	Number	(Percentage)
Hemophilia/coagulation disorder	230	(5)	7	(0)	237	(3)
Mother with/at risk for HIV infection:	4,075	(88)	4,132	(95)	8,207	(91)
Injection drug use	1,614		1,602		3,216	
Sex with an injection drug user	758		721		1,479	
Sex with a bisexual male	88		93		181	
Sex with person with hemophilia	17		15		32	
Sex with transfusion recipient with HIV infection	11		14		25	
Sex with HIV-infected person, risk not specified	641		670		1,311	
Receipt of blood transfusion, blood components, or tissue	74		80		154	
Has HIV infection, risk not specified	872		937		1,809	
Receipt of blood transfusion, blood components, or tissue	242	(5)	140	(3)	382	(4)
Risk not reported or identified	75	(2)	93	(2)	168	(2)
Pediatric subtotal	4,622	(100)	4,372	(100)	8,994	(100)

Source: Courtesy of CDC, HIV/AIDS Surveillance Report, 13(1), June 2001.

virtually all such infected infants were breast-fed, the findings suggest the passage of HIV in mother's milk.

Indeed, in 1999, researchers confirmed HIV infection via the breast milk. They studied 672 infants born without HIV infection to women in the developing African nation of Malawi. Forty-seven cases of HIV infection were apparently due to breast milk, nearly half occurring within the first five months after birth. Where inflammation of the mammary tissues occurred, the passage of HIV particles was higher. Researchers noted that discontinuing breast-feeding would lessen the possibility of HIV passage, but it would also reduce the ability of mothers to pass helpful antibodies and nutrients to their offspring.

For many years, the study of pediatric AIDS was hampered by the lack of a diagnostic test to detect HIV in the newborn's tissues. Antibody tests were the staple means of diagnosis, but positive antibody tests could have reflected either the newborn's antibodies or those passing across the placenta from the mother. Then, during the mid-1990s, the viral load test was introduced (Chapter 7), and physicians could detect the RNA or DNA associated with HIV. Availability of this test encouraged studies to determine whether AZT or other anti-AIDS drugs could be given to the mother to prevent prenatal transmission of HIV. The studies indicated that rapid implementation of AZT treatment can effectively block HIV's transmission to the fetus, and a steep decline of prenatally acquired AIDS occurred during the last half of the 1990s, as Figure 5.10 illustrates. The decline was further encouraged by improved treatments for HIV-infected newborns, treatments that delay the onset of AIDS.

Cases of pediatric AIDS in the United States are concentrated in the New York City area, probably because of the high number of female residents who are injection drug users or sex partners of injection drug users. No other state reported a number close to New York's. Through June 2000, for example, 1997 cases of pediatric AIDS were reported in the New York area since the beginning of the epidemic. The next closest metropolitan area was Miami, Florida (473 cases), then Newark, New Jersey (320 cases). Epidemiologists are quick to point out that the cases noted are only those that fit the definition for AIDS. Thousands of other babies have probably been born infected with HIV, but they show no symptoms yet.

An interesting aspect of AIDS in newborns emerged in 1996 when the highly respected journal *Science* discussed interesting new data under the provocative headline "Can Some Infants Beat HIV?" The thrust of the article was that a collaborative study in Europe indicated that some HIV-infected newborns apparently cleared the HIV from their tissues. Investigators studied 2319 children who had HIV antibodies at birth, but subsequently tested negative. Tests performed for the presence of the virus (Chapter 7) showed that nine of the children cleared the viruses as well as the antibodies from their bloodstreams. The results confirmed an earlier French study in which 12 of 188 children cleared HIV from their bodies. These studies strengthened the possibility that in some newborns, antibodies might be able to neutralize HIV before it becomes entrenched in the tissues. Another view is that HIV was "weaker" in the blood from which it was cleared. Still another possibility is that HIV remains in the infants' tissues, even though it is gone from the blood. Studies are continuing in hopes of learning more about this phenomenon.

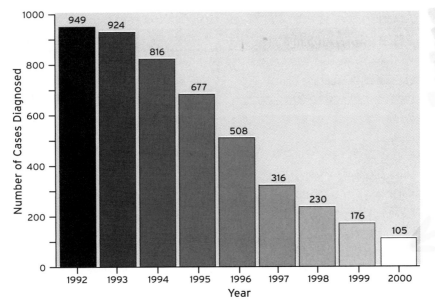

FIGURE 5.10

A histogram showing the estimated number of cases of pediatric AIDS between 1992 and 2000. The decline is partly due to the <u>treatment</u> of infected pregnant women with anti-HIV medications. *Source: Courtesy of CDC, HIV/AIDS Surveillance Report, 12(1), June 2000.*

AIDS in Africa

Africa appears to be one of the hardest-hit continents of the world. In 2001, for instance, an estimated 70 percent of the more than 35 million people with HIV infection or AIDS were living in sub-Saharan Africa. And close to 4 million Africans were infected in a single year, 2000 (compared to 44,000 in North America that same year). An estimated 17 million Africans have died since the AIDS epidemic began in the late 1970s, close to 4 million of them children. Epidemiologists estimate that 9.0 percent of all adults in Africa are infected with HIV, and in countries such as Zimbabwe and South Africa, one out of five adults (20 percent of the adult population) carries HIV. The grim statistics portend a harsh future of escalating disease in which 25 million more Africans will die of AIDS. Indeed, the UNAIDS has made estimates of life expectancy in nine sub-Saharan countries with and without AIDS. These statistics, presented in Table 5.5, show the appalling effects of the AIDS epidemic, which to many is so terrible that it eclipses the oft-used word "crisis."

Since the first reports of AIDS in Africa were published in 1983, it has become apparent that the disease exhibits a different pattern of spread than that seen in Western Europe and the United States. In Africa, most transmissions of HIV take place during heterosexual vaginal intercourse, and currently, the number of infected women there is higher than the number of infected men (Figure 5.11). By contrast, there is a four-to-one ratio of infected men to infected women in North America.

Epidemiologists cannot fully account for the majority of transmissions by heterosexual intercourse, but they believe that lesions and sores from STDs provide a gateway to the bloodstream. African men and women suffer from a high

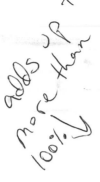
adds up to more than 100%.

TABLE 5.5 HIV/AIDS in Africa			
Estimated Percentage of Infected Adults (15-49)		**Estimated Life Expectancy with/without AIDS, 2000-2005**	
Botswana	25%	Botswana	41/70 yrs.
Kenya	12	Kenya	48/66
Malawi	15	Malawi	40/53
Mozambique	14	Mozambique	38/53
Namibia	20	Namibia	41/64
Rwanda	13	Rwanda	41/51
South Africa	13	South Africa	47/64
Zambia	19	Zambia	42/60
Zimbabwe	26	Zimbabwe	41/66
(United States	0.18)		

w/ w/out

Source: Courtesy of UNAIDS.

number of STDs, including syphilis, chancroid, gonorrhea, and genital herpes. Each of these diseases is accompanied by lesions of the genital organs, and contact with these lesions and sores may permit viral transmission by infected persons to sex partners. In one study, 54 percent of African sex workers (prostitutes) with genital lesions also were infected with HIV, whereas only 17 percent of sex workers without an apparent STD were HIV-positive.

Another possible avenue for heterosexual transmission in Africa may arise from the refusal to circumcise males. It has been suggested that leaving the penile foreskin in place encourages inflammation and formation of sores under the foreskin, thereby providing a passageway for HIV to enter or leave the body. There is also the cultural practice of "dry sex" performed in certain African communities. In this process, a woman dries her vagina with powders or cloths previous to having sex, a practice that can increase friction during intercourse and heightens sexual pleasure but also leads to abrasion of the vaginal wall and entry of free HIV and HIV-infected T-lymphocytes. The practice of dry sex probably also destroys many of the helpful bacteria in the vaginal tract and increases the likelihood that a condom will tear.

Although it is clear that condom use can interrupt the spread of HIV, traditional attitudes often mitigate against their use. For example, if a woman insists that a man wear a condom, she may imply that she is a sex worker; thus, she will press a man to have sex without using a condom as proof of her virtue. And yet in some communities, if she becomes infected with HIV, a woman will be divorced by her husband and ostracized from the community. Alternatively, if a woman suggests condom use, her husband may become angry because she is suggesting

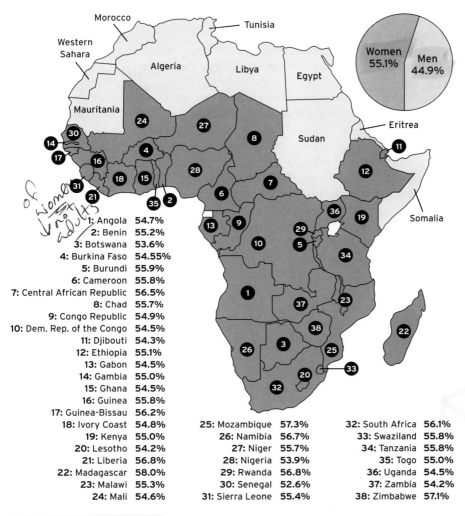

FIGURE 5.11

Percentage of adults aged 15 to 19 with HIV infection or AIDS who are women and who live in sub-Saharan countries, 1999. *Source: Adapted from UNAIDS.*

Pie chart: Women 55.1%, Men 44.9%

of women not adults (handwritten annotation)

scary (handwritten annotation)

1: Angola 54.7%
2: Benin 55.2%
3: Botswana 53.6%
4: Burkina Faso 54.55%
5: Burundi 55.9%
6: Cameroon 55.8%
7: Central African Republic 56.5%
8: Chad 55.7%
9: Congo Republic 54.9%
10: Dem. Rep. of the Congo 54.5%
11: Djibouti 54.3%
12: Ethiopia 55.1%
13: Gabon 54.5%
14: Gambia 55.0%
15: Ghana 54.5%
16: Guinea 55.8%
17: Guinea-Bissau 56.2%
18: Ivory Coast 54.8%
19: Kenya 55.0%
20: Lesotho 54.2%
21: Liberia 56.8%
22: Madagascar 58.0%
23: Malawi 55.3%
24: Mali 54.6%

25: Mozambique 57.3%
26: Namibia 56.7%
27: Niger 55.7%
28: Nigeria 53.9%
29: Rwanda 56.8%
30: Senegal 52.6%
31: Sierra Leone 55.4%

32: South Africa 56.1%
33: Swaziland 55.8%
34: Tanzania 55.8%
35: Togo 55.0%
36: Uganda 54.5%
37: Zambia 54.2%
38: Zimbabwe 57.1%

something he should have thought of first. For such instances, counselors have devised scripts that women can follow to allow their partners to save face. Using microbicides (Chapter 6), may be a useful alternative.

In addition, AIDS also can be related to practices such as ritual scarring with contaminated needles, transfusions of contaminated blood to treat diseases such as malaria, reuse of contaminated needles during immunization programs, and ritual removal of the clitoris from women. Anal intercourse among homosexual men probably accounts for some cases of AIDS, but admitting to this practice often incurs social disgrace in Africa, and homosexual men are reluctant to reveal their lifestyle.

The typical African patient with AIDS exhibits a wasting syndrome known as "slim disease." Its symptoms are similar to those seen in the United States and other parts of the world: Weight is lost rapidly, intractable diarrhea develops, fever runs high, and the patient abandons interest in eating. Within a period of two months, 30 percent of the body weight may be lost (Figure 5.12). Many patients have infection with the protozoal parasites *Cryptosporidium* and *Isospora* (Chapter 4). These parasites attack the intestinal cells and encourage the body to pour out huge volumes of fluid. Researchers have also located HIV in intestinal macrophages and have suggested that viral infection of these macrophages may reduce the defense normally available to the body and exacerbate the vigorous parasitic infection.

Among the opportunistic diseases, tuberculosis is the most prevalent in Africa (most AIDS wards in African hospitals are tuberculosis sanitaria). Kaposi's sarcoma is found in both HIV-infected and noninfected individuals. *Pneumocystis carinii* pneumonia is relatively rare in Africa. Subtype C of HIV accounts for most infections in South Africa.

The AIDS epidemic in Africa is largely confined to urban centers, where infectious disease is common. Malaria is widespread in the cities, and few Africans reach the age of 30 without suffering an attack of malaria or some other disease. Constant barrages of these diseases place the immune system under stress, a factor that may reduce its ability to resist HIV. This phenomenon, in which two diseases affect the body simultaneously, is called co-infection. The co-infection theory has gathered support in recent years and is offered as still another explanation for the pattern of distribution displayed by AIDS in Africa.

AIDS in the World

To international epidemiologists, the World Health Organization (WHO) and the United Nations Programme on AIDS (UNAIDS) are preeminent. These specialized agencies of the United Nations work to promote physical, mental, and social health in peoples of the world. Among their duties are collecting and distributing data on epidemics and establishing international programs for dealing with epidemics.

Through the end of 2000, the UNAIDS reported these staggering statistics: worldwide, over 40 million adults are living with AIDS; of these, 5.6 million became infected in the year 2001; and of almost 25 million individuals who have died of AIDS, 3 million died in 2000. Moreover, 269 countries are now involved in the pandemic. Although the rate of new infections was waning in Europe and the United States (due largely to secure blood supplies and vigorous education campaigns), the pandemic was spreading, and sub-Saharan Africa, South and Southeast Asia, and Latin America were identified as the next epicenters for explosion. Indeed, 90 percent of all people living with HIV infection or AIDS inhabit these three regions of the world (Figure 5.13 shows the global statistics).

The transmission of HIV appears to fall into three major patterns, corresponding to three different portions of the world. In western Europe, the pattern

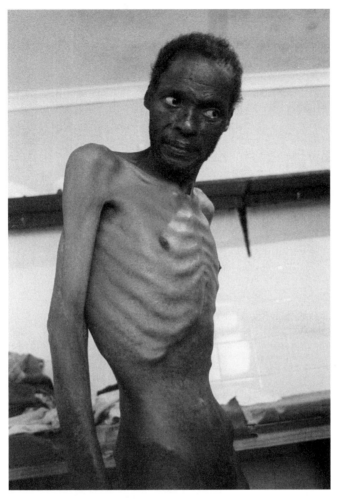

FIGURE 5.12
A patient with AIDS displaying the symptoms of "slim disease," the wasting phase of AIDS commonly observed in Africa. This photograph was taken at the Strand hospice near Cape Town, South Africa.

of transmission is similar to that in the United States, with the great majority of cases occurring in homosexual men and injection drug users. By contrast, in eastern Europe, the Middle East, North Africa, and Asia, the incidence of AIDS is relatively low. In these regions, cases are generally related to heterosexual contact with travelers who acquired HIV elsewhere, or they are associated with imported contaminated blood or implements. The third pattern of transmission is seen in Latin America and in areas of sub-Saharan Africa. HIV probably spread through these areas in the 1970s. (Blood stored in Zaire from 1959 has shown that the virus was present at that time.) Most transmission in these regions is by heterosexual contact, as we noted previously. AIDS has particular significance to the world's developing countries because persons with AIDS are often young and middle-aged business workers who represent the country's future. A substantial economic impact on certain countries is predicted for the years ahead (Chapter 10).

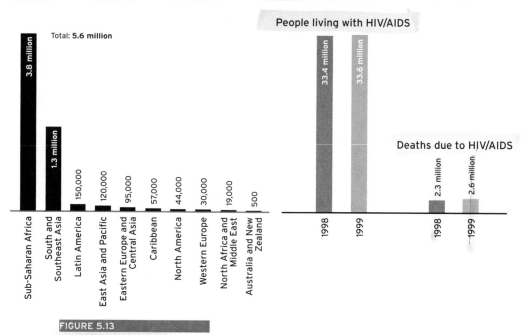

look over →

FIGURE 5.13

The global impact of AIDS shown in WHO estimates of the number of people newly infected with HIV in 1999. The inset on the right shows the one-year increase of the number of individuals living with HIV infection and AIDS and the number of deaths associated with AIDS. *Source: Adapted from World Health Organization.*

AIDS is particularly threatening to children of the world. During 1999, for instance, an estimated 570,000 children aged 14 years and younger became infected with HIV. More than 90 percent were infants borne to HIV-infected women. And of this number, nine out of ten lived in sub-Saharan Africa.

Public health officials note that during 1999, the steepest growth curve for HIV cases was recorded in states of the former Soviet Union. Since 1997 the total number of new cases has been doubling each year. Between 1997 and 1999, the proportion of people living with AIDS doubled in these countries. Most new infections were traced to infected needles used by injection drug users. Epidemiologists are concerned that the wave of illicit drug use may spread to the Middle East and with it, the AIDS epidemic (relatively few cases of AIDS are now in this area).

Across the continent of Asia, about 6.5 million people were living with HIV infection at the beginning of the new century. India and China are areas of acute concern because of their enormous populations. As of 2000, India was estimated to be second to South Africa in the total number of cases of HIV infection, and 75 percent of those cases were believed to be acquired by heterosexual contact. Unfortunately, the disease remains highly stigmatized in India, especially for women—even if monogamous women are infected by their husbands, they often bear the blame for their own illness.

The rate of HIV infection in China was low as the new century began, and most of the 18,000 total confirmed cases were related to injection drug use. Concern has been expressed for the growing sex industry in China, especially since condom use is unpopular. Infected blood is another possible mode of HIV transfer because before it was banned, selling one's blood at a commercial collection center was a common way of earning money. Researchers point out that China would be a good location for conducting vaccine trials because the country has large cohorts of uninfected people.

The worldwide problem of AIDS is compounded by underrecognition, underdiagnosis, and underreporting. Nevertheless, the WHO and UNAIDS are committed to preventing new HIV infections through education, blood screening, and treatment for injection drug users. They also seek to bring support and care to the afflicted, while linking together national and international efforts to break the chains of transmission. According to many public health epidemiologists, AIDS has no precedent in history. As long ago as 1988, Jonathan Mann, the former AIDS program director of the WHO, suggested that AIDS ". . . is changing the way the world thinks. It is becoming a key piece in the history of our time."

Other Transmission Methods

Because HIV is present in blood and semen and, in some cases, in very low levels in saliva or other body fluids, it is remotely possible that one could acquire HIV by methods other than anal or vaginal intercourse or sharing of contaminated needles. For example, any instrument coming in contact with blood or body fluid can be a potential source of HIV if very large numbers of viruses are present and if large amounts of fluid are transmitted, among other factors. Acupuncture needles are an example of such an instrument, as are tattoo needles, razors, and implements used to puncture the ears during ear piercing. It should be emphasized, however, that the risk of contracting HIV from these instruments is extraordinarily low because many concurrent factors, such as viral numbers, volume of fluid, health condition of the recipient, and inoculation site must be taken into consideration.

For HIV transmission, ordinary social kissing is not considered a high-risk behavior, but the risk increases with open-mouthed, or "French," kissing. This is because of the considerable amounts of saliva exchanged. The risk increases still further if the uninfected individual has lesions or sores of the mouth (canker sores, for example). It is well to note, however, that the fragility of the virus argues against transmission by deep kissing. (Laboratory experiments indicate that HIV survives very poorly in saliva.) In addition, the level of HIV in saliva is extremely low: In one research study, only 1 of 83 HIV-infected individuals had HIV in the saliva.

Oral-genital contact may be a risky practice, depending on the circumstances. If there are wounds, abrasions, or lesions of the mouth, for example, free viruses or HIV-infected T-lymphocytes from the semen may enter the circulatory system. Few researchers would argue that HIV cannot be spread through oral-genital contact, but the actual risk has not yet been defined. Part of the reason is that most studies contain too few patients to yield truly convincing data, and these studies were rarely designed to assess the actual time of HIV infection. There is also the daunting task of evaluating the risk of a single sexual act in the context of an individual's entire sex history.

Health care workers often come in contact with blood and may therefore be at risk for HIV infection. Emergency service personnel, physicians, morticians, dental hygienists, medical technologists, and nurses are examples of such workers. The common denominator for infection in all cases is that blood must enter the health worker's system. In addition, the amount of blood entering must be considerable. For instance, in one study of 85 health care workers who came in contact with the blood of an AIDS patient, none contracted AIDS. In a second study of 531 workers, only three developed antibodies to HIV, indicating exposure to the virus. Of the 531 exposed, 34 had sustained needlestick injuries and 12 had been exposed to splashes of blood. The three who did develop AIDS antibodies were either injection drug users or sexually active homosexuals, so they might have come in contact with the virus by other routes.

To assess the risk in health care settings and other situations, certain data must be available. For instance, the geographic location in which the incident took place should be known. (The chances of encountering contaminated blood are higher in urban San Francisco than in a rural Iowa community.) One should ask how exposure took place. (Airborne blood splashes are much less likely to transmit HIV than needlestick injuries.) What volume of blood was transmitted? (Was the skin scratched with blood present, or was there a deep penetration wound and a considerable amount of blood?) And how much virus did the blood contain? (Blood from a person with HIV infection probably contains less virus than blood from a person with AIDS.) Data such as these lend individuality to each case and help determine the likelihood that the worker has been infected.

How AIDS Is Not Transmitted

In science, it is commonly acknowledged that one should never say never. Therefore, it would be improper to suggest that AIDS absolutely cannot or never has been transmitted by any of the methods this section discusses. It is scientifically impossible to prove that something does not happen, and proving that certain methods do not allow HIV to move among individuals is no exception.

Improbable Transmissions

Epidemiologists have established that a multitude of common activities do not allow HIV to pass among individuals because such activities do not involve contact with blood or semen or involve maternal-fetal transfer (Figure 5.14). Most of these activities are listed under the broad category of casual contact. Social kissing is included here, as are shaking hands, hugging, and other forms of physical contact. HIV is not transmitted by contacting bodily secretions such as sweat, mucus (as in sneezing or coughing), or saliva (as in sharing eating utensils or a can of soda).

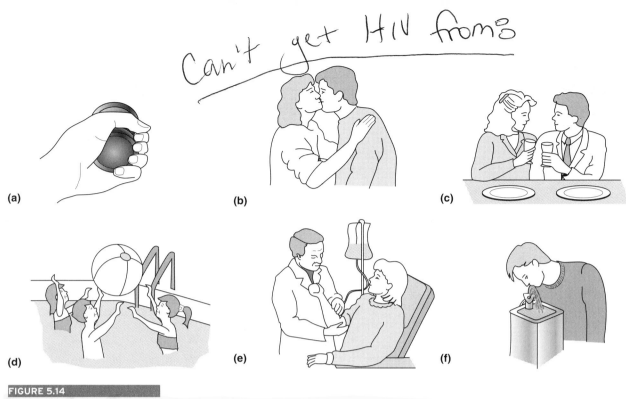

FIGURE 5.14

Methods that are not known to transmit human immunodeficiency virus. (a) Touching a doorknob; (b) a social kiss; (c) eating at a restaurant; (d) swimming at a pool; (e) donating blood; (f) drinking at a water fountain.

One does not acquire HIV by using a telephone or toilet seat or soap bar used by an AIDS patient. The virus, if once present, has probably disintegrated; even if it were still there, no opportunity exists for penetrating the recipient's bloodstream.

The list goes on. HIV is not contracted in restaurants or eating facilities or from an infected chef or waiter (unless, of course, one were to share contaminated needles or have sexual contact with that individual). HIV does not remain active in the water of a hot tub, on the surface of a deodorant stick, or on the metal of a doorknob. Swimming pools do not transmit AIDS, nor do laundry facilities, drinking fountains, or public restrooms. It is not likely that one could become infected by donating blood (Healthline 5.4), by caring for an AIDS patient, or by coming in contact with a child who has AIDS. Even people who touch the blood of an AIDS patient are at minimal risk. As one prominent researcher has suggested: "You need quite a slug of blood in your veins to become infected."

It should be understood that each case is unique, and that making blanket statements is not advised. Based on all the best evidence to date, however, there is nothing to indicate that HIV can be transmitted by any of the aforementioned ways.

1 **Q** Is it possible to contract AIDS by donating blood?

A It is virtually impossible to contract AIDS while donating blood. The needles and equipment used for blood donation are new and sterile. After one use, they are destroyed. Therefore, there is no way that a person can come in contact with HIV by donating blood.

2 **Q** Is it possible to contract AIDS by receiving a transfusion of blood?

A Since March 1985, the American Red Cross and other blood banks have routinely tested donated blood to see if it is contaminated with HIV. The test, while highly accurate, is not perfect. It detects the presence of antibodies to the virus to determine if the blood is infected. But it can take up to 12 weeks, and in rare cases longer, for those antibodies to appear. Therefore, it is possible that someone recently infected with AIDS could donate blood, and the presence of the AIDS antibodies would not be detected. A 1995 study published by the Food and Drug Administration (FDA) suggests that the chance of receiving a unit of contaminated blood is 1 in 225,000.

3 **Q** I received a blood transfusion in 1983. Could I have come in contact with the AIDS virus?

A Unfortunately, yes. Some individuals acquired HIV while receiving blood before blood testing was instituted in March 1985. If you believe you are infected or if you wish to be tested for HIV, you should contact your doctor or visit an anonymous testing site.

The Mosquito Connection

Throughout recorded history, mosquitoes and other arthropods have been responsible for spreading many epidemics. Plague was spread by fleas, typhus by lice, and malaria by mosquitoes. In addition, ticks transmit the agents of Lyme disease and Rocky Mountain spotted fever.

In all these instances, the disease organisms greatly increase their numbers within the arthropod, then exit from it efficiently. For malaria and yellow fever, the respective parasites (a protozoan and a virus) multiply in the mosquito, then concentrate in its salivary gland. When the mosquito takes its next blood meal, the parasites pass with its saliva into the victim's blood.

No such model exists for AIDS. Since AIDS has been known in the United States, researchers have been unable to locate multiplying HIV in mosquitoes or other arthropods; nor have they observed the viruses in a place where they could exit the arthropod host. It should also be noted that mosquitoes suck blood—they do not inject blood from one person into another. To be sure, residual blood might remain after a bite on a mosquito's needlelike injecting tube (the proboscis), but entomologists point out that a mosquito continually washes its proboscis with saliva, thereby cleansing it. Moreover, the amount of blood on the proboscis is roughly a thousandth of what might be encountered in a needlestick.

Additional evidence that no animal intermediate is involved in HIV transmission comes from Africa. It is well known that African children play outside in mosquito-infested areas. Children would constitute a large percentage of African AIDS cases if the disease were mosquito-borne. Statistics show, however, that children represent a relatively small percentage of Africans with AIDS. Many African children suffer from malaria, but comparatively few suffer from AIDS.

Scientists have shown that HIV can remain active within mosquitoes for a period of several hours after they have been fed blood with a high concentration of the virus. This observation, however, does not support the notion that mosquitoes transmit HIV in nature because the virus neither multiplies within a mosquito nor concentrates at a point where it can leave the mosquito. While these activities occur with many microbial agents, they do not appear to do so for HIV. Barring some fundamental biochemical change in the virus or the mosquito, an HIV-mosquito connection is unlikely to emerge in future years.

AIDS in Schools and Colleges

Although the incidence of AIDS in school-age children and teenagers is relatively low, the potential exists for young people to be the next victims of the AIDS epidemic, because young people experiment with drugs and sexuality, two modes for the transmission of HIV. As the number of sexual experiences and sex partners increases, the odds increase that an individual will come in contact with an HIV-infected person. Public health officials suggest that having sexual contact with a certain individual essentially brings a person in contact with all other individuals with whom that individual has had sexual contact. It is quite conceivable that HIV-infected T-lymphocytes or free viruses could be moving through any person-to-person chain, despite the fact that all appear to be in good health.

Through December 2000, over 25,000 cases of AIDS had been diagnosed in U.S. teenagers (Table 5.6). The data show that in males, most cases occur in sexually active homosexuals and hemophiliacs. Only 4 percent occurred from heterosexual contact. In females, by comparison, 52 percent resulted from sexual contact—in most cases, through sex with an injection drug user. Teenage girls were more likely than boys to contract AIDS through injection use only. In both males and females, a substantial number of cases resulted from unidentified risks.

School-sponsored HIV prevention programs are an efficient way of helping reduce behaviors associated with HIV transmission. In 1996, the CDC reported the results of a survey to determine the percentage of state education departments requiring instruction in certain health-related topics. Also surveyed were 502 school districts in 50 states and the District of Columbia. The results, shown in Table 5.7, indicate that almost 80 percent of the states and almost 85 percent of the school districts require instruction in HIV prevention. Although the statistics are notable, health officials have resolved to bring the number of states up to at least 95 percent. In doing so, they hope to reduce in school-age students the risk for acquiring HIV.

Nor are college-age students free from risk. According to a 1990s estimate, one in 300 college students was infected with HIV. To be sure, this percentage is low (0.3 percent), but in a sexually active, drug-experimenting population on campus, the potential for rapid spread of HIV is unmistakable. In the early 1990s, the American College Health Association found that half of the 3600 colleges in the United States had virtually no AIDS education program. Fortunately, many campuses have taken an aggressive approach to preventing AIDS since then. On one campus, for example, cigarette machines were replaced by condom machines; on another campus, students wore sweatshirts that proclaimed: "No Glove, No Love." By the end of the decade, the number of AIDS-prevention programs in colleges and universities has increased substantially.

Ignorance and feelings of invincibility are but two of the obstacles that must be overcome in AIDS education programs for schools and colleges. An unexpectedly large number of students, for instance, continue to believe that HIV can be contracted from toilet seats and mosquitoes and by donating blood. Students are reluctant to ask questions for fear that others will think they have AIDS or are drug users. They refrain from talking about sex or considering condom use out of embarrassment. And the idea of sickness and death simply does not occur to most of them. To the great majority of young people, AIDS is not of crisis proportions. Health officials agree, but they add the word "yet."

TABLE 5.6 — AIDS in Teenagers (Aged 13 to 19) by Sex and Exposure Category, through June 2001

	Cumulative Total	
Male exposure category	**Number**	**(Percentage)**
Sexually active homosexual men	1,324	(52)
Injection drug use	119	(5)
Sexually active homosexual men who inject drugs	116	(5)
Hemophilia/coagulation disorder	103	(4)
Heterosexual contact:	174	(7)
Sex with injection drug user	27	
Sex with person with hemophilia	2	
Sex with transfusion recipient with HIV infection	0	
Sex with HIV-infected person, risk not specified	145	
Receipt of blood transfusion, blood components, or tissue	12	(0)
Risk not reported or identified	684	(27)
Male subtotal	2,532	(100)
Female exposure Category		
Injection drug use	245	(7)
Hemophilia/coagulation disorder	0	(0)
Heterosexual contact:	1,669	(50)
Sex with injection drug user	269	
Sex with bisexual male	122	
Sex with person with hemophilia	23	
Sex with transfusion recipient with HIV infection	3	
Sex with HIV-infected person, risk not specified	1,252	
Receipt of blood transfusion, blood components, or tissue	20	(1)
Risk not reported or identified	1,426	(42)
Female subtotal	3,360	(100)
Total	**5,893**	

Source: Courtesy of CDC, HIV/AIDS Surveillance Report 12(1), June, 2000.

The Epidemiology of AIDS

TABLE

5.7

Percentage of States and School Districts Requiring Education in HIV Prevention and Other Health-Related Topics, 1996

Topic	States Requiring Topic (Percentage)	School districts Requiring Topic (Percentage)
Alcohol- and other drug-use prevention	75.0	86.0
Conflict resolution and violence prevention	38.5	61.0
Dietary behaviors and nutrition	68.9	80.1
HIV prevention	78.7	83.0
Injury prevention and safety	62.2	74.5
Physical activity and fitness	65.2	81.9
Pregnancy prevention	43.9	72.1
Sexually transmitted disease prevention	65.1	80.9
Suicide prevention	37.8	66.7
Tobacco-use prevention	71.7	83.2

Source: Courtesy of CDC, MMWR 45(35), September 6, 1996.

[handwritten: → highest on the list]

LOOKING BACK

Discovering that an epidemic is in progress and defining the circumstances under which it spreads are tasks for epidemiologists. For the AIDS epidemic, epidemiologists have concluded that AIDS is a bloodborne disease due to a fragile virus that is passed among individuals by blood-to-blood or semen-to-blood contact. Pregnant women can also pass the virus to the developing fetus or after birth, possibly through breast milk. Through 2000, 82 percent of all cases in the United States occurred in men, 18 percent in women, and 1 percent in children under the age of 13. The 1990s saw a gradual shift of the AIDS epidemic away from homosexual men and toward blacks, Hispanics, and women.

In homosexual men, human immunodeficiency virus (HIV) is passed primarily by anal intercourse because bleeding of the rectal tissue permits entry of the virus. In this case, a risk exists for both the insertive and receptive partner. Injection drug users pass HIV by allowing their blood to mix with that of another person in a contaminated needle and syringe when "works" are shared. Over 25 percent of AIDS cases in the United States occur in this way. Heterosexual couples may be at risk because during vaginal intercourse, viruses may enter through lesions or abrasions on the genitals. Both males and females are at risk, and special risks exist among the elderly. Newborns acquire HIV from their mothers via placental transfer, but drug therapy can reduce the possibility of such transfer.

In Africa, the major method for spreading the virus among heterosexuals is by vaginal intercourse. Epidemiologists believe that ulcers from sexually transmitted diseases allow entry into the bloodstream. The number of reported cases in Africa far exceeds that in the United States, and the major manifestation of AIDS in African patients is the wasting syndrome. In the world at large, 269 countries had reported AIDS cases by 2002, and over 40 million people had AIDS. Travelers and imported blood may be involved in the spread.

Other methods of AIDS transmission generally involve substantial exposures to contaminated blood, and certain data should be used to assess the risk of exposure. Health care workers are at risk because of their contact with blood and body fluids, but such factors as type of exposure and volume of fluid transmitted determine the risk of HIV transfer. Virtually no risk is involved in such activities as social kissing, contact with AIDS patients, or a mosquito bite. In schools and colleges, special attention is warranted because young people experiment with drugs and sexual relationships.

REVIEW

This chapter has dealt with the spreading of the AIDS epidemic among different groups of individuals and in different parts of the world. To test your knowledge of these concepts, select the letter of the phrase that best completes each of the following statements. The correct answers are listed in Appendix A.

1. All of the following are part of the job of an epidemiologist except
  a. discovering that an epidemic is in progress.
  b. developing a drug for use in the epidemic.
  c. defining circumstances under which a disease spreads.
  d. studying the pattern of distribution of a disease.

2. In a male, the presence of a sexually transmitted disease (STD) such as gonorrhea or chlamydia can contribute to HIV transmission because
  a. the bacterial agents enhance the aggressiveness of HIV.
  b. the body's antibacterial antibodies react with HIV.
  c. STDs can cause erosion of the urethra and provide an entry path for HIV.
  d. HIV attaches to the bacteria and is transmitted when they are transmitted.

3. HIV could conceivably pass through the lining of a woman's uterus if she is exposed to the virus
  a. during the time of ovulation.
  b. when her levels of progesterone are highest.
  c. during the menstrual period.
  d. during the time of lowest estrogen levels.

_a_   4. All of the following are methods by which HIV is known to be transmitted except
    a. social kissing.
    b. placental transfer from mother to fetus.
    c. contact with contaminated blood in syringes.
    d. anal intercourse.

_d_   5. As of 2000, the total number of cases of AIDS in the United States stood at
    a. more than 2.5 million.
    b. less than 200.
    c. approximately 10 million.
    d. almost 800,000.

_d_   6. Whereas the percentage of AIDS cases involving homosexual men is dropping, the percentage continues to rise in
    a. teenagers.
    b. injection drug users.
    c. health workers.
    d. doctors and surgeons.

_a_   7. Direct blood-to-blood or semen-to-blood transfer of HIV is necessary for the transmission of AIDS, because
    a. the AIDS virus is a very fragile virus.
    b. blood and semen contain cofactors that stimulate the development of AIDS.
    c. the AIDS virus is a very resistant virus.
    d. contact with oxygen in the atmosphere kills the AIDS virus.

_d_   8. The transmission of HIV can be limited by all of the following methods except
    a. using a condom during sexual encounters.
    b. disinfecting needles used to inject drugs.
    c. limiting the number of sexual partners.
    d. using mosquito repellents.

_a_   9. In the Western Hemisphere, confirmed cases of AIDS have been reported
    a. in nearly every country.
    b. only in the United States and Canada.
    c. primarily in Mexico and the Caribbean islands.
    d. in all countries except those in South America.

_b_   10. The typical AIDS patient in Africa exhibits symptoms that typify
    a. the AIDS-dementia complex.
    b. the HIV wasting syndrome.

c. an extreme case of cytomegalovirus disease.

d. an asymptomatic HIV infection.

_a_ **11.** Research evidence has shown that mosquitoes
  a. do not transmit HIV.
  b. transmit HIV only among injection drug users.
  c. serve as an important intermediary host for HIV.
  d. pass along HIV in their saliva.

_c_ **12.** The HIV antibodies detected in a newborn's blood most likely have come from.
  a. the newborn's immune system.
  b. the father's sperm cells.
  c. the mother's blood system.
  d. the food taken in during the first few days.

_a_ **13.** During vaginal intercourse, the risk of HIV infection increases if
  a. the woman has vaginal lesions.
  b. HIV antibodies are present in the semen.
  c. the man uses a condom.
  d. the woman uses birth control pills.

_a_ **14.** If mosquitoes were capable of transmitting HIV,
  a. many more adults would have AIDS.
  b. fewer injection drug users would have AIDS.
  c. the number of cases of pediatric AIDS would be higher.
  d. fewer homosexual men would have AIDS.

_b_ **15.** In Africa, the most predominant method for HIV transmission appears to be
  a. ritual scarring and reuse of needles.
  b. heterosexual vaginal intercourse.
  c. imported contaminated blood.
  d. social kissing.

FOR ADDITIONAL READING

Adler, N. E., et al. 1993. "Socioeconomic inequalities in health." *JAMA* 269: 3140–3145.

Altman, L. K. 1990. "Advances in treatment change face of AIDS." *New York Times,* June 12.

Anderson, J. E., et al. 1999. "Prevalence of sexual and drug-related HIV risk behaviors in the U.S. population." *J. Acquire. Immune Defic. Syndr.* 21: 148–156.

Balter, M. 1993. "East Europe: A chance to stop HIV." *Science* 262: 1964–1966.

Begley, S. 2000. "Ten million orphans." *Newsweek*, January 17.

Binswanger, H. P. 2000. "Scaling up HIV/AIDS programs to national coverage." *Science* 288: 2173–2178.

Branegan, J., et al. 2001. "Death stalks a continent." *Time*, February 12.

CDC. 1994. "Heterosexually acquired AIDS–United States, 1993." *MMWR* 43(9): 155–160.

———. 1994. "HIV prevention practices of primary-care physicians—United States, 1992." *MMWR* 42(51): 988–992.

Cohen, J. 2001. "AIDS gains foothold in key Asian groups." *Science* 294: 282–284.

Conover, T. 1993. "Trucking through the AIDS belt." *The New Yorker*, August 16.

Diaz, T., et al. 1993. "AIDS trends among Hispanics in the United States." *Am. J. Public Health* 83: 504–509.

Edlin, B. R., et al. 1994. "Intersecting epidemics: crack cocaine use and HIV infection among inner-city young adults." *N. Eng. J. Med.* 331: 1422–1427.

Mann, J. M., and D. J. M. Tarantola. 1998. "HIV 1998: The global picture." *Scientific American*, July.

McGeary, J. 2001. "Death stalks a continent." *Time*, February 12.

Normile, D. 2000. "China awakens to fight projected AIDS crisis." *Science* 288: 2312–2314.

Pennisi, E. 1995. "AIDS becomes more of an equal opportunity epidemic." *ASM News* 61: 236–241.

Preventing HIV Transmission

LOOKING AHEAD

As the AIDS epidemic continues to spread, individuals can take certain measures in their personal lives and at work to protect themselves and others from contracting the human immunodeficiency virus (HIV). This chapter describes some of the available measures. On completing the chapter, you should be able to . . .

- Recognize how behaviors during sexual activity can be altered to prevent the passage of HIV.

- Understand the methods for preventing HIV transmission among those who use injection drugs.

- Describe the universal precautions recommended for all health care workers and be familiar with particular precautions suggested for surgical procedures, dentistry, embalming, and medical laboratories.

- Specify the precautions recommended by public health officials for those who work in public safety professions.

- Discuss the reasons why AIDS education is necessary in schools and survey the methods for implementing such education.

INTRODUCTION

In the 1840s, a cholera epidemic broke out in Europe. It spread quickly and reached England in June 1849. The district near Golden Square in London was among the worst affected areas—more than 500 people died in one ten-day period that August. A physician named John Snow lived near Golden Square. Snow had studied cholera for years, and he saw in the epidemic an opportunity to test some of his ideas. Most scientists of his time believed that infected air was the probable cause of cholera, but Snow believed water was the culprit. With meager resources but much determination, he began a systematic study of the source of the cholera.

Snow discovered that most people living near Golden Square drew their water from a well on Broad Street. A hand pump operated the well, and anyone could work it. Snow examined the well closely and found that it was being contaminated by sewage overflowing from a nearby tenement. And a person living in the tenement had died recently of cholera. The relationship between the well and the disease was unmistakable.

On September 7, 1849, Snow presented his findings to the local community council. The members listened attentively but were skeptical. How, they asked, did Snow intend to interrupt the epidemic? Snow thought for a moment, then replied with the now-classic solution: "It's simple—take the handle off the Broad Street pump." The next day the handle was gone, and soon the epidemic subsided in that area.

Of course, not all epidemics are quite so easy to interrupt. For AIDS, scientists know what causes the disease (in fact, Snow did not know the cause of cholera), and they know how HIV spreads through a population. But halting the spread of AIDS requires more than knowledge alone. It demands changes in social customs and cultural practices, and it requires the willingness of people to adapt their behaviors. As we shall see in this chapter, there are many ways of interrupting the spread of AIDS, but they require more than simply removing the handle of a water pump.

Personal Protection

Prior to World War II, doctors had to contend with a variety of sexually transmitted diseases (STDs), including syphilis, gonorrhea, chancroid, and lymphogranuloma. But with the widespread use of antibiotics after the war, the incidence of syphilis and gonorrhea declined, and that of most other STDs dropped as well.

Then came the 1960s and the sexual revolution. It was a time of affluence and defiance of traditional values. Birth control pills, contraceptive devices, and vasectomies offered sexual liberation to go along with social and economic freedoms. And antibiotic resistance surfaced. Not surprisingly, the incidence of STDs soared. Today, the United States is in the grip of an epidemic of STDs. Public health officials estimate that one of four Americans between the ages of 15 and 55 will contract an STD at some time in his or her life; 10 million Americans visit clinics and doctors' offices annually to be treated for an STD; more than $2 billion is spent each year in health care costs for STDs.

Moreover, the list of STDs has continued to expand. In the United States, gonorrhea remains one of the most reported infectious disease, and syphilis accounts for roughly 35,000 new cases annually (Figure 6.1). During the 1990s, chlamydia became more common, affecting 3 to 5 million Americans each year, and genital herpes affects

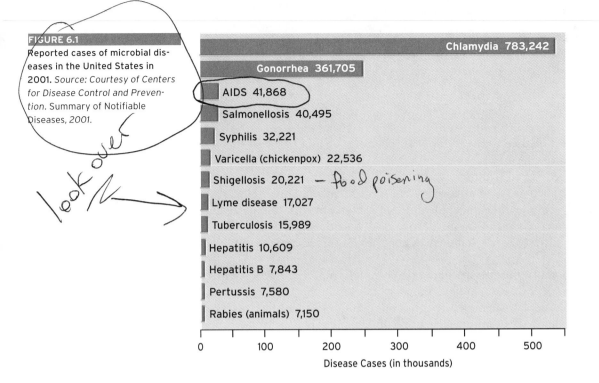

Chlamydia 783,242

Gonorrhea 361,705

AIDS 41,868

Salmonellosis 40,495

Syphilis 32,221

Varicella (chickenpox) 22,536

Shigellosis 20,221 — food poisoning

Lyme disease 17,027

Tuberculosis 15,989

Hepatitis 10,609

Hepatitis B 7,843

Pertussis 7,580

Rabies (animals) 7,150

look out

0   100   200   300   400   500

Disease Cases (in thousands)

several million people annually. The fungal disease candidiasis and the protozoal disease trichomoniasis each account for over a million cases per year. Hepatitis B is now considered an STD, and lymphogranuloma and chancroid are again being seen in patients. The latest addition to the list is AIDS.

The common denominator among STDs is the fragility of the infectious agent. The responsible microorganism—whether it causes gonorrhea, syphilis, chlamydia, or AIDS—prefers the warm, moist environment of the human body and rapidly dies or is inactivated when exposed to an environment outside the body. The agent is able to infect only when passed directly from person to person in a moist environment. And because it infects organs of the reproductive system, the usual method of transfer involves physical contact between these organs during vaginal intercourse or anal intercourse.

Public health officials advise that couples should not have to worry about AIDS, so long as they have been mutually faithful since the 1970s (when HIV is believed to have entered the United States) and avoid other risk factors, such as contaminated needles associated with injection drug use. In addition, individuals at risk through body fluid contact can avoid HIV infection as well as other STDs by practicing sexual abstinence.

By comparison, those who continue to have multiple sexual contacts place themselves and their partners at risk for HIV infection and AIDS. Sexual contact with sex workers (prostitutes) increases the risk further, because prostitutes have innumerable sexual contacts. The presence of another STD pushes the risk even higher, since lesions and sores from the STD permit entry of HIV (Chapter 5). Epidemiological studies indicate that vaginal intercourse permits transmission of HIV and that oral-genital contact may be a risky practice as well. As indicated in Chapter 5, anal intercourse involves the highest risk because tearing and bleeding of the rectal tissue permits HIV access to the blood stream. The next paragraphs explore how the possibility of HIV transmission can be reduced.

Safer Sex Practices

The foolproof way to avoid contact with HIV through sexual activity is to avoid sexual activity with infected persons or to have a lifelong monogamous relationship. Because this suggestion is not realistic for many people, public health officials trying to prevent the spread of AIDS have encouraged modifications of sexual behaviors. These modifications are collectively known as safer sex practices. The implication is that they can reduce the risk of HIV transmission, but they cannot eliminate the risk completely (they are "safer" sex practices, not "safe" sex practices, the latter term implying a 100-percent guarantee).

Among the most important safer sex practices is the use of condoms. Anything that creates a barrier between the semen and the internal tissues of sexual partners can lessen the risk of HIV transfer. The purpose of a condom is to form such a barrier. A condom (or "rubber") is a soft, stretchable sheath placed over the penis during sexual intercourse, whether vaginal, oral, or anal. The condom acts as a barrier to collect semen and prevent it from entering the sexual partner's body (Figure 6.2). Extensive studies have demonstrated conclusively that condoms

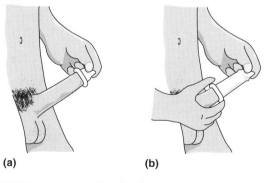

(a)   (b)

FIGURE 6.2

A condom creates a barrier between the semen and the internal tissues of the sexual partner and lessens the risk of HIV transfer. (a) The condom is put on when erection is achieved. (b) The condom is rolled directly onto the penis, leaving a reservoir for catching the semen.

BOX
6.1

No Excuses

Excuses for not using condoms are usually so persuasive that couples find it hard to answer them effectively, and they often give in to unprotected sex. Here are some excuses for not using condoms and some reasonable replies:

She: "I use the pill; you don't have to use a condom."

He: "Let's use one anyway; either of us could be infected with something and it will help prevent passage."

She: "You carry condoms around? Was this all a trick to get me into bed?"

He: "I keep one with me because I care about your health and mine, and you never know where a night is going to end up."

He: "I don't have any infection. And I haven't had sex for months."

She: "Thanks for letting me know. I don't have anything either but I could be harboring something without having any symptoms. Let's use a condom to be sure."

She: "It's hard to feel anything when you wear a condom."

He: "It's hard for me too, but there are lots of other feelings, and the protection's worth it."

He: "I might lose my erection if we stop right now."

She: "Not necessarily; I'll help you put it on. We'll make it a part of the whole thing."

He: "It's messy, and it smells bad."

She: "A little mess isn't so bad when you consider the alternative—AIDS!"

She: "They're unnatural and a fake."

He: "Maybe so, but getting sick is even worse."

She: "I'm insulted! Do you think I'm some sort of slut?"

He: "I didn't say that. I'm just trying to be careful for both of us. I want you to be sure I don't give you anything."

She: "Real men aren't afraid of getting sick; they don't use condoms."

He: "Maybe I'm a little more caring than those other guys."

He: "I love you. I wouldn't make you sick. I don't need a condom."

She: "I believe you love me and that you wouldn't intentionally make me sick. But AIDS can be in your body without your knowing it. So if you really love me you'd be aware of my needs and care for me."

He: "Just this once, no condom."

She: "All it takes is once; AIDS is forever!"

can decrease the risk of STDs, including HIV infection, by decreasing the transmission of infectious agents. In 1993, for example, the Centers for Disease Control and Prevention (CDC) reported that HIV failed to be transmitted among 123 couples who used condoms when one person was infected. In laboratory tests, microorganisms as small as viruses (including HIV) fail to pass the barrier (Box 6.1).

Several types of condoms are available commercially. In the laboratory, studies under mechanical conditions simulating sexual intercourse indicate that latex condoms can prevent the passage of all infectious agents, including HIV. Natural skin (membrane or "lambskin") condoms are believed to be less effective. This is probably because latex condoms are consistently thick and of quality (although the latex can cause allergic reactions), while natural skin condoms made from lamb's intestinal tissue can vary in quality and are generally more porous. In addition, fresh condoms are preferable to older ones because heat and aging can weaken the material. To alert consumers, boxes of condoms are labeled with an expiration date (Figure 6.3).

For greatest effectiveness, the condom must be used correctly and in every sexual encounter when there is doubt about the health status of the partner. Some helpful guidelines for condom use to decrease the risk of HIV infection are as follows:

1. A condom must be worn each time one has genital, anal, or oral sexual contact, and the condom must be put on as soon as erection is achieved and before the penis is inserted into the partner. Care should be taken to avoid damage with the fingernails or other sharp objects.

2. The condom should be rolled directly onto the penis. It should not be unrolled from the ring then stretched over the penis. A reservoir tip for catching semen should be present; if not present, a small amount of space should be left at the tip.

3. A spermicidal cream or foam containing nonoxynol-9 or a water-based jelly (such as KY) can be used to lubricate the tip of the condom before it is put on (it should be noted, however, that nonoxynol-9 kills helpful bacteria in the woman's vaginal tract and may change the chemical

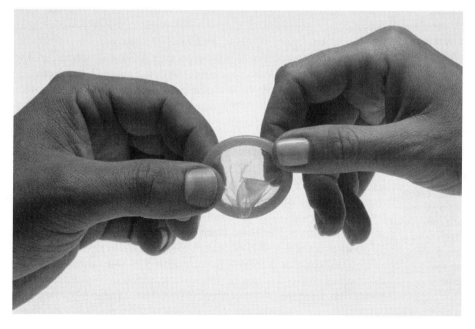

FIGURE 6.3

A condom reduces the risk of HIV transfer for both the wearer and his sexual partner. Latex condoms are believed to be more effective than natural skin condoms because they are uniformly thick and of controlled quality. For greatest protection, condoms should be used in all sexual encounters.

1 Q My girlfriend and I are sexually active, and I'd like to use condoms. Where can you get them?

A Condoms are sold at drugstores and supermarkets and in some vending machines. They do not require a prescription for purchase and are relatively inexpensive.

2 Q Should women carry condoms?

A AIDS poses a risk to women who are exposed to the infected semen of men. It is therefore in a woman's own best interest to insist that a man use a condom. Women who anticipate having sexual intercourse should carry condoms. They should also investigate female condoms as a method of protection.

3 Q How can you bring up the topic of condom use with your partner?

A Using a condom is a sensitive issue that couples may find difficult to talk about. But condoms are meant to prevent the passage of HIV and other infectious agents and to prevent unwanted pregnancies. Viewed in this positive context, using a condom is a sign of respect, and it is an advantage to both individuals in a sexual relationship.

4 Q If a couple has been engaging in unprotected sexual intercourse, is it too late to start using a condom?

A It is never too late to begin using condoms. If, for example, one partner becomes infected by sharing a contaminated needle today, HIV could be passed to the other partner the next time they have sexual intercourse. Using a condom would limit that possibility.

environment there so that pathogenic bacteria could thrive and cause urinary tract infections). Use of petroleum lubricants such as petroleum jelly, vegetable oil, or massage or body lotions is not advised because they can promote condom failure by reducing its strength.

4. The condom should be removed soon after ejaculation to avoid leaking of semen from the condom as the penis becomes limp. It is also a good idea to hold the rim of the condom during withdrawal to prevent its slipping off.

5. Condoms are for single-time use. They are not intended for reuse and should be discarded properly. Washing the hands and the penis after sexual intercourse is also recommended.

Condoms reduce the risk of infection for both the wearer and his sex partner (Healthline 6.1). For the wearer, condoms lessen the exposure of the penis to infectious secretions and infected cells of the partner's reproductive organs or rectum. For the receptive sex partner, condoms prevent deposit of infectious semen, contact with infected discharge from the male reproductive tract, and exposure to lesions on the penis. Though the actual effectiveness of condom use in prevention of STDs is difficult to assess, several case-control studies indicate a lower rate of STDs in condom users and, thus, fewer health-related problems. Indeed, many colleges have decided to remove all their cigarette machines and replace them with condom machines. "Why kill people," said one administrator, "when you can help save their lives?"

Other safer sex practices involve activities where no body fluids are exchanged, that is, activities taking place outside the body. Among these practices are massaging various sensitive parts of the body (the back, scalp, neck, and face are examples); rubbing the bodies together and stroking the partner's genital organs, as long as the penis does not come in contact with the vagina or rectum; masturbation, either of self or of the sexual partner; and kissing various body parts. It should be noted, however, that deep, or "French," kissing could involve some slight risk if mouth or gum sores are present and if large amounts of saliva are exchanged (Chapter 5).

The effectiveness of safer sex practices is underscored by the results of the CDC study cited earlier and by results of a study published in 1988 by Margaret A. Fischl of the University of Miami. In the study, Fischl reported on 58 heterosexual married couples. In each couple, one spouse was infected with HIV. Over the duration of the study, 13 couples abstained from sexual intercourse and none of the 13 spouses transmitted HIV; 23 couples engaged in sexual intercourse using condoms, and HIV was transmitted in only three cases; and 22 couples engaged in sexual intercourse without condoms, with the result that 14 spouses were infected with HIV (Table 6.1).

look over

TABLE 6.1 The Relationship of Sexual Activity to Development of HIV Antibody among 58 Spouses of HIV-Positive Individuals*

Sexual Activity	Total Number	HIV+	HIV−	Percentage Converted
Abstinence	13	0	13	0
Sexual contact with condoms	23	3	20	13
Sexual contact without condoms	22	14	8	64

* Spouses did not display HIV antibodies at the beginning of the study.

Source: Fischl, N. A., et al. "Heterosexual Transmission of Human Immunodeficiency Virus (HIV): Relationship of Sexual Practices to Seroconversion." Third International Conference on AIDS. Washington, D.C., 1988, p. 178.

Another approach to safer sex practices is for women to use a vaginal foam or gel that will block HIV transmission. A promising advance is the development of a vaginal microbicide, a substance that women can use to protect themselves against HIV and other sexually transmitted microorganisms. Such a product would have to be nontoxic and nonirritating; it would have to withstand changing acidity levels in the vagina; it would need to fulfill aesthetic requirements for female consumers; and it could not kill the lactobacilli and other beneficial bacteria normally found in the vaginal tract.

One promising microbicide now in development is a protein that blocks HIV's entry into cells lining the vaginal tract by latching onto the viral gp120 envelope protein. This blocking protein does not react with vaginal bacteria or sperm cells because they lack the attachment site, and it cannot be used as a therapeutic drug because its molecule is too large to pass into the bloodstream. Another possible microbicide is reported to block HIV's replication in T-lymphocytes found in the vagina. A third microbicide prevents semen from raising the acidity of the vaginal fluid (as it normally does); the vagina thus can maintain an acidity that is inhospitable to HIV. Corporate excitement for such products is diminished by the reality that most users in the world would be impoverished women, so poor profit returns might be anticipated. Nevertheless, research on microbicides continues as another avenue through which sex can be made safer.

For Injection Drug Users

Injection drug users who share drug paraphernalia are at high risk for AIDS because they are exposing their blood to the blood of an infected individual when they share needles and syringes. HIV need not pass through any cell layers or penetrate a lesion to reach the bloodstream (as it must during passage by sexual activity).

Ironically, the social structure of injection drug users may promote the sharing of syringes and needles. For example, the ethics of cooperation within small friendship groups is applied to the sharing of drug paraphernalia, which drug users call their "works." To refuse to share one's works can damage the reputation and reliability of the owner. Limited supplies of drug paraphernalia can also encourage sharing. Sharing is promoted by the rental of "houseworks" at places where injection drug users congregate (the so-called shooting galleries). After being used, the houseworks are returned to the owner for the next rental. Reusing contaminated needles and syringes under such conditions easily spreads HIV from a small group of friends into a larger population of injection drug users. An infected individual might then have sexual intercourse with a nonuser and transfer the virus to that person.

Clearly, the best way to avoid HIV from contaminated needles is to avoid using drugs. For those who choose to inject drugs, the safer practice is to avoid sharing drug paraphernalia. Although this practice may lead to social isolation, the benefits may outweigh the risk of contracting HIV.

It is also possible to decontaminate the syringe and needle with household bleach and hot water. Bleach contains chlorine, and the chlorine reacts with proteins in the HIV capsid and envelope to alter the chemical structure of these structures and thereby inactivate the virus. The syringe should be filled with bleach, then flushed out a few times. After this filling and flushing, the syringe should be filled with hot (preferably boiled) water a few more times to rinse it thoroughly (Figure 6.4). A 10-percent bleach solution (one part bleach added to nine parts water) inactivates HIV. More concentrated solutions may also be used, but they may leave a chlorine residue in the syringe that could be toxic to the body. Also not advised is using a lighted match to heat the needle, because HIV can be trapped within clots of blood left in the syringe. Furthermore, placing the needle and syringe in boiling water is inadequate, because the hot water may not completely fill the implements.

Among the more controversial issues of contemporary society is whether municipalities should participate in needle exchange programs. In such a program, used needles (and syringes) are traded at no cost for sterile ones at designated locations and times. Opponents of these exchange programs argue that they condone and encourage drug use; proponents counter that they help interrupt the AIDS epidemic among injection drug users.

One of the first needle exchange programs in the United States was put into operation in New Haven, Connecticut, in 1992. A van, painted with vivid stripes and a rising sun, plied the streets of the city four times a week. Identifying themselves by code names, drug users came to the van and exchanged their needles for "survival kits" containing clean needles, bottles of bleach and water, and condoms. Rather than accelerating inner-city drug abuse, the program has apparently slowed the rate of infection, increased addict referrals to treatment programs, increased police empathy for addicts (police cars are steered clear of the van to avoid giving the impression of entrapment), and gained the trust of addicts. The van has become a visible expression of the city's desire to help its underprivileged

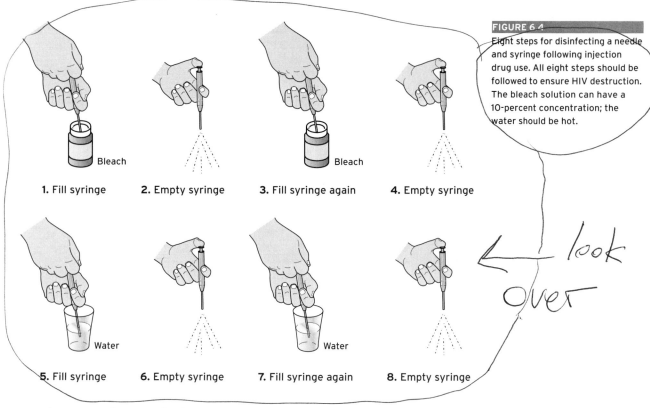

FIGURE 6.4

Eight steps for disinfecting a needle and syringe following injection drug use. All eight steps should be followed to ensure HIV destruction. The bleach solution can have a 10-percent concentration; the water should be hot.

1. Fill syringe
Bleach

2. Empty syringe

3. Fill syringe again
Bleach

4. Empty syringe

5. Fill syringe
Water

6. Empty syringe

7. Fill syringe again
Water

8. Empty syringe

population. And to avoid subjectivity, the city utilized scientists at nearby Yale University to evaluate the program. Experimental programs in New York City and Washington, D.C. soon followed.

The number of needle exchange programs continued to grow through the 1990s and into the new century as moral and philosophical support came from the CDC, National Institutes of Health, and American Medical Association. By 2002, more than 165 programs were operating at over 500 sites (including sidewalk tables, health clinics, cars, and storefronts) in over 30 states, and organizations were actively campaigning for more programs (Figure 6.5). Over 20 million syringes were being exchanged each year, and on-site counseling and testing for HIV were being offered at most of the sites. Although many of the programs receive state, county, and/or city funding, the major stumbling block to their growth is that federal funding is not permitted by law. In response, program supporters continue to point out that preventing HIV infection among injection drug users costs about $20 per user per year, a notable difference from the estimated $120,000 it costs to treat an HIV-infected person until death.

Needle exchange programs continue to face lack of funding and perennial resistance from communities who do not want such programs to operate in their backyards. Supporters point out that the latter objection could be addressed by using mobile vans, as in New Haven, Connecticut. Also, while the federal funding debate continues, programs could be helped by state approval of syringe sales at

AIDS activists continue to campaign for condom supply and needle exchange programs as a way of reducing HIV transmission among injection drug users. By 2000, about 150 needle exchange programs were operating in the United States.

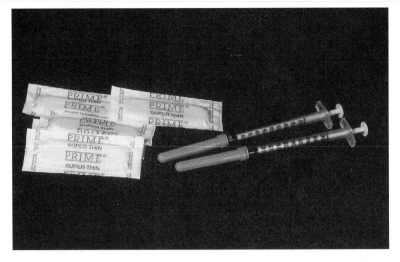

local pharmacies. In New York, for example, the sale of syringes won approval during 2001; a ten-pack costs $2 to $6 at local pharmacies. That year, New Hampshire and Rhode Island also removed the requirement for a prescription to purchase syringes and needles.

Interrupting the spread of AIDS among injection drug users has a corollary benefit to society, because injection drug users are the major link by which HIV enters the heterosexual population. Through June 2001, for instance, public health epidemiologists attributed 85,738 cases of AIDS to heterosexual contact. Of that number, 30,607 cases, or 36 percent, were linked to injection drug users. Clearly, the education campaigns directed at injection drug users merit public support. Such campaigns include counseling about "safer shooting" practices, distribution of bleach vials for cleaning syringes, and expedited admission of infected individuals to drug treatment. Programs such as these are currently under way in several U.S. cities (Healthline 6.2).

Protecting Health Care Workers

Epidemiologists reviewing the scientific literature of recent years have concluded that HIV transmission within health care settings is extremely rare but, nevertheless, possible. As the AIDS epidemic continues to spread, the possibility increases that health care workers will be exposed to blood and body fluids from patients infected with HIV. And the number of health care workers is considerable. An estimated 4.7 million people in the United States (including students and trainees) are considered health care workers because their activities involve contacts with patients or with blood or other body fluids from patients. These workers may be involved in surgery, emergency room care, dentistry, laboratory, or morgue service. Even laundry service workers are considered health care workers.

The transmission of HIV among health care workers can occur by any of several means. These include cuts with sharp objects (scalpels, razors), contamination of open wounds, exposure of mucous membranes, and of particular concern, self-injection with blood-contaminated needles ("needlestick").

Epidemiologists point out that infection control procedures can significantly reduce the number of accidental occupational exposures to HIV. Fundamental to infection control is the assumption that all patients are potentially infected with HIV in their blood and other body fluids. An assumption such as this must be made because a medical history and routine examination cannot reliably identify all patients infected with HIV and because testing for HIV may require the consent of the individual (Chapter 7). This consent is not necessarily forthcoming from the patient.

Universal Precautions

Recommendations for protecting health care workers were first made by the CDC in 1983. As the years passed, CDC officials realized that the wisest course for these workers was to consider all patients potentially infectious. Public health officials therefore promulgated a series of "universal blood and body fluid precautions," known simply as "universal precautions." Universal precautions are employed to protect the health care worker from infection by the patient, as well as the reverse, and to prevent the spread of HIV among patients through contaminated devices or surfaces. The precautions apply to blood, semen, and other body fluids, but they do not apply to feces, saliva, tears, and urine, because the amount of HIV is extremely low in most cases. Among the universal precautions are the following:

1. Health care workers should use barrier precautions such as gloves to prevent skin and mucous membrane exposure to blood or other body fluids from a patient. Gloves should be worn for touching blood and body fluids, mucous membranes, or nonintact skin of all patients; for handling items or surfaces soiled with blood or body fluids; and for performing venipuncture and other procedures where access to the patient's blood is required. Gloves should be changed after contact with each patient. Masks and protective eyewear or face shields should be worn during procedures that are likely to generate airborne droplets of blood or other body fluids, to prevent exposure of mucous membranes of the mouth, nose, and eyes. Gowns or aprons should be worn during procedures that are likely to generate splashes of blood or other body fluids.

2. Hands and other skin surfaces should be washed immediately and thoroughly if contaminated with blood or other body fluids. Hands should be washed immediately after gloves are removed.

Healthline 6.2

1 **Q** I quit using drugs some years ago. Could I have been infected before I quit?

A Unfortunately, yes. HIV has been in the United States at least since the late 1970s. Anyone using injection drugs from that time on could have been infected if he or she shared needles and syringes.

2 **Q** Can I kill HIV by heating my needle with a match?

A Using a match is better than not doing anything, but the heat will probably cause the blood to clot and trap the virus. Rinsing out the needle and the syringe in bleach is the more effective way of disinfecting it.

3 **Q** I've heard that when you're on drugs, you're more likely to spread AIDS by sexual contact than when you're not on drugs. Why?

A When injection drug users get high and have sex, they are less likely to think about using condoms. Also, prostitutes often pay for an expensive drug habit by trading sex for money. AIDS is therefore more likely to be spread by injection drug users than by nonusers.

3. Health care workers should take precautions to prevent injuries caused by needles, scalpels, and other sharp instruments or devices when performing procedures, cleaning used instruments, disposing of used needles, and handling sharp instruments after procedures. To prevent needlestick injuries, needles should not be recapped, purposely bent or broken by hand, removed from disposable syringes, or otherwise manipulated by hand. After they are used, disposable syringes and needles, scalpel blades, and other sharp items should be placed in puncture-resistant containers for disposal; the puncture-resistant containers should be located as close as practical to the use area. Large-bore reusable needles should be placed in a puncture resistant container for transport to the reprocessing area. The container should be placed out of reach of small children.

4. To minimize the occurrence of mouth-to-mouth resuscitation, mouthpieces, resuscitation bags, or other ventilation devices should be available for use in areas in which the need for emergency resuscitation is predictable.

5. Health care workers who have open lesions or fluid-yielding skin inflammations should restrain from all direct patient care or handling of patient-care equipment until the condition resolves.

6. Pregnant health care workers should be especially familiar with the precautions and adhere to them strictly to minimize the chances of HIV transmission.

The universal precautions promulgated by the CDC are intended to supplement (but not replace) recommendations for routine infection control, such as hand-washing and glove use to prevent microbial contamination of the hands. Epidemiologists at the CDC point out that specifying the type of barrier protection for every clinical situation is impractical and that health care workers must exercise their own good judgment.

Invasive Procedures

Invasive procedures are those that involve surgical entry into the tissues, cavities, or organs of a patient. They also involve repair of major traumatic injuries in such areas as the delivery room, the emergency room, or the physician's or dentist's office (Figure 6.6). In such a case, universal precautions are advised, with the addition of the following precautions:

1. All health care workers who participate in invasive procedures must routinely use appropriate barrier precautions to prevent skin and mucous membrane contact with blood and other body fluids of all patients. Gloves and surgical masks must be worn for all invasive procedures. Protective eyewear or face shields should be worn for procedures that commonly result in the generation of droplets, splashing of blood or other body fluids, or the generation of bone chips. Gowns or aprons made of materials that provide an effective barrier should be worn during invasive procedures that are likely to result in the splashing of blood or other body fluids. All health care workers who perform or assist in vaginal or cesarean deliveries should wear gloves and gowns when handling the placenta or the infant until blood and amniotic fluid have been

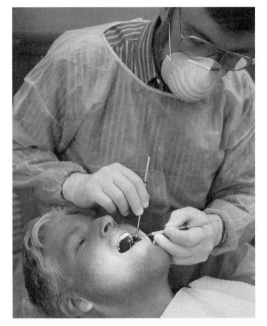

FIGURE 6.6
Among the chief recommendations in the universal precautions is the use of barrier precautions when participating in invasive procedures such as surgery and dentistry. Gloves, gowns, and masks are essential barrier precautions.

removed from the infant's skin and should wear gloves during post delivery care of the umbilical cord.

2. If a glove is torn or a needlestick or other injury occurs, the glove should be removed and a new glove used as promptly as patient safety permits; the needle or instrument involved in the incident should also be removed from the sterile field.

Dentistry

Epidemiologists at the CDC have recommended that special precautions be implemented for dentistry because contamination of the saliva with blood from the gums is predictable. Moreover, trauma to the hands of dental professionals is common, and blood spattering may occur. Infection control procedures also protect the patient's oral membranes from possible exposure to blood from breaks in the skin of the dental worker's hands. Among the special precautions for dentistry are the following:

1. All dental workers should wear gloves for contact with oral mucous membranes of all patients and should wear surgical masks and protective eyewear or chin-length plastic face shields during dental procedures in which splashing or spattering of blood, saliva, or gingival fluid is likely. Rubber dams, high-speed evacuation, and proper patient positioning, when appropriate, should be used to minimize generation of droplets and splatter.

2. Handpieces should be sterilized after use with each patient since blood, saliva, or gingival fluid may be aspirated into the handpiece or waterline.

Handpieces that cannot be sterilized should be flushed; the outside surface cleaned and wiped with a suitable chemical germicide, then rinsed. Handpieces should be flushed at the beginning of the day and after use with each patient. Manufacturers' recommendations should be followed for use and maintenance of waterlines and check valves and for flushing of handpieces. The same precautions should be used for ultrasonic scalers and air/water syringes.

3. Blood and saliva should be thoroughly and carefully cleaned from material that has been used in the mouth (e.g., impression materials, bite registration), especially before polishing and grinding intraoral devices. Contaminated materials, impressions, and intraoral devices should also be cleaned and disinfected before being handled in the dental laboratory and before they are placed in the patient's mouth.

4. Dental equipment and surfaces that are difficult to disinfect (e.g., light handles or X-ray-unit heads) and that may become contaminated should be wrapped with impervious-back paper, aluminum foil, or clear plastic wrap. The coverings should be removed and discarded, and clean coverings should be put in place after use with each patient.

As a general principle, the CDC recommends that dental workers consider the blood, saliva, and gingival fluid from all patients to be potentially infectious. The special precautions are formulated on this basis.

That dental practices can transmit HIV was vividly demonstrated in the early 1990s when six patients of a Florida dentist were identified with HIV infection. Investigators found that all six patients had the same strain of HIV as the dentist, and epidemiologists could not identify any risk factors (such as injection drug use or heterosexual contact with an infected individual) that could account for HIV transmission. Five of the patients had root canal therapy or dental extraction. One patient, Kimberly Bergalis, was the first to link her infection to treatment via a series of letters to the Florida Health Department. Bergalis died in 1992; two years before, the dentist had died.

Through 2002, there have been no other documented instances of HIV transmission from health care workers to patients. CDC epidemiologists have investigated dozens of instances among health care practitioners (including surgeons, obstetricians, physicians, and other dentists) where HIV transmission may have occurred. In each case, they concluded that a risk factor (such as injection drug use) was involved, indicating that when transmission to a patient occurs, there is some underlying risk practice or factor.

Autopsy and Embalming

Autopsy and embalming procedures carry special risk because of the workers' exposure to HIV-infected tissue of internal organs. For all persons performing or assisting in postmortem procedures, the CDC recommends adherence to the universal precautions, with special reference to the wearing of gloves, masks, protective eyewear, gowns, and waterproof aprons. Particular attention should be paid to decontamination of all instruments and surfaces with appropriate chemical germicides both during and after postmortem procedures.

Epidemiologists have suggested additional precautions during procedures that involve transporting and embalming the body of an HIV-positive person or AIDS patient. Funeral directors, for example, are advised to spray body wrappings liberally with disinfectant, then add a layer of plastic wrapping or place the body in a pouch. At the funeral home, disinfectant should be sprayed and swabbed on the entire body, especially the orifices and genital organs. A stronger-than-normal solution of embalming fluid is recommended, and the drainage vessel should remain closed for an extended time to ensure that the fluid has contacted any viral particles in the blood. During drainage, care should be taken to avoid blood splash on the embalming table and, if possible, in the waste sink. Before treating the body cavity, epidemiologists suggest that several hours pass to maintain embalming fluid pressure within the blood vessels and keep the fluid within the blood. When the cavity is treated, use of an extra measure of fluid is recommended in both thoracic and abdominal cavities. Extreme caution must be used when handling any visceral organs or tissues, and the embalmer should exercise care to avoid abrasions and scratches from such things as cut bones of the rib cage. After suturing, all incisions should be thoroughly sealed.

Medical Laboratories

A medical laboratory is a specialized facility where urine, feces, blood, and other patient specimens are analyzed biologically and chemically by skilled technologists and technicians. Laboratory workers receive blood and other specimens on a regular basis and are expected to perform the protocols desired by attending physicians and to report the results. CDC epidemiologists recommend that laboratory workers follow the universal precautions, supplemented with additional specified precautions, as follows:

1. All specimens of blood and body fluids should be put in well-constructed containers with secure lids to prevent leaking during transport. Care should be taken when collecting each specimen to avoid contaminating the outside of the container and the laboratory form accompanying the specimen.

2. All persons processing (such as removing tops and vacuum tubes) blood and body fluid specimens should wear gloves. Masks and protective eyewear should be worn if mucous membrane contact with blood or body fluids is anticipated. Gloves should be changed and hands washed after completion of specimen processing.

3. For routine procedures, such as histologic and pathologic studies or microbiologic culturing, a biological safety cabinet is not necessary. However, biological safety cabinets (Class I or II) should be used whenever conducting procedures that have a high potential for generating airborne droplets. These include activities such as blending, treating with ultrasonic vibrations, and vigorous mixing.

4. Mechanical pipetting devices should be used for manipulating all liquids in the laboratory. Mouth pipetting must not be done.

5. Use of needles and syringes should be limited to situations in which there is no alternative, and the recommendations for preventing injuries with needles outlined under universal precautions should be followed.

6. Laboratory work surfaces should be decontaminated with an appropriate chemical germicide after a spill of blood or other body fluids and when work activities are completed.

7. Contaminated materials used in laboratory tests should be decontaminated before preprocessing or placed in bags and disposed of in accordance with institutional policies for disposal of infective waste.

8. Scientific equipment that has been contaminated with blood or other body fluids should be decontaminated and cleaned before being repaired in the laboratory or transported to the manufacturer.

9. All persons should wash their hands after completing laboratory activities and should remove protective clothing before leaving the laboratory (Figure 6.7).

Decontamination Procedures

In the vast majority of health care settings, the standard sterilization and disinfection procedures are adequate for decontaminating patient care equipment. Because HIV is fragile, it is inactivated rapidly after exposure to commonly used chemical germicides, even when the germicides are used in lower concentrations than normal.

In addition to commercially available germicides, a solution of household bleach (sodium hypochlorite) is an inexpensive and effective germicide. The solution should be prepared daily in a concentration from 10 percent (1 part bleach to 9 parts water) to 1 percent (1 part bleach to 99 parts water). The concentration

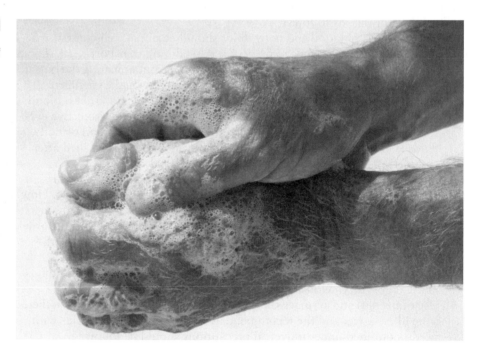

FIGURE 6.7

Hand-washing is one of the simplest yet most effective methods of preventing the spread of HIV. Any health care activity should always be followed by hand-washing, regardless of how major or minor the activity has been. If *there were* a single rallying cry among public health officials attempting to stem the spread of AIDS and other diseases, it would be "Wash your hands!"

depends on how much blood, mucus, or other organic material is present—the higher concentration for the higher measure of contamination. Unfortunately, many surfaces and instruments are corroded by bleach solutions, so commercially available germicides may be preferable.

Extensive studies of the survival of HIV in the health care environment indicate that the virus rapidly becomes inactive on exposure to the air. Of course, conditions vary (e.g., temperature, pH, amount of blood present, number of viruses present), but the general principle is that no changes in sterilization, disinfection, or housekeeping procedures are warranted when HIV is present. Standard decontamination procedures assume "worst case" conditions of extreme viral, bacterial, or other microbial contamination; therefore, extraordinary attempts to eliminate HIV are not required. For example, surfaces in patient care settings are usually cleaned on a regular basis as well as when spills occur. These decontamination procedures help prevent HIV transmission. Table 6.2 summarizes the methods for preparing equipment used in health care settings to limit HIV contamination.

For decontaminating spills of blood and other body fluids, a chemical germicide approved for use as a "hospital disinfectant" is recommended. The germicide should be applied to the spill by first surrounding the spill, then working in toward the center. Paper toweling should be placed on top of the liquid and a period of several minutes should elapse before the area is wiped clean to give the chemical time to react with the microorganisms. Fresh germicide should be used to treat the area a second time. Gloves should be worn at all times. For laundry, normal hygienic and commonsense procedures should be followed when dealing with soiled linens. Linen, for example, should be bagged where it was used, and bags that prevent leakage should be used. Similarly, infected gauze pads and other forms of waste that may contain HIV require no special procedure but should be handled as they would be to deal with any infectious microorganisms.

Exposures to HIV

Several medical centers have conducted ongoing studies of health care workers exposed to possible infection through contact with blood or body fluids from AIDS patients. In virtually all of these studies, the risk of transmission was found to be extremely low. For instance, researchers at the National Institutes of Health (NIH) tested 983 health care workers who were exposed to possible HIV infection through contact with patients or infected materials: 137 had suffered needle-stick injuries; 345 had experienced mucous membrane exposure; the remainder had miscellaneous exposures. None of the workers displayed evidence of HIV infection six months after exposure. Another study was conducted at the University of California, where 212 workers were tested after contact with infected blood; after six months, only one person had evidence of HIV infection.

One of the most comprehensive and long-range of such studies was performed by CDC researchers beginning on August 15, 1983, and terminating on April 20, 1989. In the study, 1449 health care workers were followed for a minimum of 1 year and tested for evidence of HIV exposure at intervals of 6 weeks and 3, 6, and 12 months after exposure. The workers came from throughout the

6.2 Suggested Methods for Processing Patient Care Equipment in Health Care Settings

Sterilization:	Destroys:	All forms of microbial life, including high numbers of bacterial spores.
	Methods:	Steam under pressure (autoclave), gas (ethylene oxide), dry heat, or immersion in EPA-approved chemical "sterilant" for prolonged period of time, e.g., 6-10 hours or according to manufacturers' instructions. Note: liquid chemical "sterilants" should be used only on those instruments that are impossible to sterilize or disinfect with heat.
	Use:	For those instruments or devices that penetrate skin or contact normally sterile areas of the body, e.g., scalpels and needles. Disposable invasive equipment eliminates the need to reprocess these types of items. When indicated, however, arrangements should be made with a health care facility for reprocessing of reusable invasive instruments.
High-Level Disinfection:	Destroys:	All forms of microbial life **except** high numbers of bacterial spores.
	Methods:	Hot water pasteurization (80-100°C, 30 minutes) or exposure to an EPA-registered "sterilant" chemical as above, except for a short exposure time (10-45 minutes or as directed by the manufacturer).
	Use:	For reusable instruments or devices that come into contact with mucous membranes (e.g., laryngoscope blades, endotracheal tubes).
Intermediate-Level Disinfection:	Destroys:	*Mycobacterium tuberculosis*, vegetative bacteria, most viruses, and most fungi, but does **not** kill bacterial spores.
	Methods:	EPA-registered "hospital disinfectant" chemical germicides that have a label claim for tuberculocidal activity; commercially available hard-surface germicides or solutions containing at least 500 ppm free available chlorine (a 1:100 dilution of common household bleach—approximately $1/4$ cup bleach per gallon of tap water).
	Use:	For those surfaces that come into contact only with intact skin, e.g., stethoscopes, blood pressure cuffs, and splints, and have been visibly contaminated with blood or bloody body fluids. Surfaces must be precleaned of visible material before the germicidal chemical is applied for disinfection.

TABLE			
6.2	**Suggested Methods for Processing Patient Care Equipment in Health Care Settings (Continued)**		
Low-Level Disinfection:	Destroys:	Most bacteria, some viruses, some fungi, but not *Mycobacterium tuberculosis* or bacterial spores.	
	Methods:	EPA-registered "hospital disinfectants" (**no** label claim for tuberculocidal activity).	
	Use:	These agents are excellent cleaners and can be used for routine housekeeping or removal of soiling in the **absence** of visible blood contamination.	
Environmental Disinfection:		Environmental surfaces that have become soiled should be cleaned and disinfected using any cleaner or disinfectant agent that is intended for environmental use. Such surfaces include floors, woodwork, ambulance seats, countertops, etc.	

IMPORTANT: To assure the effectiveness of any sterilization or disinfection process, equipment and instruments must first be thoroughly cleaned of all visible soil.

Source: Centers for Disease Control and Prevention.

United States, and had suffered needlestick injuries (80 percent), cuts with sharp objects (8 percent), contamination of open wounds (7 percent), and mucous membrane exposure (5 percent). They suffered exposures in different locations in the health care facilities and under different working conditions (Figure 6.8). Of 1172 health care workers with complete data as of April 1989, only four developed HIV infection, a total of less than 1 percent.

In its surveillance report on AIDS for 1995, the CDC summarized the number of cases of HIV infection and AIDS occurring in health care workers as a result of occupational exposure. As of December 31, 1994, over 440,000 cases of AIDS had been reported in the United States, and 42 health care workers (less than one hundredth of 1 percent of the total) were infected in documented occupational transmission. Another 91 workers (two hundredths of 1 percent of the total) were possibly infected during their work. Fifteen of the 42 cases occurred in laboratory technicians and 13 in nurses.

A more recent report was issued in June 2001. In that report, the CDC noted that the risk of HIV transmission through contact among health care workers is about 0.3 percent; through mucous membrane exposure, it is about 0.09 percent. The CDC has also received reports of 56 health care workers who contracted HIV while at work and 138 who may have done so through occupational exposure. Data such as these indicate that the risk of HIV transmission to health care workers during the normal course of their duties is extremely low. However, the findings do not justify a cavalier disregard of prudent precautions. This point was driven home when CDC officials reported three cases of HIV transmission via

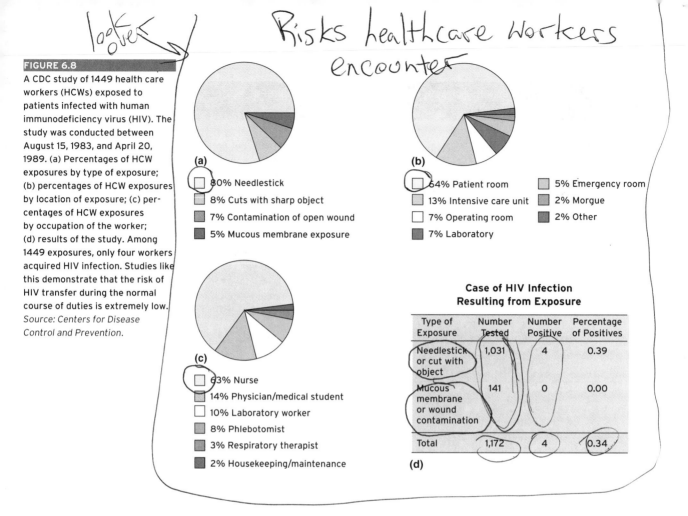

(handwritten: looK over, Risks healthcare Workers encounter)

FIGURE 6.8

A CDC study of 1449 health care workers (HCWs) exposed to patients infected with human immunodeficiency virus (HIV). The study was conducted between August 15, 1983, and April 20, 1989. (a) Percentages of HCW exposures by type of exposure; (b) percentages of HCW exposures by location of exposure; (c) percentages of HCW exposures by occupation of the worker; (d) results of the study. Among 1449 exposures, only four workers acquired HIV infection. Studies like this demonstrate that the risk of HIV transfer during the normal course of duties is extremely low.
Source: Centers for Disease Control and Prevention.

(a)
- 80% Needlestick
- 8% Cuts with sharp object
- 7% Contamination of open wound
- 5% Mucous membrane exposure

(b)
- 64% Patient room
- 13% Intensive care unit
- 7% Operating room
- 7% Laboratory
- 5% Emergency room
- 2% Morgue
- 2% Other

(c)
- 63% Nurse
- 14% Physician/medical student
- 10% Laboratory worker
- 8% Phlebotomist
- 3% Respiratory therapist
- 2% Housekeeping/maintenance

Case of HIV Infection Resulting from Exposure

Type of Exposure	Number Tested	Number Positive	Percentage of Positives
Needlestick or cut with object	1,031	4	0.39
Mucous membrane or wound contamination	141	0	0.00
Total	1,172	4	0.34

(d)

skin exposure to blood. In one case, a hospital worker was exposed to blood when she pressed gauze against the arm of an AIDS patient who was bleeding. In the second case, blood spilled onto the arms and hands of a worker manipulating a machine used to separate blood components. In both of these cases, workers had skin lesions or chapped skin, and neither was wearing gloves. In the third case, a rubber stopper popped off a glass tube, splattering blood onto the skin and into the mouth of a worker. CDC recommendations for reporting an occupational exposure are listed in Table 6.3.

Cases like these are rare, but they illustrate the need for caution in the health care setting (Box 6.2). The take-home message is brief and straightforward: Observe universal precautions and be careful!

Protecting Public Safety Workers

The general infection-control procedures outlined by the universal precautions apply not only to health care settings but also to any environment where workers contact other individuals and where microbial transmission can occur. Public safety workers perform their assignments in such environments. They hold positions as emergency medical technicians, firefighters, and law enforcement and correctional facility officers. Approximately 600,000 Americans are employed in these capacities.

Working in the public safety sector carries some risk of exposure to HIV. Exposure can be unpredictable, so protective measures should be used, even when the risk is not obvious. Because public safety workers perform their duties under extremely variable conditions, control measures must necessarily be simple and uniform to ensure compliance.

Fire and Emergency Medical Services

Among the workers considered in the general category of fire and emergency medical services are firefighters, paramedics, emergency medical technicians, and advanced-life-support personnel. Individuals in these professions perform their duties in prehospital, uncontrolled environments where time for decision making is extremely limited. Recommendations are made with these conditions in mind and under the basic premise that workers must be protected from exposure to blood and other body fluids that are potentially infectious. Accordingly, CDC epidemiologists recommend the following:

1. Disposable gloves should be a standard component of emergency response equipment and should be put on by all personnel prior to initiating any emergency care tasks involving exposure to blood or other body fluids to which universal precautions apply. Extra pairs should

TABLE 6.3	CDC Recommendations for Content of a Report on an Occupational Exposure to HIV
Date and time of exposure	
Details of the procedure being performed, including where and how the exposure occurred; if related to a sharp device, the type and brand of device and how and when in the course of handling the device the exposure occurred	
Details of the exposure, including the type and amount of fluid or material and the severity of the exposure (e.g., for a percutaneous exposure, depth of injury and whether fluid was injected; for a skin or mucous membrane exposure, the estimated volume of material and the condition of the skin [e.g., chapped, abraded, intact])	
Details about the exposure source (e.g., whether the source material contained HBV, HCV, or HIV; if the source is HIV-infected, the stage of disease, history of antiretroviral therapy, viral load, and antiretroviral resistance information, if known)	
Details about the exposed person (e.g., hepatitis B vaccination and vaccine-response status)	
Details about counseling, postexposure management, and follow-up	

BOX
6.2

"An Ounce of Prevention . . ."

The report of HIV infection or AIDS in a fellow worker at a health care facility can be an unsettling experience. Other employees will need reassurance that the workplace is safe and that the infection was probably acquired in the worker's private life. Still, some fear may remain that the workplace is dangerous, especially if it is a health care facility in which AIDS patients receive treatment. To minimize this concern and to reduce the risk of infection, a plan can be implemented to deal with potential or actual HIV infection among employees. The plan could include the following:

Education

Guest speakers, including specialists at the facility, can be invited to address health care workers on the various ramifications of AIDS. Reading materials can be supplied on the cause, transmission, diagnosis, and treatment of AIDS with emphasis on precautions taken while handling blood-contaminated materials. Besides reassuring employees, the sessions demonstrate management's concern about their well-being and its willingness to confront AIDS-related issues.

Protective Materials

Management can provide protective supplies to further demonstrate its commitment to employee safety via materials expenditures. Needle drop boxes and gloves (in small, medium, and large) can be placed in all work areas, and masks, goggles, and gowns can be made available. Containers of 10-percent bleach solution can be placed throughout the facility in case of spills. And employees can be taught precautionary safeguards such as glove replacement and how to clean up as spill.

Precautions Policy

A policy can be developed that stresses prevention first, but also guidance and support when workers contract or believe they may have contracted an infectious disease. Incorporation of employee concerns, legal considerations, and suggestions from human resource groups is essential to such policy development. The policy should include such issues as AIDS education, how employees who test positive for HIV will be evaluated, precautions against infection, insurance coverage, and rights to privacy.

Working with AIDS patients is often a stressful situation. But health care workers can act more intelligently if they know enough to protect themselves. Both responsible management and employee compliance can contribute to stress reduction.

always be available. Considerations in the choice of disposable gloves should include dexterity, durability, fit, and the task being performed. For situations where large amounts of blood are likely to be encountered, gloves should fit tightly at the wrist, to prevent contamination of hands by blood seepage around the cuff. For multiple trauma victims, gloves should be changed between patient contacts, if the emergency situation allows. More extensive personal protective equipment measures are indicated for situations in which broken glass and sharp edges are likely to be encountered, such as when extricating a person from an automobile wreck.

2. Masks, eyewear, and gowns should be carried in all emergency vehicles that respond to medical emergencies or victim rescues. These protective barriers should be used in accordance with the level of exposure encountered. Minor lacerations or small amounts of blood do not require the same barrier use as is required with victims who are bleeding heavily, either externally or internally. Masks and eyewear (including safety glasses) should be worn together or faceshields should be used, and these should be put on by all personnel before beginning work in any situation where splashes of blood or other body fluids are likely to occur. If large splashes or quantities of blood are present or anticipated, impervious gowns or aprons should be worn. An extra change of work clothing should be available at all times.

3. For artificial ventilation of trauma victims, disposable airway equipment or resuscitation bags should be used. Disposable resuscitation equipment and devices should be used only once. If reusable, they should be thoroughly cleaned and disinfected after each use, according to the manufacturer's recommendations. In addition, mechanical respiratory assist devices (for example, bag-valve masks, oxygen demand valve resuscitators) should be available on all emergency vehicles and to all emergency response personnel during any medical emergency or victim rescue. Pocket mouth-to-mouth resuscitation masks designed to isolate emergency response personnel (the so-called double lumen systems) from contact with victims' blood and blood-contaminated saliva, respiratory secretions, and vomitus should be available all personnel who provide emergency treatment. Table 6.4 summarizes recommended personal equipment that should be used for protection in the prehospital setting.

Law Enforcement Officers

Law enforcement officers risk exposure to HIV if they encounter blood while performing their duties. At a crime scene, for instance, police officers may need to handle blood-contaminated materials or help remove a body. In correctional facilities, officers may encounter contaminated syringes and needles during searches, or they may have to subdue disruptive inmates. Epidemiologists make certain recommendations. For law enforcement officers to reduce the risk of acquiring HIV in the normal course of a day's events. They point out, however, that an extremely diverse range of potential situations exists, and the informed judgment of the officer is paramount when unusual events present themselves. Among the guidelines are the following:

1. Law enforcement officers are exposed to a range of fights and assaults, during which they may be exposed to blood or blood-contaminated materials. In cases such as these, appropriate protection should be worn if feasible and as conditions permit. For instance, gloves should be put on

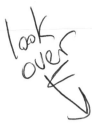

TABLE 6.4 Examples of Recommended Personal Protective Equipment for Worker Protection against HIV Transmission in Prehospital Settings*

Task or Activity	Disposable Gloves	Gown	Mask	Protective Eyewear
Bleeding control with spurting blood	Yes	Yes	Yes	Yes
Bleeding control with minimal bleeding	Yes	No	No	No
Emergency childbirth	Yes	Yes	Yes, if splashing is likely	Yes, if splashing is likely
Blood drawing	At certain times	No	No	No
Starting an intra-venous (IV) line	Yes	No	No	No
Endotracheal intubation, esophageal obturator use	Yes	No	No, unless splashing is likely	No, unless splashing is likely
Oral/nasal suction-ing, manually cleaning airway	Yes	No	No, unless splashing is likely	No, unless splashing is likely
Handling and cleaning instru-ments with micro-bial contamination	Yes	No, unless soiling is likely	No	No
Measuring blood pressure	No	No	No	No
Measuring temperature	No	No	No	No
Giving an injection	No	No	No	No

* Defined as settings where delivery of emergency health care takes place before arrival at hospital or other health care facility.

Source: Centers for Disease Control and Prevention.

and a change of clothing should be available if blood is splattered (Healthline 6.3).

2. Exposure to HIV may occur during cardiopulmonary resuscitation (CPR), so protective masks and airways should be available to officers and training should be given in their use.

3. During searches and evidence handling, an officer may come in contact with HIV, especially through a puncture wound with a blood-contaminated needle. Therefore, individual discretion should be used to determine if a prisoner should empty his or her own pockets, and protective gloves should be worn for all body cavity searches. Long-handled mirrors and flashlights should be used to search hidden areas such as above ceilings or under car seats. Purses should be searched by turning them over and emptying the contents onto a table. Puncture-proof containers should be available for sharp objects.

Prison populations in all states include individuals at high risk for AIDS. For example, injection drug users often continue their drug use while in prison, and illegal tattoo machines are available among prisoners. Homosexual practices also occur in prisons. Corrections officers thus can come in contact with HIV-infected persons on a regular basis and should take appropriate precautions.

An interesting dilemma has arisen regarding the education of inmates. In the outside community, risk reduction measures for HIV exposure are emphasized, but such measures are not feasible in prisons. Condom use, for example, is strongly advised in the community, but within prison confines, homosexual practices are prohibited and punished, so the risk reduction afforded by the use of condoms cannot be encouraged. Similarly, needle disinfection is advocated in the community, but drug use in prison is not tolerated, so risk reduction measures for needle users are not promulgated. The discrepancies between recommended public health measures and prison practices have evoked legal issues. For example, inmates argue that they should be taught how to avoid the risky consequences of their behavior, but prison officials often disagree. These questions are currently being tested in the court system.

AIDS Education in the Schools

Public health experts generally agree that education is the most valuable tool against the spread of HIV infection and AIDS. But, they advise, an AIDS education program must be carefully constructed. It must, for example, deal with the public health threat of AIDS while taking positive health behavior into account. In addition, it must consider an array of moral, religious, and legal values.

Education programs can be effective in preventing the spread of HIV, because the virus is transmitted almost exclusively by behaviors that individuals can modify. With this in mind, the CDC has promulgated a number of guidelines for school health education to

Healthline 6.3

1

Q Have any AIDS researchers contracted HIV infection during the course of their work?

A Yes. In the fall of 1987, federal officials reported that two laboratory researchers had contracted HIV, apparently in the course of their work. In both cases, the workers came in contact with liquid containing HIV. The first worker sustained a cut through a glove and was apparently contaminated with HIV; the second had numerous cuts and abrasions of the hand through which the virus may have passed.

2

Q I am an EMT (emergency medical technician) whose hands are chronically chapped. Would you recommend that I wear gloves?

A While there is virtually no evidence that HIV can penetrate intact skin, the risk of transmission increases if the hands are chronically chapped. For your job, public health officials recommend that gloves be worn as often as possible.

3

Q As a police officer, I cannot always stop and put on a pair of gloves when I anticipate contacting blood. What should I do?

A Precautions suggested for public safety workers such as EMTs, police officers, and firefighters must be used on a commonsense basis. The situation dictates whether gloves or other protective devices can be used. If contact with blood is made, the skin should be washed thoroughly with hot, soapy water. A general antiseptic should then be applied if available.

prevent the spread of AIDS. It stipulated, however, that the specific scope and content of AIDS education in schools should be determined locally and should be consistent with parental and community values. Essentially, the proposed curriculum was designed to ensure that students understand the nature of the AIDS epidemic and the specific actions they can take to prevent HIV infection.

The CDC guidelines advocate that school systems advise students to abstain from sexual intercourse and intravenous drug use as ways of avoiding HIV. Those students who engage in sexual intercourse or inject drugs should be encouraged not to do so. For students unwilling to adopt less risky behaviors, the school program should advise them to (1) avoid sexual intercourse with infected persons, (2) use condoms, (3) seek treatment for drug addiction, (4) avoid sharing needles, and (5) seek HIV counseling if they suspect they are infected.

In the AIDS education curriculum, students should learn the biology of AIDS as well as the emotional and social factors that influence the spread of HIV (Figure 6.9). Accordingly, in the early elementary grades, teachers should allay the fears of young children that they will become infected. Emphasis should be placed on the facts that AIDS is hard to get, that AIDS primarily affects adults, and that researchers are actively seeking a cure for the disease.

Once students reach the late elementary and middle school grades, the curriculum could encompass discussions about the nature of viruses, including their transmission and disease potential. Brief information can be communicated about the symptoms of AIDS, the estimated infected population, the ubiquitous nature of the disease, methods for transmitting the virus, and how the virus is not transmitted.

For students at the junior and senior high school levels, the breadth of AIDS education can be considerable. The three major methods of transmission can be studied in depth, and risk factors can be explored, including how risks are increased and reduced. Protective devices for sexual intercourse and precautions for injection drug use can be discussed, and consideration for others can be emphasized. Counseling should be encouraged to increase student understanding of AIDS and to explain how testing can be performed to give students a clearer understanding of their HIV status.

Another AIDS-related educational issue in secondary school: concerns the use of blood in school laboratories (Box 6.3). But, among the most controversial issues that secondary schools must address is whether to distribute condoms to students. Proponents point to their desire to save lives, but opponents are equally vociferous about sending the message that promiscuous sex is condoned. Proponents counter that students must have parental permission to obtain condoms and must take the initiative to get them in an appropriate place such as a nurse's office, while opponents counter that providing condoms will give the incorrect impression that wearing them makes sex completely safe. Proponents counter that parents can opt their children out of the program, while opponents ponder the psychological effects of such a decision on the child. As the debates continue, school officials continue to advocate AIDS education programs.

It bears mention that any AIDS education campaign must be carefully thought out, as illustrated by a serious mistake made in the mid-1980s in Mexico. A government campaign was warning teens to avoid casual sex, but it also reassured them that casual contact would not spread AIDS. The campaign did not seem to be working until a psychologist found out why: In the local vernacular, "casual sex" and "casual contact" were both interpreted to mean the same thing— sex without commitment. What had begun as a campaign to stop AIDS instead was helping to spread it. The lesson was clear: Halting the AIDS epidemic requires attention to local customs, traditions, and language.

LOOKING BACK

Preventing the spread of AIDS is a task that can be accomplished by individuals at risk for acquiring human immunodeficiency virus (HIV). Individuals, for example, can interrupt the passage of HIV by avoiding sexual intercourse with multiple partners and by not using injection drugs. Those who continue to have multiple sexual partners should use devices such as condoms to form a barrier between semen and the tissues of the sexual partner. Condoms protect both the wearer and his sexual partner.

Safer sex practices can also be utilized to prevent semen passage and, by inference, HIV passage. Activities taking place outside the body are considered safer sex practices. Women can use vaginal foams and gels as well as microbicides that block HIV entry to cells. Those who use injection drugs can interrupt the spread of AIDS by disinfecting drug paraphernalia with a chemical such as bleach and

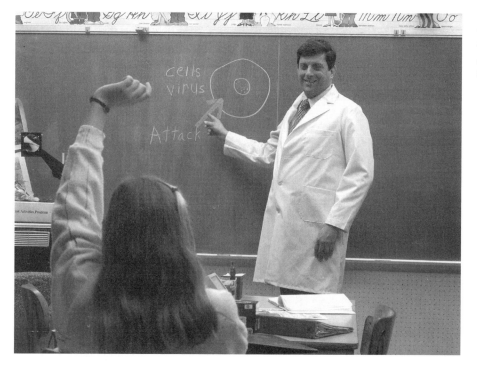

FIGURE 6.9
The breadth of AIDS education in the schools should be considerable, especially in view of the susceptibility of students to HIV.

BOX
6.3

End of the Blood Typing Lab?

"I couldn't believe all the students in this A/P lab who took alcohol swabs and set them down on the lab tables instead of discarding them right into the hazardous waste bag . . . And then this one girl pricked herself with another girl's used lancet!! I asked her if she realized what she did and she said 'Yes, but (Laura) is a good Christian girl.'"

Letter from a student

One of the outfalls of the AIDS epidemic has been a serious reconsideration of the use of human blood in the high school and college teaching laboratory, particularly in the exercise involving blood typing. In this exercise, blood is obtained from each student by pricking a fingertip with a lancet. Drops of blood are then placed on a slide and combined with anti-A, anti-B, and anti-Rh sera to determine which antigens are present on the red blood cells and what the blood type is.

Although it is statistically unlikely that a student is unknowingly carrying HIV, nevertheless it is possible. If so, then HIV transmission during blood typing could conceivably occur in the following ways: blood lancets may inadvertently be placed in wastebaskets where they pose a hazard to custodians and other students; students may bleed excessively and deposit fresh blood on the desk or other surface where other individuals can contact it; cotton or gauze is often used to wipe excess blood from the fingertip, and cotton or gauze dropped in a wastebasket can be dangerous to others; slides containing blood may be dropped and broken, and the broken pieces may pierce the skin and inoculate HIV if present; the procedure of slide cleaning may bring the technical staff in contact with contaminated blood, and if skin blisters or cuts are present, HIV transmission could occur.

For teachers and professors who consider it essential to demonstrate the principles of blood typing, alternative methods may suffice. For example, screened blood from a local blood bank may be employed. Computer simulations are also available, and video software can be purchased for showing in class. Disposable blood typing cards can be obtained from biological supply companies to eliminate slide washing at the end of the exercise. Regardless of whether instructors choose to discontinue blood typing or be more cautious than in the past, they should at the very least consider the value of reducing the risk of HIV transmission.

by refusing to share drug paraphernalia. Needle exchange programs are also an efficient way of reducing HIV transfer.

To interrupt the spread of HIV among health care workers, the CDC has promulgated universal precautions that all such workers should observe. Barrier measures, hand-washing, injury precautions, and care for abraded skin are among the key recommendations. Special precautions are also promulgated for invasive procedures, dentistry, autopsy and embalming, and medical laboratories.

Some risk of HIV transmission exists for public safety workers, especially when contact is made with blood. Risk reduction recommendations are therefore made by the CDC for firefighters, emergency medical personnel, and law enforcement and correctional officers. Gloves and other barrier protections are suggested. Informed judgment and common sense are paramount when unusual events present themselves.

One method for preventing the spread of AIDS is through education in the schools, beginning in the elementary grades and proceeding through the high school years. Student surveys indicate a desire to know about AIDS and reveal certain misperceptions that require correction. Among the more controversial issues facing secondary schools is whether to distribute condoms to students.

REVIEW

Having completed this chapter, you should be familiar with methods by which the spread of HIV can be interrupted. To test your knowledge, place a T to the left of a statement if it is true or an F if it is false. Correct answers are listed in Appendix A.

__F__ **1.** A lighted match is an excellent way for injection drug users to sterilize their needles.

__T__ **2.** One method by which health care workers can be exposed to HIV-contaminated blood is through needlestick injuries.

__T__ **3.** The universal precautions promulgated by the CDC are recommendations for all health care workers.

__F__ **4.** A condom prevents the passage of bacteria from the semen to the man's sex partner but does not prevent the passage of viruses.

__T__ **5.** The agents of sexually transmitted diseases, including AIDS, are generally unable to withstand exposures to the outside environment that other microorganisms can tolerate.

__F__ **6.** In controlled laboratory studies, natural lambskin condoms were found to be more effective for preventing HIV passage than latex condoms.

__T__ **7.** Law enforcement officers may be exposed to HIV-contaminated blood when they suffer needlestick injury while conducting a search.

__F__ **8.** AIDS education in the lower school grades should begin with descriptions of HIV and include a thorough grounding in sex education, including condom use.

__T__ **9.** One of the most effective germicides for destroying the AIDS virus is a solution of bleach in water at a concentration of 1 percent to 10 percent.

_T_ **10.** Health care workers should assume that all patients are infected with HIV in their blood and other body fluids.

_F_ **11.** Disposable gloves need not be carried in emergency response equipment because technicians rarely encounter accident victims who are infected with HIV.

_F_ **12.** One widely adopted way of interrupting the spread of AIDS among prison inmates is to distribute clean, sterile needles to drug addicts.

_F_ **13.** Medical laboratory technicians should pipet liquids by mouth because the probability of dealing with HIV-contaminated fluids is very low.

_T_ **14.** Funeral directors and embalmers should be concerned about exposure to HIV because the virus may be present in the blood, other body fluids, and organs of the deceased.

_T_ **15.** Abstinence from sexual intercourse and avoiding injection drug use are effective methods for avoiding exposure to HIV.

FOR ADDITIONAL READING

Adler, T. 1995. "Debugging blood: protecting people from tainted blood." *Science News* 147:92–95.

Bell, D. M. 1997. "Occupational risk of human immunodeficiency virus infection in healthcare workers: An overview." *Am. J. Med.* 102 (suppl. 5B): 9–15.

Benowitz, S. 1997. "Politics polarizing issues in needle-exchange programs." *The Scientist*, February 3.

Blumenthal, R. N., et al. 1999. "Collateral damage in the war on drugs: HIV risk behaviors among injection drug users." *Intl. J. Drug Policy* 10: 25–38.

Brainard, J. 1998. "HIV's quiet accomplice?" *Science* 154: 158–160.

Centers for Disease Control. 1987. "Recommendations for prevention of HIV transmission in health-care settings." *MMWR* 36(25): 3–18.

———. 1988. "Guidelines for effective school health education to prevent the spread of AIDS." *MMWR* 37(52): 1–14.

———. 1989. "Guidelines for prevention of transmission of human immunodeficiency virus and hepatitis B to health-care and public safety *workers.*" *MMWR* 38(56): 1–37.

Ciesielski, C., et al. 1992. "Transmission of human immunodeficiency virus in a dental practice." *Ann. Inter. Med.* 116: 798–805.

Coates, T. J., and C. Collins. 1998. "Preventing HIV infection." *Scientific American*, July.

Hein, K. 1998. "Aligning science with politics and policy in HIV prevention." *Science* 280: 1905–1907.

Levy, J. 1993. "Pathogenesis of human immunodeficiency virus infection." *Microbiol. Revs.* 57: 183–289.

Lifson, A. R. 1995. "Do alternate modes of transmission of human immunodeficiency virus exist? A review." *JAMA* 259: 1353–1356.

Rogers, A. S., et al. 1993. "Investigation of potential HIV transmission to the patients of an HIV-infected surgeon." *JAMA* 269: 1798–1801.

Rosendahl, I. 2001. "Needle-exchange programs gain ground." *Medical Laboratory Observer,* July.

Valdiserri, R. O., D. R. Holtgrave, and R. M. Brackbill. 1993. "American adults' knowledge of HIV testing availability." *Am. J. Public Health* 83: 525–528.

Wang, S. A., et al. 2000. "Experience of health care workers taking post-exposure prophylaxis after occupational HIV exposures." *Infect. Control Hosp. Epidemiol.* 21: 780–785.

HIV Testing and Diagnosis

LOOKING AHEAD

In contemporary medicine, laboratory tests provide essential information relative to a physician's diagnosis and help ensure that the diagnosis is correct. This chapter surveys some of the procedures used in laboratory testing for HIV infection and AIDS. On completing the chapter, you should be able to . . .

- Summarize the general approach used by physicians to diagnose HIV infection and AIDS.
- Describe the various laboratory tests available to assist the diagnosis of HIV infection and understand the scientific basis for each test.
- Conceptualize how different laboratory tests seek to detect antibodies produced against HIV or chemical components of HIV.
- Summarize how gene probes work and specify the value of the polymerase chain reaction in HIV testing.
- Discuss the meaning of viral load, describe how the viral load is determined, and summarize some advantages of knowing an HIV infected person's viral load.
- Understand the limits of laboratory tests for HIV infection and AIDS and specify some of the drawbacks to each test.
- Summarize the controversies surrounding interpretation and use of the results from laboratory tests with special reference to voluntary testing and mandatory testing.

INTRODUCTION

For many centuries, physicians practiced heroic medicine to save patients from the ravages of disease. They prescribed frightening courses of blood-lettings and purges, and they subjected patients to enormous doses of strange medicines and concoctions, ice-water baths, starvation, and other drastic remedies. These treatments probably made an already bad situation worse by reducing the body's natural defenses to the point of exhaustion.

Then, during the 1820s, a group of physicians in Boston and London experimented to see what would happen if they withheld treatment from patients and let nature take its course. Surprisingly, they found survival rates of untreated patients similar to and sometimes better than those of treated patients. As word of their experiments gradually spread, many of the worst features of heroic medicine began to disappear. A more conservative, nonmeddling approach to disease developed, and physicians sharpened their skills as diagnosticians. Their job was to recognize a certain illness, distinguish it from other illnesses, explain it to the family, and attempt to predict what would happen in the future. Then they would care for the patient within the limits of what was known.

Today's physicians understand the role of microorganisms in disease, and they have available numerous therapies and preventatives to help control disease. Nevertheless, their skills as diagnosticians must remain acute because they are usually the first health care providers we seek out when we are ill. And, in the effort to interrupt the AIDS epidemic, HIV testing is a key diagnostic tool because physicians can identify those who harbor the human immunodeficiency virus and counsel them on measures to prevent its spread. Also, partner notification may follow diagnosis when circumstances warrant, and infected individuals can be evaluated for drug treatment for HIV and preventative therapy for opportunistic diseases. Finally, the statistics generated from HIV testing and diagnosis help agencies plan medical and social support programs while providing a framework for interrupting the spread of the AIDS epidemic.

In this chapter, we shall discuss the laboratory methods used for detecting HIV and helping physicians identify HIV infection and AIDS. Considering the advanced state of biotechnology, these methods tend to be complex. We shall also explore the implications of HIV testing and the conflicting views on how test results should be used. These are among the more controversial issues associated with the AIDS epidemic.

HIV Antibody Tests

To even the casual observer, it is obvious that the most direct diagnostic method for HIV infection is identifying the human immunodeficiency virus in the body tissues. As we shall discuss presently, such a test is available, but the more cost-effective way of detecting HIV infection is to locate antibodies produced against the virus rather than the virus itself. These antibody methods are accurate and reliable, within certain limitations.

Any laboratory test for detecting antibodies is called a serological test, because it involves a patient's serum (Healthline 7.1). The patient who tests positive has the antibodies sought by the test and is said to be seropositive. By contrast, the patient who tests negative lacks the antibodies and is termed seronegative. One other bit of diagnostic jargon: A patient seroconverts when the serum tests positive.

1 Q I've heard that the typical AIDS tests do not directly determine if HIV is in your body. What do they really determine?

A The AIDS tests most often used are not direct tests for HIV. Rather, they are tests for HIV antibodies, the proteins produced by the body's immune system when HIV enters the body. The theory is that when a person has been exposed to HIV, the blood contains HIV antibodies. Therefore, a positive test means that antibodies are present and that exposure has taken place sometime in the past. The test is thus an indirect test.

2 Q Does a positive HIV antibody test mean you have AIDS?

A No, a positive test merely means that you have been exposed to HIV and that some form of the virus is very likely still in your body. No one can predict whether you will develop AIDS. The test only indicates that you currently have HIV infection. Of course, if you have other recognizable symptoms of AIDS, then the test confirms the diagnosis.

3 Q After I took an AIDS test, the physician said that I had not seroconverted and that I was seronegative. What do those words mean?

A Serum is the clear fluid of the blood where antibodies are dissolved; it is used to test for HIV antibodies. When the serum gives a positive reaction (HIV antibodies are present), the person has seroconverted and is said to be seropositive. By contrast, if no reaction occurs (no HIV antibodies), the doctor uses the term "seronegative," as in your case, and says you have not seroconverted.

In most cases, serological tests are used to detect the presence of disease. They are based on the supposition that when the body is exposed to an infectious agent, such as HIV, the immune system reacts through the process of either antibody-mediated immunity or cell-mediated immunity (Chapter 3). Certain tests, such as the tuberculosis skin test, are designed to detect the products of cellular immunity, but most bacterial and viral tests identify the products of antibody-mediated immunity—the antibodies. Since serological tests do not detect the infectious agent itself, they are indirect tests.

For the diagnosis of HIV infection and AIDS, a number of antibody-based serological tests are available to the physician. Two such tests, the enzyme-linked immunosorbent assay and the western blot analysis, are routinely used to detect and confirm HIV antibodies in the blood. Though the theories behind the tests are somewhat involved, performing the tests is routine for trained, licensed technicians.

Enzyme-Linked Immunosorbent Assay (ELISA)

Currently, the most widely used diagnostic test for HIV infection is an antibody-based test called the enzyme-linked immunosorbent assay, or ELISA. Through July 2002, the Food and Drug Administration (FDA) had licensed five different manufacturers to produce ELISA kits for the U.S. Market. Laboratories may use any of the eight kits for their diagnostic tests.

Each of the ELISA kits uses the same general procedure: A sample of a patient's serum is added to HIV antigens (protein fragments of HIV). These antigens are bound to beads or coated along the walls of tiny wells (Figure 7.1). The mixture is incubated for a period of time to permit antibodies in the serum to attach to (immunosorb to) the HIV antigens. Next, enzyme molecules linked to antibodies are added to the mixture. The antibodies, in this case, are produced by horses injected with human antibodies. The horse's immune system views the human antibodies as foreign substances and produces antibodies against them. These "antihuman" antibodies are then isolated from the horse's blood and chemically linked to a highly specific enzyme for use in the test.

Once the enzyme-linked antibodies have been mixed in, the reagents are permitted to react. Then the residual enzyme-linked antibodies are washed away. Next, the technician adds a substrate, that is, a chemical compound that will react with the enzyme, When the substrate reacts with the enzyme, a color change takes

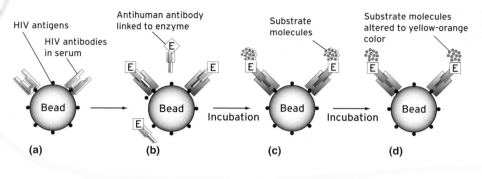

FIGURE 7.1

A positive ELISA test. (a) HIV antigens are bound to microscopic beads. A serum sample containing HIV antibodies is added to the beads and the mixture is shaken. The HIV antibodies bind to the HIV antigens. (b) A sample of enzyme-linked antihuman antibodies is added. The enzyme-linked antibodies bind to the HIV antibodies on the surface of the beads. (c) Substrate molecules are added. (d) Enzyme molecules on the bead surface alter the substrate molecules and change their color to a yellow-orange that can be detected by a color-sensing instrument. The reaction shows that HIV antibodies are in the serum sample.

place; depending on whether the color change occurs, the technologist can infer whether the serum had HIV antibodies or lacked them. Figure 7.1 displays how a positive test works.

The ELISA test is complex, but you should make the effort to understand what is taking place (Healthline 7.2). Given the medical and social significance of a positive ELISA test, the results must be accurate (i.e., it must be possible to unambiguously distinguish negative results from positive results), and interpretation of the results must be correct. In one survey, when 601 test laboratories ("participating laboratories") performed the ELISA test on samples identical to those tested by 15 established laboratories ("referee laboratories"), the results showed a very close correlation. This observation indicates that the ELISA test can be performed by different laboratories with accurate results.

Clinical data submitted by ELISA kit manufacturers to the FDA indicate that both the sensitivity and the specificity of their kits exceed 99 percent. *Sensitivity* refers to the probability of a positive test resulting when the serum sample has antibodies; for ELISA, the sensitivity is greater than 99 percent. *Specificity* refers to the probability of a negative test when the serum sample lacks antibodies; for ELISA, the specificity is also greater than 99 percent. Indeed, the American Red Cross Blood Services laboratories have reported that a 99.8 percent specificity was consistently achieved during testing of donated blood for transfusion purposes.

In current laboratory practice, a sample of serum that tests negative (or "nonreactive") is considered free of HIV antibodies. If a sample tests positive (or "reactive"), the results are reported as "initially reactive," and the sample is retested twice (Figure 7.2). If both retests yield negative results, the sample is reported as "nonreactive for HIV antibodies." However if either or both retest yields positive results, the sample is reported as "repeatedly reactive for HIV antibodies." Under these conditions, the ELISA test results should be validated by an independent supplemental test. In the United States, the validation test most often used is the western blot analysis. We shall examine that test next.

A ELISA stands for enzyme-linked immunosorbent assay. It is a laboratory test in which the fluid part of the blood (the serum) is mixed with specific reagents to see whether HIV antibodies are present in the blood. A color change at the end of the test signals that the antibodies are present (the test is "reactive," or "positive");·no color change indicates the absence of antibodies (the test is "nonreactive," or "negative").

2 Q Suppose the ELISA test gives a positive result. What happens then?

A Should the ELISA test give a positive result, the test will be repeated in duplicate. If both succeeding tests yield negative results, then the test result is reported as "negative." If, however, either or both yield positive results, then a confirmatory test is used to validate the results.

3 Q What test is used to validate the ELISA test?

A In the United States, the western blot analysis is currently the test of choice for validation. This test, like the ELISA test, is AIDS antibody test, but it is more expensive and difficult to perform, and it detects multiple and more specialized HIV antibodies. If the results of the western blot analysis are positive, then the HIV-positive status is confirmed; if negative, then the ELISA test may have to be repeated.

Western Blot Analysis

The western blot analysis is a variation of a procedure devised in the 1970s by British investigator E. M. Southern. Southern used his procedure to separate fragments of DNA and identify them. He began with a standard laboratory technique called gel electrophoresis. The basic principle of gel electrophoresis is that molecules dissolved in a gel of agarose will respond to an electrical field and move through the gel according to fragment size (Figure 7.3). Usually, the smaller fragments move faster than the larger fragments. Once separated, the DNA fragments are transferred to filter paper by placing the gel in contact with the paper. The paper draws the fragments out of the gel, literally blotting them exactly as they were positioned in the gel. This procedure came to be known as the Southern blot technique.

When this technique was adapted to study fragments of RNA instead of DNA, it was whimsically named the "northern" blot procedure. Further adaptation was needed when analyzing protein molecules such as those from viruses, so researchers modified the technique and devised the "western" blot analysis. (There is no "eastern" blot analysis yet.)

The western blot analysis is used as a confirmatory test when an ELISA test has given a positive result. In the laboratory, HIV proteins from laboratory cultures are separated by gel electrophoresis. Such proteins as gp41 and gp120 are used. Then the proteins are transferred to a special nitrocellulose paper by blotting the paper against the gel. Next, a person's serum is diluted and added to the paper. If HIV antibodies are present, they bind to their complementary viral proteins (that is, gp41 antibody binds to gp4l protein, while gp120 antibody binds to gp120 protein).

Because these reactions are invisible, the product of the reaction is made visible by adding a staining reagent. The reagent consists of stain combined with commercially prepared antihuman antibodies. These antibodies react with human HIV antibodies. The stain gathers where HIV antibodies have accumulated, and distinctive bands of color appear on the paper when the person is seropositive (Figure 7.4). The bands correspond to different HIV proteins separated from one another in the electrophoresis step. Obviously, if no HIV antibodies were in the serum, no reaction with HIV antigens would take place, and no stain would be attracted to the nitrocellulose paper. The absence of stained bands indicates that the person is seronegative.

For the western blot analysis, antibodies reacting with at least three specified HIV antigens must be detected for the test to be considered positive (Table 7.1). Thus, the western blot analysis is more specific than

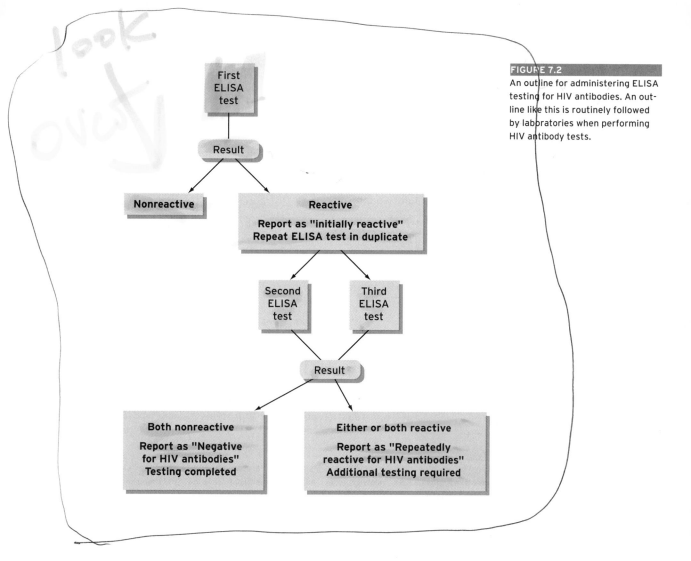

look over

FIGURE 7.2

An outline for administering ELISA testing for HIV antibodies. An outline like this is routinely followed by laboratories when performing HIV antibody tests.

First ELISA test

Result

Nonreactive

Reactive

Report as "initially reactive"
Repeat ELISA test in duplicate

Second ELISA test

Third ELISA test

Result

Both nonreactive

Report as "Negative for HIV antibodies"
Testing completed

Either or both reactive

Report as "Repeatedly reactive for HIV antibodies"
Additional testing required

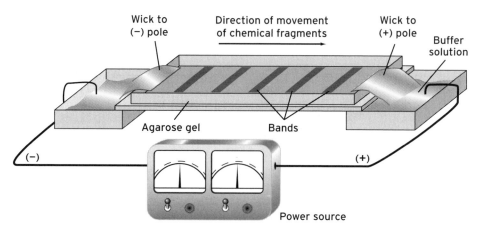

Wick to (−) pole

Direction of movement of chemical fragments

Wick to (+) pole

Buffer solution

Agarose gel

Bands

(−)

(+)

Power source

FIGURE 7.3

An electrophoresis apparatus such as that used in the western blot analysis. An electrical power source maintains positive (+) and negative (−) charges in two buffer solutions. Wicks connect the agarose gel to the buffer solutions. Chemical fragments move through the electrically charged gel according to their sizes. Bands form where the movements of different size fragments come to an end.

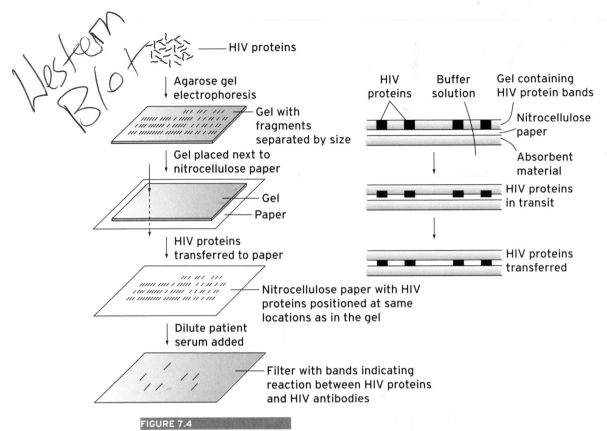

Western Blot

— HIV proteins

Agarose gel electrophoresis

Gel with fragments separated by size

Gel placed next to nitrocellulose paper

Gel

Paper

HIV proteins transferred to paper

Nitrocellulose paper with HIV proteins positioned at same locations as in the gel

Dilute patient serum added

Filter with bands indicating reaction between HIV proteins and HIV antibodies

HIV proteins   Buffer solution   Gel containing HIV protein bands

Nitrocellulose paper

Absorbent material

HIV proteins in transit

HIV proteins transferred

FIGURE 7.4

The western blot analysis. (a) HIV proteins (antigens) are separated by agarose gel electrophoresis, as shown in Figure 7.3. The proteins form bands in the electrophoresis gel. (b) When the gel is placed next to a nitrocellulose paper in a buffer solution, the solution carries the proteins to the paper and deposits them there (right side of diagram). (c) The result is a paper containing the proteins positioned in the same place as they are on the gel. (d) Finally, a sample of diluted patient serum is added. If HIV exposure has taken place, different HIV antibodies will react with different HIV proteins, and when a staining reagent is added, the stain will gather where the antibody-protein reaction has taken place and form distinctive bands of color. The bands indicate that the person is seropositive. No bands of color will develop if the person is seronegative.

the ELISA test (where a mixture of "generalized" HIV antibodies is detected). For western blot analyses that are inconclusive (e.g., only one or two HIV antigens detected), the results are reported as "indeterminate."

As with the ELISA test, the sensitivity and specificity of the western blot analysis exceed 99 percent, as long as certain criteria are met. However, if a laboratory chooses to use different western blot reagents or unlicensed tests or less stringent interpretive methods, then the 99-percent levels of sensitivity and specificity may not hold, since these are determined under carefully controlled conditions. Laboratories can also ensure the reliability of test results by training their personnel carefully, establishing quality controls, and participating in perfor-

Organization	Criteria
Association of State and Territorial Public Health Laboratory Directors/CDC	Any two of: • p24 • gp41 • gp120/gp160*
FDA-licensed Du Pont test	p24 and p31 and gp41 or gp120/gp160
American Red Cross	≥ 3 bands—1 from each gene-product group: • *gag* and • *pol* and • *env*
Consortium for Retrovirus Serology Standardization	≥ 2 bands: p24 or p31, plus • gp41 or • gp120/gp160

*Distinguishing the gp120 band from the gp160 band is often very difficult. These two glycoproteins can be considered as one reactant for purposes of interpreting western blot test results.

Source: Centers for Disease Control and Prevention.

mance evaluation programs administered by public health agencies. Standardization of test kits and attention to technical proficiency also boost confidence in test results.

False Positives and Negatives

Since the ELISA test was introduced in 1985, its results, validated by the western blot analysis, have been used to make many medical and personal decisions. For example, millions of donated pints of blood have been screened using the tests, and only those units testing negative for HIV antibodies are used for transfusion. Donated organs have also been tested and assumed safe for transplant if HIV antibody tests are negative. And the shaping of personal behaviors (e.g., whether to use a condom) has been influenced by the results of HIV tests.

Yet it is common knowledge that the antibody tests are not absolutely perfect. Since 1985, several cases of AIDS have been related to transfused blood previously tested negative for HIV antibodies. Moreover, several individuals who believed they had HIV infection on the basis of antibody tests were later found to have no trace of the virus when their tissues were examined. It is possible, therefore, that HIV antibody tests (ELISA and western blot analysis) can give false negative and false positive results. A false negative result (or false negative) is one that indicates HIV is absent when, in fact, it is present in the body. A false posi-

1 Q Could I be infected with HIV and still give a negative result on an HIV antibody test?

A Yes. In a few cases, a person has been infected with HIV but the immune system has not had enough time to produce sufficient HIV antibodies to show up as a positive test result. The test will therefore give a negative result, a so-called false negative. Under these circumstances, one could mistakenly believe that no HIV is present and infect others.

2 Q Does a positive antibody test necessarily mean that I am infected with HIV?

A A positive test result does not have to signify infection with HIV. In a few cases, the laboratory has erred in performing the test, or it may be possible that HIV antibodies have neutralized all the HIV that entered the body. In the latter case, the person will continue to have a positive result because the antibodies remain long after the viruses have disappeared. The test result is a false positive.

3 Q What does "anonymous testing" mean?

A Some states offer free testing for individuals who perform high-risk behaviors so that those persons can learn if they have suffered HIV exposure. At the testing center, the person is given a number, then the technician takes a small amount of blood for testing. Some days later, the test results are listed by number and given to the person having that number, along with counseling on the meaning of the results. No names or addresses are ever requested or used.

tive result (false positive) occurs when evidence indicates the presence of HIV in the body when, in fact, none is present (Healthline 7.3).

How is it possible for an individual to be seronegative yet harbor HIV? One possibility is that serological tests detect antibodies produced in response to HIV, and there is a time gap between the entry of the virus into the body and the appearance of antibodies. For instance, researchers have found that the time necessary to produce enough antibodies for a positive test can be six to ten weeks. Should an infected person go for HIV testing two or three weeks after being infected, the test results will probably be negative, even though HIV is present.

Another possible reason for a negative test may be the heterogeneity of HIV. Studies have shown that HIV undergoes numerous mutations in the lymphoid tissues and that numerous strains of HIV may be present in a single individual. In response, the body will produce numerous types of antibodies with different molecular configurations, and these may not be detected by the ELISA test. The test may therefore give a negative result because it is not detecting the type(s) of antibodies that are present.

False positives develop when tests signal the presence of HIV antibodies even though none are present. ELISA tests may give false positives, but the western blot analysis eliminates virtually all of them. A possible reason for a false positive may lie in the test itself. The viruses for the ELISA test are cultivated in human cells, and a certain amount of cellular debris can remain with the viral fragments when they are isolated. This debris can attract human antibodies; when the latter accumulate on the bead, they can attract the enzyme-linked antibodies. A positive result ("reactive") will erroneously be observed. Another reason for a false positive may be the presence of other antibodies in a person's blood. For example, certain non-HIV antibodies are known to react slightly with HIV antigens. A person's serum may also give a positive result because of a previous HIV infection that is now gone.

False positives and negatives may also be associated with technical errors in the tests or with the person performing the tests. In the ELISA test, for example, improper washings carried on during test performance may contribute to errors, as may contaminations of samples or color reagents or both. Receiving news of a positive test can be extremely traumatic. Thus, the need for more reliable test results has encouraged public health officials to urge the development of tests that detect the virus itself.

Other Antibody Tests

For validation of the ELISA test, other tests (with imposing names) are available. Some laboratories use a test called the indirect immunofluorescence assay, while other laboratories employ the radioimmunoprecipitation assay.

The indirect immunofluorescence assay (IFA) is used by clinical laboratories for detecting antibodies against many viruses, including those of influenza, herpes simplex, and AIDS. For AIDS, the test begins by combining a patient's serum sample with HIV-infected cells attached to glass slides. If HIV antibodies are present in the serum, they bind to the HIV antigens present on the cellular surfaces (Figure 7.5). The remaining serum is then washed away.

The test continues with the addition of antihuman antibody linked to a fluorescent compound. If HIV antibodies are present on the cell surfaces, the fluorescent-tagged antibodies will accumulate there. When viewed under a special microscope that projects ultraviolet radiation, the test cells glow with a green light in a positive test. The person has seroconverted. If no light is given off, no HIV antibodies are present in the serum sample. The person has failed to seroconvert.

Compared to the western blot analysis, the IFA has equivalent sensitivity and specificity but is easier to perform. In addition, the results of IFA can be obtained in as little as 30 minutes, compared with the overnight incubation generally required for the western blot analysis. However, the western blot test is FDA-licensed and therefore carries the weight of FDA approval. Also, the western blot test is available in a kit and is therefore within the budget of most clinical laboratories.

The *radioimmunoprecipitation assay* (RIPA) is considerably more complex than any of the other tests for HIV antibodies that we have encountered in this chapter. It is very expensive and somewhat hazardous to perform, because multiplying viruses are used. The test may be employed under certain conditions, for

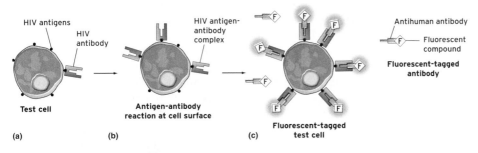

FIGURE 7.5

The indirect immunofluorescence assay. (a) Experimentally infected test cells containing HIV antigens are placed on a glass slide and combined with patient's diluted serum. (b) If the serum contains HIV antibodies, the antibodies combine with the antigens at the cell surface to form an antigen-antibody complex. (c) A sample of antihuman antibodies carrying a fluorescent compound such as fluorescein isothiocyanate is added to the cells. The antihuman antibody combines with the HIV antibody on the cells' surfaces and causes the fluorescent label to accumulate. When viewed under a special microscope, the cells will fluoresce with a green glow.

example, when testing organ tissues prior to transplant. To perform the RIPA, purified HIV particles are bound with radioactive isotopes, then incubated with a serum sample from the person being tested. If HIV antibodies are present, they will bind to the radioactive HIV antigens. The antigen-antibody complexes are separated by gel electrophoresis and are then identified when the radioactivity accumulates as bands in the gel. The radioactivity permits detection of ultraminute amounts of HIV antibodies, and confidence in the results tends to be high. The substantial cost and sophisticated nature of the RIPA, however, preclude its wider use.

Home and Simplified Tests

At the other end of the spectrum of HIV diagnostic testing is a simplified home test. Sold under the trade name Confide, the test requires that a person obtain three drops of blood using an antiseptic wipe and lancet in the kit. The individual blots the blood onto a test card, which is coded with a unique identification number. The card is then mailed to a laboratory for ELISA testing; the person calls an 800 number a few days later and uses the identification number to learn the result. If the result is positive, the call is always rotated to a counselor.

The efficacy of the home test has been demonstrated in numerous research studies. In one study, subject-drawn blood spot samples were compared with professionally-drawn samples, and close to 100 percent of the subject samples were found adequate. The test has been approved by the FDA since 1996 and is available in most pharmacies. Its accuracy, the availability of HIV therapies for those testing positive, and the public health benefits of knowing who is HIV-infected have contributed to its use.

A number of simplified tests that do not require blood samples are also now in use (Figure 7.6). One such test called OraSure requires that an oral tissue sample be taken using a special absorbent pad of cotton held by a stick resembling a toothbrush. The pad is used to scrape a tissue sample from between the gum and cheek. Then the pad is placed in a vial of preservative (to help retard bacterial growth), which is sealed and sent to a clinical laboratory to test for HIV antibodies by the western blot analysis. Persons so tested are given information regarding the reliability of the test and the alternative procedures that use blood samples. They are also counseled about the need for confirmatory tests if a positive result is obtained. The test has been FDA-approved since 1996.

Still another test requires a urine sample for analysis. The test has been available to physicians since its approved by the FDA in 1996. Patients provide a urine sample, and a physician sends it to a laboratory for antibody testing. Although the level of accuracy is lower than for blood tests, the urine test is believed to increase the number of people found to be HIV-infected because more individuals are willing to be tested (since no blood is drawn). Thus, it will help epidemiologists track the AIDS epidemic and get patients into therapy sooner. Also, the test does not require the assistance of a person trained in venipuncture, which reduces the risk of occupational exposure as well as cost. Research studies indicate that a combination of blood and urine tests detects more HIV-positive individuals than either test alone, possibly because antibodies may be present in one body fluid and not in the other.

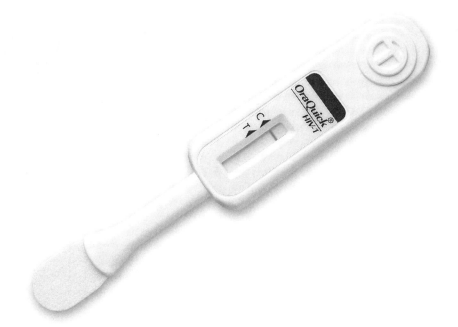

FIGURE 7.6
A simplified home test for detecting HIV antibodies.

The newest antibody tests are the rapid-screening HIV tests. Though only one such test is FDA-approved as yet (and it is reasonably complex), the rapid-screening tests detect HIV antibodies in a matter of minutes and at the point of health care. Such tests could be useful in inner-city emergency rooms, where patients who do not have regular physicians could be tested quickly. The tests would also find use in HIV-infected women who are pregnant and whose first contact with the health care system comes at the time of delivery. Indeed, one CDC model has shown that in a single year, health officials cold learn the HIV status of nearly 700,000 more people if rapid-screening tests were widely available. Moreover, as Table 7.2 shows, if clinic personnel were encouraged to recommend HIV testing for all urgent-care patients, more HIV infections could be detected. Mobile testing units in urban settings and in developing countries with primitive clinical testing facilities also stand to benefit from such tests. At least five such tests were under development during 2002.

HIV Antigen (Viral Load) Tests

Though serological tests are widely used to assist diagnoses and to screen blood, they are indirect tests of HIV infection and, as such, fail to give the clearest picture of viral presence. Furthermore, they are subject to false negatives because a person can remain seronegative for weeks or longer after exposure to HIV. And they do not establish how much virus is in the body (the viral load) or which tissues the virus has infected or which variant of the virus is present. For these reasons, diagnosis is better served by tests directed specifically at HIV or chemical fragments of HIV, commonly known as HIV antigens.

7.2 Number of Individuals Tested for HIV at a Georgia Clinic When Testing Was Routinely (1999) and Not Routinely (2000) Recommended			
Test process	Testing Not Routinely Recommended (1999)	Testing Routinely Recommended (2000)	Increase from 1999 to 2000
Clinic visits	19,626	19,911	285
HIV tests conducted	1,100	2,787	1,687
Newly detected infections*	47	74	27
HIV-positive patients who learned they were infected	28	55	27
HIV-positive patients who entered into care	13	26	13
*Positive HIV test result (western blot).			
Source: Courtesy CDC, MMWR, 50(29), June 29, 2001.			

But detecting HIV and/or HIV antigens is not easy. The standard technique for pinpointing retroviruses, for example, is to identify the presence of the enzyme reverse transcriptase, but this technique has not been used as a diagnostic test because it is very complicated and expensive and it identifies all retroviruses, not just HIV. Applying other established diagnostic techniques for detection of HIV antigens has also proven difficult because HIV may exist as a provirus in T-lymphocytes, and the number of infected cells may be too low. In addition, tests available to detect infected cells are not sensitive enough to give confidence in their results when screening large numbers of blood samples.

The diagnostic tests that detect HIV antigens are directed at both proteins and nucleic acids (Healthline 7.4). Proteins such as p24 are a logical target of diagnostic tests (as we shall discuss presently), but investigators have shown that HIV-infected cells may not be synthesizing the viruses, so viral proteins may not be present. They also caution that infected T-lymphocytes cultured in the laboratory and tested for viral proteins do not always reflect the level of viral infection in the individual. Thus, a test for detecting viral nucleic acids is considered more dependable. Such a test is called the viral load test. Using the technologies of gene probes, gene amplification, and the polymerase chain reaction, the viral load test has gained wide acceptance among physicians and scientists. We discuss this test next.

Gene Probes

Gene probes and the polymerase chain reaction (PCR) are central to the viral load test. They are outgrowths of research in molecular biology that began in the

1950s. With the discovery of new enzymes, new apparatus, and new technologies, scientists found they could reproduce DNA in a test tube, fragment it, determine its composition, change its structure, exchange pieces of it, and map its genes. As the age of molecular biology unfolded, scientists applied newfound principles to diagnosis, devising the antibody tests we have discussed previously and developing the gene probes and viral load tests we explore here.

A gene probe is a single-stranded segment of DNA that can recognize and bind to a complementary segment of DNA on a large DNA molecule. The probe may be labeled with a radioactive isotope that will signal when binding has taken place (Figure 7.7). Underlying the technology is the fact that DNA (such as the DNA of an HIV provirus) exists as two strands opposing one another much like the sides of a ladder. To perform the viral load test and hunt for proviral DNA, infected T-lymphocytes are secured and broken open. All the cellular DNA (including the proviral DNA) is then isolated and split apart, thereby separating the two strands. Now the radioactive gene probe is added. Like a left hand seeking its unique matching right hand, it mingles among all the DNA strands until it locates a complementary strand. Binding to the complementary DNA strand, the probe brings along its radioactive label, and the signal is given that proviral DNA has been found. In an uninfected individual, no such union takes place (there is no proviral DNA). Hence, no radioactivity accumulates, and no signal is sent.

The viral load test typifies the important relationship between basic research and practical applications. The test requires a gene probe, which is, as we have seen, a single-stranded DNA molecule to complement the HIV proviral DNA. Synthesizing such a probe mandated that scientists analyze and decipher the chemical structure of HIV's DNA, a task that required a considerable expenditure of time and research funds. Gene probes now exist for the RNA in HIV, as well as for the proviral DNA. Thus, gene probes can be used to determine the viral load in the bloodstream and other body fluids, as we shall see presently.

The Polymerase Chain Reaction

One major problem with the viral load test is securing enough DNA to perform the test (for example, only 1 in 10,000 T-lymphocytes may be infected with HIV). This problem has been addressed by using a technology called gene amplification to increase the amount of DNA.

Gene amplification employs a procedure called the polymerase chain reaction (PCR). The technology was developed by Nobel laureate Kary

Healthline 7.4

1 **Q** I've heard about an AIDS test called the viral load test. What is that?

A The viral load test is one in which fragments of RNA from HIV are multiplied many times over to produce enough fragments for a test. Then a gene probe chemically searches for and combines with the RNA fragments. Calculations are used to determine the number of copies of HIV RNA in a milliliter of blood, Which is equivalent to the number of HIV particles in a milliliter of blood.

2 **Q** Why is a viral load test better than the AIDS antibody tests?

A The HIV antibody tests (ELISA, western blot analysis, and others) search for indirect evidence of HIV by identifying antibodies produced in response to HIV's presence. By contrast, the viral load test searches for RNA fragments of HIV and thus is a direct test for HIV's presence. A direct test is considered more reliable than an indirect test.

3 **Q** Why is the viral load test better for detecting HIV in newborns than the AIDS antibody tests?

A Newborns receive antibodies from their mothers through the placenta and umbilical cord, and the AIDS antibody tests may be detecting the mother's antibodies rather than those of the child who is exposed to HIV. It is therefore advisable to use a direct test such as the viral load test to determine whether HIV is actually present in the newborn.

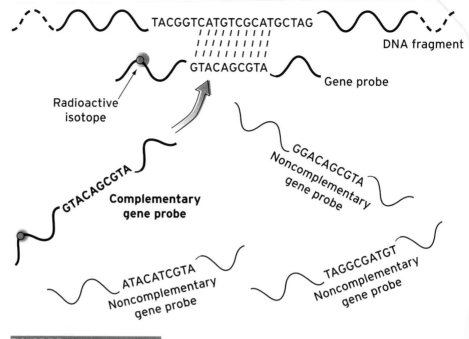

TACGGTCATGTCGCATGCTAG — DNA fragment

GTACAGCGTA — Gene probe

Radioactive isotope

GTACAGCGTA
Complementary gene probe

GGACAGCGTA
Noncomplementary gene probe

ATACATCGTA
Noncomplementary gene probe

TAGGCGATGT
Noncomplementary gene probe

FIGURE 7.7

Gene probe activity. A gene probe is a single-stranded segment of DNA. When combined with separated DNA strands, the gene probe will seek out its complementary DNA segment and bind with it. If the probe is attached to a radioactive isotope, the radioactivity will accumulate at the binding site and signal that a reaction has taken place. The diagram shows only the nitrogenous bases involved in the union of the DNAs.

Mullis at the Cetus Corporation in California in 1984. Gene amplification is performed with double-stranded DNA obtained from T-lymphocytes (and presumably containing HIV proviral DNA). The DNA is separated to yield two strands by carefully heating the material to a specific temperature. After strand separation, a mixture of nucleic acid building blocks (nucleotides) is added, together with an enzyme called DNA polymerase and a short piece of DNA "primer." The primer specifies the segment to be copied. Then the temperature is reduced slightly, but not enough for the two DNA strands to recombine (Figure 7.8). Now, the DNA polymerase synthesizes new complementary strands of DNA, using the building blocks, the primer, and the single strands of DNA as templates. A copy of each separated DNA strand is created. Where there were two DNA strands, there are now four.

The polymerase chain reaction is repeated dozens of times, each cycle taking 1 to 2 minutes. It is performed in a highly sophisticated automated processor and results in a million fold amplification of the genes, because each copied DNA segment serves as a source for millions of additional copies. By incorporating this technology with that of a gene probe, the medical equivalent of a needle in a haystack can be located.

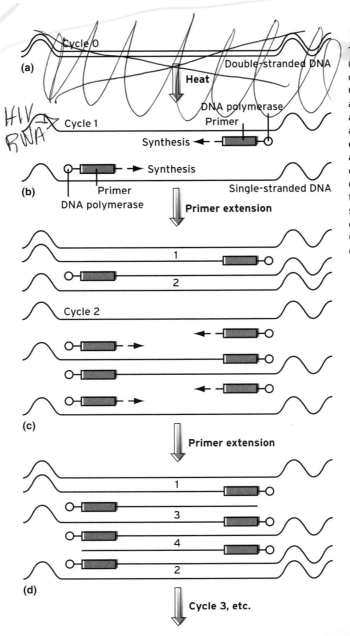

HIV RNA

FIGURE 7.8

The polymerase chain reaction. (a) Heat is used to separate the double-stranded DNA molecule. In Cycle 1, a mixture of nucleotides, an enzyme called DNA polymerase, and a piece of DNA primer are added. (b) The DNA polymerase extends the primer using the available nucleotides to yield two double-stranded DNA molecules. (c) The process is repeated, and at the end of Cycle 2, four double-stranded DNA molecules are produced. Repeating the process in Cycle 3 yields a total of eight double-stranded DNA molecules.

The PCR systems available today are able to amplify RNA as well as DNA and to provide enough RNA to do a viral load test for free HIV particles. To perform the test, the RNA (if present) is used as a template to synthesize DNA, with the enzyme reverse transcriptase serving as a catalyst. Then the same DNA amplification and gene probe procedures are performed as above. The results are commonly expressed as copies of HIV RNA per milliliter (mL). In 1996, the FDA approved the first commercial test to measure viral loads in patients.

Advantages of the Viral Load Test

Because the viral load test identifies viral nucleic acid, it helps clinicians determine which babies are actually HIV-infected and assists epidemiologists in following the AIDS epidemic in newborns. As noted in Chapter 5, antibodies found in newborns are most likely derived from the mother via the placenta. The viral load test makes it possible to detect infected cells directly. In one study, for example, CDC investigators tested blood samples from 200 infants born in New York. Half of the infants had mothers who were positive for HIV antibodies. By using the viral load test, researchers succeeded in locating HIV infection at or near the time of birth in all but one of the children. In adults as well, tracking the viral load has become as valuable as following the clinical signs of AIDS.

A safer blood supply is another benefit from the viral load test. Because the test can detect as few as 100 HIV particles in a milliliter of blood, it is far superior to hunting for HIV antibodies. Moreover, the viruses can be detected as few as 10 days after infection. Unfortunately, the current high cost of the viral load tests precludes their use on every unit of donated blood. To resolve this dilemma, blood banks employ a process called minipooling. In one example of minipooling, a blood bank combines samples from 16 blood donations in a primary pool, then combines samples from 8 such primary pools in a master pool (thereby bringing together 128 samples). A sample from the master pool is subjected to the viral load test, and if it is positive for HIV RNA, each of the primary pools is tested until the infected blood donation is located. If the test on the master pool sample returns a negative result, all 128 units are declared safe for transfusion. In this way, the viral load test can be utilized, costs can be controlled, and the risk of HIV transfer through donated blood (now about 1 in 750,000) can be significantly lowered, perhaps to zero.

Measuring viral loads has also helped revolutionize our understanding of HIV's behavior. For example, by using the viral load test, scientists have shown that soon after infection there is no true latent period, as once believed, but an explosion of viral activity in the bloodstream; then, with the onset of the immune response, viral multiplication stabilizes and remains constant for a long period of time (Figure 7.9). Furthermore, researchers have discovered that the viral load in a person with HIV infection can be used as a barometer of how quickly he or she will progress to AIDS. For instance, experimental results obtained in 1996 by John Mellors and his colleagues at the University of Pittsburgh indicate that if the viral load is less than 4500 HIV RNA copies per mL (cpm), the median progression time to AIDS is 10 years; if the viral load is 4501 to 13,000 cpm, the median time to progress to AIDS is 7.7 years; if the viral load is 13,001 to 36,300 cpm, the median time is 5.3 years; and if the viral load is more than 36,300 cpm, the median time is 3.5 years. These results establish that the viral load is directly related to the rate of disease progression and provides a valuable measurement for discriminating disease stages.

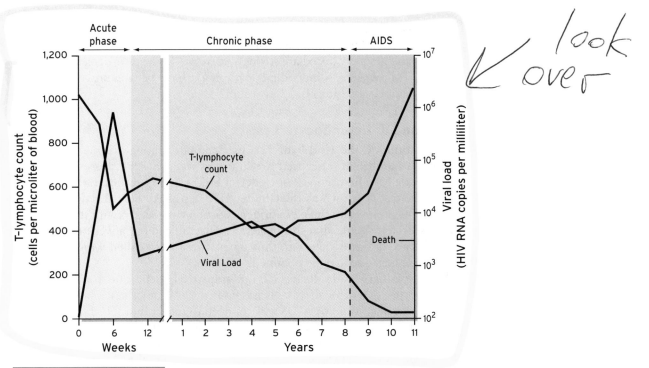

FIGURE 7.9

The relationship between viral load and the T-lymphocyte count in an AIDS patient. Note that early in the disease, the viral load rises dramatically as the T-lymphocyte count drops. This same pattern is seen in the later stages in the disease as the patient progresses to AIDS. *Source: Adapted from Anthony Fauci et al., Annals of Internal Medicine, Vol. 124, 1996.*

Moreover, knowing how to measure the viral load has helped define new principles of HIV therapy (as we discuss in Chapter 8). For example, viral load measurements can be used to determine the effectiveness of the HIV treatment (e.g. the viral load drops as treatment proceeds) or the failure of the treatment (e.g. the viral load returns to pretreatment levels). A viral load of 400 cpm was arbitrarily established as the level at which HIV is "undetectable" in the patient (although there are calls to reduce that number), and treatment guidelines aim to maintain the HIV level below 400 cpm. Finally, viral load measurements provide researchers in drug development with an easier way of evaluating clinical outcomes of their tests, as we explore in Chapter 8. For these reasons, viral load determinations have been paired with T-lymphocyte counts (Chapter 4) for guiding the decision-making process in diagnosis and therapy. Indeed, in 1996, the first evidence of the effectiveness of combination therapies (Chapter 8) came as a result of viral load studies.

As of 2002, the FDA had approved three viral load test kits for marketing in the United States, one each from Roche Diagnostics, Bayer Corporation, and Organon Teknika. The standard test from each manufacturer detects 400 cpm or higher, and each company makes an ultrasensitive test that detects a level as low as 50 cpm. Results from different laboratories that use the three commercially available tests produced are strongly correlated. The tests detect RNA only from HIV-1, however, so individuals who might have been exposed to HIV in Africa should be tested for HIV-2 as well.

Protein and T-Lymphocyte Tests

The HIV antibody and viral load tests predominate among diagnostic applications, but a number of other tests are in use as well. In 1996, for example, the FDA approved the first blood test to detect HIV antigens rather than HIV antibodies. The test is known as the Coulter HIV-1 p24 Antigen Assay. It screens blood for the presence of the p24 antigen, a protein associated with the capsid of HIV. Research indicates that this protein is detectable about a week earlier than antibodies are typically detected, thus narrowing the so-called window period when a false negative may be obtained.

Among other available tests is an improved technique for measuring T-lymphocytes. A test for these cells has gained significance since January 1993 when the case definition for AIDS was changed to reflect the CD4 T-lymphocyte count in patients (Chapter 4). The count of T-lymphocytes in a patient has traditionally been taken by a process known as flow cytometry. In this test, live blood cells flow in single file through a measuring device where they scatter laser light, allowing a count to be taken. Only one blood sample can be measured at a time in a flow cytometer, and samples of blood must be no more than two days old. In 1995, the FDA approved a new test that employs blood samples up to five days old. The test passes blood cells over a plate coated with antibodies that react with the CD4 receptor sites. A visualization reaction similar to that in ELISA is then used to complete the test.

Implications of HIV Testing

One of the more volatile current issues concerns who should be tested for HIV infection. On the federal level, testing has been mandatory for members of the armed forces since 1985, and Congress passed a bill in 1987, requiring testing of immigrants. In state legislatures, more than 100 bills are introduced each year mandating various forms of HIV testing. Premarital testing appears to be the most popular approach to mass screenings, but there are many questions to be resolved: Should the infected person be notified of the presence of HIV or simply informed that the marriage application has been turned down? And what should the intended spouse be told (Healthline 7.5)?

Health officials have used such terms as "universal," "mandatory," "compulsory," "routine," and "voluntary" to describe various plans. Of these adjectives, universal, mandatory, and compulsory evoke the strongest reaction. Proponents of universal testing maintain that it will help define the extent of the AIDS epidemic. They also point out that such testing will help identify those infected so that they and their partners can take precautions to limit the spread of HIV. In addition, universal testing can help discover who is in need of early treatment to slow the progression of AIDS and HIV-related diseases and indicate where available resources should be concentrated.

Opponents of universal testing are equally adamant about why it would be of little value. They admit that testing high-risk groups makes sense, but, they ask, how does one define a person at high risk? For example, is a male homosexual automatically at risk? Not necessarily, because a homosexual man with a very limited number of partners is at considerably less risk than a heterosexual man with multiple partners. They also see the value of testing people who use venereal disease clinics but point out that the threat of an AIDS test might scare away people who need the care offered by the clinic. Moreover, they note, testing must be done repeatedly if it is to be effective, because a negative test is only valid until the next sexual encounter with a possibly infected individual.

There is also the important discrimination factor. For example, testing of hospital patients might yield valuable information on each person's health picture and relieve stress felt by health care workers, but a positive HIV test might also make it impossible for a person to secure health or life insurance (Chapter 10). Proponents of testing counter that patients could be tested anonymously with the results available only to physicians. This might help epidemiologists while minimizing the possibility of discrimination, but opponents counter that failing to alert those who test positive would be unethical.

Most public health officials agree that identifying HIV-positive individuals can help curtail the spread of AIDS, but only if testing is combined with counseling. Those testing positive are often in a state of shock on learning the test results. Guilt, depression, and attempted suicide may follow. These individuals need to know how to live with the implications of the diagnosis. Counseling should emphasize what the test results mean and should suggest lifestyle changes necessary to prevent infecting others, including safer sex practices.

The next question that arises is: Who else is entitled to know that an individual has tested positive for HIV? For the control of sexually transmitted diseases (STDs, including syphilis, gonorrhea, chlamydia, and others), a traditional public health approach has been to notify and offer treatment to sexual contacts of the infected person. The logical extension would be to apply the same approach in cases of HIV infection, but opponents point out that STDs are generally curable, while HIV infection is

Healthline 7.5

1

Q I've thought about taking an AIDS test, but I'm not sure. How can I decide whether I should be tested?

A There are several questions you can ask yourself to help make the decision. For example, do you live in or near an urban center where there is a high incidence of AIDS? Do you engage regularly in high-risk behaviors (share needles in injection drug use, have multiple sex partners, perform anal intercourse)? The risk of these behaviors is increased if you are in or near a geographical region where there is a high incidence of AIDS. Receiving several blood transfusions between the late 1970s and 1985 might also be a factor worth considering.

2

Q Suppose I decide to be tested. How do I proceed?

A There are several avenues you can take to have an AIDS test performed. If you have a regular physician, contact that person. A call to the local health department or to an AIDS hotline can be a way of obtaining information. You might also consider a visit to a public clinic where the test can be performed.

3

Q Who has to know about the results of my AIDS test?

A Different states have different regulations about the confidentiality of AIDS test results. The physician-patient relationship is one level of confidentiality that must be maintained. Many health departments offer confidential AIDS testing; others make anonymous testing available. Before you agree to be tested, you should be informed about what will be done with the results. And the information should be clearly spelled out.

not; plus, they note, STDs do not carry the same stigma as HIV infection and AIDS. Thus, cooperation might not be forthcoming from the person who has tested positive. Health officials also point out that pressing an individual for names of sexual partners often elicits false names. Eventually, discrimination may surface, and the person testing positive may be denied work, housing, or insurance.

A similar dilemma exists for U.S. immigrants whose application for admission to the United States is denied because of HIV infection or AIDS. Who should be notified, and what should be done with the test results? Questions such as these continue to confront public health officials as they grapple with the question of who should be tested.

Mandatory Testing

As the controversial issues concerning HIV testing are debated in the United States, laws have been instituted to mandate testing for certain groups. Since 1990, for example, all those desiring to donate blood or plasma must undergo an HIV test, as must all individuals wishing to donate sperm for artificial insemination or organs or tissues for transplantation purposes. The purpose is to prevent HIV transmission. Blood donors are asked to read an informational pamphlet describing the test, answer a series of medical questions, and sign a consent to donate blood and be tested. Donors are notified only if their test results are positive, and they are invited for counseling and additional evaluation. For living donors of tissues and organs, a similar procedure is followed. For deceased donors of tissues and organs, the question of whom to inform remains unresolved.

HIV testing is also mandatory for military recruits anticipating active duty and for those entering the foreign service a federal service agency such as the Peace Corps or Job Corps. Health officials reason that military personnel must receive numerous immunizations, and these can be dangerous to the receiver's health if immune suppression due to HIV is taking place. There also is a possibility that duty in a remote part of the world may expose the recruit to exotic organisms that could attack an HIV-infected body with unusual severity. Moreover, someone in the military might be called on in an emergency to donate blood to a wounded comrade, and the situation might not lend itself to pretransfusion HIV testing. For those entering the foreign service, similar reasons apply, plus there is a diplomatic responsibility to ensure that American representatives do not pose a danger to people in the countries in which they serve.

Other groups now tested for evidence of HIV infection are immigrants and all individuals sentenced to federal prisons. For immigrants applying for visas to the United States, the results are made available as positive or negative, but the government of the immigrant's origin is not informed. Those testing positive may be denied entry to the United States. In addition, an illegal alien who tests positive is declared ineligible for legal resident status or amnesty, but the alien is not deported because confidentiality is maintained. Federal prison inmates are tested by law on admission to the correctional facility and within 30 days of release on parole. Persons testing positive receive counseling and medical care while in prison, and probation officers counsel inmates on appropriate behaviors when release is anticipated. Most prisons now provide special care facilities for those with AIDS, but not for those with HIV infection.

Another important issue concerns the mandatory testing of newborns. Beginning in 1988, federal legislation required that all newborns be tested, but the law stipulated that the results were not to be made available to mothers. Approximately 2 million infants were tested annually, and the results were used to give a map of where HIV was spreading among heterosexuals (without violating any confidentiality), since newborns have the same antibodies as their mothers. Then, in 1995, a congressional bill was introduced requiring that the results be given to the mother, in effect making the test mandatory for both mother and child. The response by the government was to cancel the national newborn testing program.

In the late 1980s, laws requiring mandatory testing were enacted in the states of Illinois and New York for those contemplating marriage. The spouses-to-be were each informed of the partner's results, but the couple could marry whether or not they tested positive for HIV infection. Vocal proponents of the test pointed out that in 1988, 23 cases of HIV infection were detected in Illinois, cases that otherwise might have been missed. Equally vocal opponents noted that a total of about 150,000 people took the test that year, and the low number of positives (23) showed the low risk of acquiring HIV in that population. They also pointed out the fact that couples were using their feet to vote their opposition to the law: The number of marriage ceremonies taking place in states neighboring Illinois and New York rose sharply. By 1991, the laws were repealed in both states.

Since 1990, all 50 states and the District of Columbia require health care providers to report new cases of AIDS to their state health departments. In addition, in 1999, the CDC recommended that surveillance for HIV infection be performed in all states to track the AIDS epidemic more accurately. By that time, 34 states had already implemented HIV surveillance by patients' names (Figure 7.10). Included in the recommendation was a new case definition of HIV infection that incorporates the HIV antibody tests as well as the viral load test and any other test licensed for diagnosing HIV infection in the United States. Anonymous or confidential testing was deemed acceptable for the surveillance effort.

Voluntary Testing

Experiences gained during the years of the AIDS epidemic have encouraged the U.S. Public Health Service (through the CDC) to recommend HIV testing and counseling for certain groups of individuals. Included in the recommendations are the principles that counseling should take place before and after testing when possible, that personal information will be held confidential, and that a person may decline testing without consequence, except where testing is required under mandate of law (e.g., blood donors, prisoners, and immigrants).

One group for which testing is recommended includes persons who may have sexually transmitted diseases. The CDC suggests that individuals who report for treatment at health clinics, offices of private physicians, or any other health care

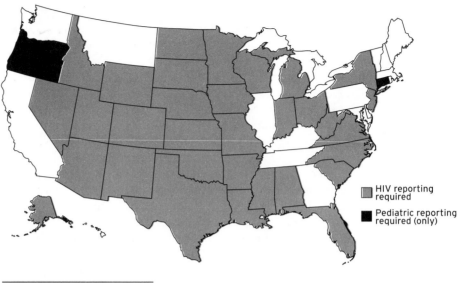

HIV reporting required

Pediatric reporting required (only)

FIGURE 7.10

States of the United States requiring name-based surveillance for HIV infections as of 2001. *Source:* United Nations Programme on HIV/AIDS.

setting should routinely receive HIV testing and counseling, but only if they consent. Another group includes all injection drug users or persons seeking treatment for injection drug abuse. For these individuals, treatment programs should be sufficiently available to allow those seeking assistance to enter promptly, and each person should be counseled on how to modify his or her behavior to prevent the spread of HIV. Outreach programs are also encouraged to educate injection drug users on the risk of AIDS and to recommend treatment for substance abuse.

Testing is also recommended for any persons who consider themselves at risk, such as health care workers who have suffered needlestick injury with contaminated blood (Healthline 7.6). Women of child-bearing age with identifiable risk are also singled out by the CDC. Such women include those who have used injection drugs, have engaged in prostitution, or have sexual partners who are bisexual, injection drug users, or hemophiliacs. In addition, testing is suggested for women of child-bearing age living in communities or born in countries where the HIV infection rate is high and for women who received blood transfusions after HIV entered the United States and before blood was being screened for HIV (that is, between 1978 and 1985). The purpose of this recommendation is to counsel women to avoid a pregnancy that could transfer HIV to the newborn. For women already pregnant, testing can help identify the presence of HIV and ensure proper medical care for them and their newborns. Counseling on family planning and future pregnancies can also be provided.

Furthermore, voluntary testing is advised for persons undergoing medical evaluation or treatment, because selected clinical signs may point to HIV infection. For example, individuals may have HIV infection if they display generalized lymphadenopathy, dementia, chronic fever or diarrhea, unexplained weight loss, or diseases such as herpes simplex, candidiasis, or tuberculosis. When medical evaluation is conducted in a hospital, the hospital may wish to suggest routine testing on admission.

Crucial to the effort to widen the scope of HIV counseling and testing is the public's perception that patient information will be held confidential and that persons found positive will not suffer discrimination. Confidentiality can be increased by improving the record-keeping practices of a health department, hospital, or other health care setting and by protecting the records within the parameters of state law. Inevitably, certain "need to know" situations will arise, and inappropriate disclosures and unauthorized releases of information will occur. However, public health policy should carefully consider ways to reduce the harmful impact of such disclosures.

There is also a difference between "counseling" and "effective counseling." In 2001, the CDC published revised guidelines for HIV counseling, which delineated an effective set of open-ended questions that promote client-centered HIV counseling and suggested certain risk-reduction steps that would more effectively change behavioral patters. Table 7.3 outlines these questions.

In the final analysis, the transmission of HIV can be reduced by an expanded program of counseling and testing, but the success of such a program depends on the level of participation. Individuals are more likely to participate when they believe they will not suffer discrimination in employment, school admission, housing, and medical services. No known medical evidence suggests that ordinary social situations permit the spread of HIV; thus, discrimination is not warranted. Diagnosis through various modes of testing can be a powerful ally in the effort to control AIDS, but diagnosis must be used as it was intended. And that precludes discrimination.

LOOKING BACK

Diagnosis has substantial importance in the effort to interrupt the AIDS epidemic because infected individuals can be identified, and measures can then be taken to counsel them on preventing the spread of HIV, while encouraging them to seek treatment. Among the most important laboratory procedures used to assist diagnosis are the HIV antibody tests. These are indirect tests based on the supposition that the body's immune system pro-

Healthline 7.6

1 **Q** While at work at the hospital recently, I was stuck by a needle contaminated with blood from an AIDS patient. Should I be tested for HIV exposure?

A Yes, your blood should be taken immediately and tested for HIV exposure, most likely by using the HIV antibody test. If negative, another test should be performed in six weeks. If the test results continue to be negative, the test will be repeated 12 weeks, 6 months, and 1 year after your injury. This is to ensure enough time for antibodies to appear in your blood. If, after one year, the tests are still negative, then it can be concluded that HIV transmission did not occur.

2 **Q** If my HIV antibody test is positive, can I still become pregnant?

A Technically, you can become pregnant, but physicians would advise against it because you would be endangering the life of your baby. A positive test means that it is likely that HIV has entered your body and is in your blood. From the blood, HIV can cross the placenta and enter the tissues of the developing fetus. It is quite possible that your child will be born infected and eventually develop AIDS.

3 **Q** Can life insurance companies require an AIDS test before issuing life insurance?

A Life insurance companies are regulated by individual states. In most states, insurance companies are now permitted to require an AIDS test before allowing you to purchase life insurance. If you test positive, the company can deny you insurance or sell it to you at a very high cost.

TABLE 7.3 — Types of Questions That Interfere With and Promote HIV Counseling

Closed-ended questions, which might interfere with client-centered HIV prevention counseling	Open-ended questions, which promote client-centered HIV prevention counseling
Have you ever injected drugs? OR	What are you doing that you think may be putting you at risk for HIV infection?
Have you (for a male client) ever had sex with a man? OR Have you (for a female client) ever had sex with a bisexual man?	What are the riskiest things that you are doing?
	If your test comes back positive, how do you think you may have become infected? When was the last time you put yourself at risk for HIV? What was happening then?
Have you ever had sex when you were under the influence of alcohol or drugs?	How often do you use drugs or alcohol? How do you think drugs or alcohol influence your HIV risk?
Do you (always) use condoms when you have sex? OR	How often do you use condoms when you have sex?
Can you always use condoms when you have sex?	When/with whom do you have sex without a condom? When with a condom? What are you currently doing to protect yourself from HIV? How is that working? What kinds of things do you do to protect your partner from getting infected with HIV? (for HIV-infected clients) Tell me about specific situations when you have reduced your HIV risk. What was going on that made that possible?
Can you always use clean works (i.e., needles, syringes, cottons, or cookers*) when you inject?	How risky are your sex/needle-sharing partners? For example, have they been recently tested for HIV?

*Cottons are filters used to draw up the drug solution. Cookers include bottle caps, spoons, or other containers used to dissolve drugs.

Source: Courtesy of CDC, MMWR, 50(RR), November 9, 2001.

duces antibodies in response to exposure to an infectious agent such as HIV. The viral load test is another key diagnostic procedure. It is a direct test used to detect the RNA of HIV or the DNA associated with proviral HIV.

Two HIV antibody tests are the ELISA test and the western blot analysis. In the ELISA test, patient's serum is added to HIV antigens, and a color change indicates that antibodies are present in the serum. For the western blot analysis, HIV antigens are separated in a gel and the patient's serum is added. If HIV antibodies exist in the serum, they will react with the separated antigens and form bands detected by a staining reaction. Both tests have 99-percent sensitivity and specificity, but both can give false negatives and false positives. For example, an infected individual may not have had sufficient time to produce enough antibodies for the test to detect, and a false negative may result. Other serological tests are also available for confirmatory testing, and some are available as FDA-approved home tests. For the latter, the individual provides a blood, saliva, or urine sample for testing.

The HIV antigen test (or viral load test) is a direct test providing evidence of HIV in the cells and tissues. A gene probe composed of DNA seeks out and combines with DNA from HIV proviruses obtained from infected lymphocytes. Because too little viral DNA may be available for a reliable test, it is advantageous to amplify the DNA through a procedure called the polymerase chain reaction (PCR). In this technique, enzymes and primers are added to DNA from a patient's cells to increase the content of any viral DNA present. The gene probe is then more efficient. Contemporary tests detect HIV RNA and give results in terms of a number of copies of HIV RNA in a milliliter of blood. The viral load test has yielded new insights on pediatric AIDS and HIV's behavior, and it has helped define new principles of HIV therapy.

Considerable controversy exists about who should be tested for HIV and what should be done with the test results. When confidentiality is broken, various forms of discrimination can ensue. At present, mandatory testing is required for military recruits, prison inmates, and certain other groups. Voluntary testing is requested of those in high-risk groups and selected others to help interrupt the AIDS epidemic.

REVIEW

Having completed this chapter on diagnosis and testing, you should be able to conceptualize the laboratory methods for detecting HIV and AIDS and summarize the uses, advantages, and shortcomings of the procedures. To test your knowledge, enter the word or words that best completes each of the following statements. Appendix A contains the correct answers.

1. _ELISA_ is the acronym used for the laboratory test most widely used to detect HIV antibodies.

2. _false negative_ characterizes the result of an HIV antibody test when the person is infected but does not have sufficient antibodies to give a positive test.

3. _electrophoresis_ is the technique in which an electric current is used to separate HIV proteins (antigens) used in the western blot analysis.

4. _T-lymphocytes_ are the cells that must be obtained from a patient to perform a gene probe.

5. _Viral load_ is the amount of HIV in the body when a test for HIV RNA is performed.

6. _Serological_ is the name given to any test that determines the presence of antibodies in a patient.

7. _Western blot analysis_ is the validation test most frequently used when the ELISA test is positive.

8. _False positive_ is the result that can occur if an uninfected person has antibodies that react with HIV antigens in a laboratory test.

9. _Antigens_ are the main targets of HIV fragment tests.

10. _Polymerase chain reaction_ is the reaction used to amplify the amount of DNA in an HIV test using a gene probe.

11. _Food & Drug Administration_ is the agency of the United States government that licenses HIV diagnostic tests.

12. _Radioimmunoprecipitation assay_ is the process wherein blood banks combine samples of donor bloods for HIV testing.

13. _Serum_ is the material obtained from a patient to perform an ELISA test.

14. _Mother_ is the source of the antibodies in a newborn's blood that make an HIV antibody test inefficient.

15. _Gene probe_ is a fragment of DNA that seeks out and binds with a complementary DNA fragment such as that from an HIV provirus.

16. _6-10 weeks_ is the approximate time after exposure to HIV required for a person's immune system to make enough antibodies to give a positive ELISA test.

17. _99%_ is the level of specificity and sensitivity exceeded by both the ELISA test and western blot analysis.

18. _Primer DNA_ is the material other than polymerase enzymes and nucleotides that must be added to DNA to carry out the PCR.

19. _ELISA_ is the serological test in which a color change signals that HIV antibodies are present in the serum of the patient.

20. *Military* is a one group for which HIV testing is mandatory in the United States.

FOR ADDITIONAL READING

Altman, L. K. 1997. "Sex, privacy, and tracking HIV infections." *New York Times,* November 4.

Burgisser, E. C., et al. 2000. "Swiss HIV cohort study. Performance of five different assays for the quantification of viral load in persons infected with various subtypes of HIV-1." *J. Acquir. Immune Defic. Syndr.* 23: 138–144.

Centers for Disease Control. 1987. "Interpretation and use of the western blot assay for serodiagnosis of human immunodeficiency virus type I infection." *MMVM* 38(5–7): 1–7.

———. 1987. "Public health service guidelines for counseling and antibody testing to prevent HIV infection and AIDS." *MMWR* 36(31): 509–515.

———. 1988. "Update: serologic testing for antibody to human immunodeficiency virus." *MMWR* 36(52): 833–840.

———. 2001. "Revised guidelines for HIV counseling, testing, and referral." *MMWR* 50: RR-19.

Chew, C. B., et al. 1999. "Comparison of three commercial assays for the quantification of HIV-1 RNA." *J. Clin. Virol.* 14: 87–94.

Cimons, M. 1996. "FDA approves HIV home tests, viral load assay." *ASM News* 62(8): 396–397.

Cohen, J. 1992. "Searching for markers on the AIDS trail." *Science* 258: 388–391.

Day, M. 1997. "Playing safer." *New Scientist,* July 16.

Ho, D. 1996. "Viral counts count in HIV infection." *Science* 272: 1124–1125.

Kilmarx, P. H., et al. 1998. "Living with HIV: Experiences and perspectives of HIV-infected sexually transmitted disease clinic patients after posttest counseling." *Sex. Transm. Dis.* 25: 28–37.

Mellors, J. W. 1998. "Viral load tests provide valuable answers." *Scientific American,* July.

Phairj, P., and S. Wolinsky. 1992. "Diagnosis of infection with the human immunodeficiency virus." *Clin. Infect. Dis.* 15: 13–16.

Root-Bernstein, R. 1990. "Misleading reliability." *The Sciences,* March/April.

Saag, M. S., et al. 1996. "HIV viral load markers in clinical practice." *Nat. Med.* 2: 625–629.

Shearer, W. T., et al. 1997. "Virtal load and disease progression in infants infected with HIV." *N. Eng. J. Med.* 336: 1337–1342.

Voelker, R. 1996. "New studies say viral burden tops CD4 as a marker of HIV infection." *JAMA* 275(6): 421–423.

Treating HIV Infection and AIDS

LOOKING AHEAD

The development of therapeutic agents for treating HIV infection and AIDS has increased the length and quality of patients' lives and has strengthened optimism that additional therapies can be found. This chapter discusses some of the available approaches to treating patients. On completing the chapter, you should be able to . . .

- Explain the principles that apply to treatment of HIV infection and AIDS, including inhibitory mechanisms of AIDS drugs and unique problems associated with AIDS therapies.

- Identify the mode of action, benefits, and possible side effects of the drug azidothymidine (AZT).

- Name and discuss several other reverse transcriptase inhibitors used to treat AIDS.

- Explain the positive impact that protease inhibitors have have in fighting the AIDS epidemic.

- Summarize the biochemical activities of fusion inhibitors, entry inhibitors, antisense molecules, and other drugs currently in developmental stages for use against HIV infection and AIDS.

- List some therapies available for treating the opportunistic diseases associated with AIDS.

- Describe the methods for testing the effectiveness of experimental drugs prior to release for patient use and discuss some of the ethical considerations involved in drug testing.
- Explain some alternative therapies for treating AIDS patients, such as bone marrow transplants and gene therapy.

INTRODUCTION

Yellow fever stands out as one of the most savage diseases ever to strike the United States. During the 1700s, for example, historians chronicled thirty-five separate epidemics. The disease raged through the country like a firestorm, and no city was hit harder than Philadelphia.

In 1793, Philadelphia was the capital of and largest city in the United States. When yellow fever broke out among the 40,000 residents, the panic rivaled that in Europe during the plague years. Thousands fled the city, and those who remained lived in fear. Officials posted warning notices where infected people lived and assigned guards to quarantine the sick. Uninfected individuals sought protection by wearing cloth masks soaked in garlic juice, vinegar, or camphor. For the sick, physicians prescribed blood-lettings, purges, and ice water baths. In the end, most of the 24,000 people remaining in the city contracted the disease. Almost 5000 perished.

Yellow fever continues to occur in contemporary times, even though physicians know considerably more about it than they did 200 years ago. They know, for example, that yellow fever is caused by a virus, which attacks the liver and causes bile to seep into the bloodstream. They understand that yellow fever is transmitted by mosquitoes and that epidemics can be interrupted by controlling mosquito populations. And, unfortunately, they realize that for the person having yellow fever, the possibility of a cure is not much better than it was 200 years ago.

A similar pattern applies to many diseases. For instance, the agents of hepatitis, polio, rabies, mononucleosis, measles, herpes, and many other viral diseases are well known; the modes of transmission for these diseases have been identified; and epidemiologists can interrupt their spread. But drugs for treatment are relatively rare and, in many cases, unknown. Indeed, for viral diseases, therapeutic drugs are the exception rather than the rule.

For the first dozen years of the AIDS epidemic, physicians were generally pessimistic about the development of therapeutic drugs. In recent years, however, their pessimism has been replaced by optimism. Combinations of the drug azidothymidine (AZT) and protease inhibitors have proven helpful for lessening the symptoms of HIV infection and prolonging life. In addition, many other drugs are in various stages of development, and the search for therapeutic agents is well funded and has a high priority at several universities and pharmaceutical companies. Numerous novel approaches to therapy are also being pursued by researchers. The result has been a sense of hope not felt by the victims of yellow fever in Philadelphia. We shall examine the basis for this optimism in the pages ahead.

General Principles of AIDS Treatment

Through the early and mid-1980s, health care professionals viewed AIDS as an acute, almost immediately lethal crisis. Toward the end of the 1980s and into the 1990s, however, this viewpoint changed. During these years, new therapies for AIDS came into use; and with their acceptance, the length and quality of life of AIDS patients has improved. For those with access to reasonably good health care, AIDS has become a chronic disease, with an estimated 12-year course, on average. Greater physician expertise, coupled with a higher level of patient motivation and improved therapies, has changed the dim prospects once facing AIDS patients.

At the forefront of this change are a number of therapeutic drugs. Before examining their nature and mode of action, we shall explore some principles that apply to drug therapy, discuss the approaches taken by drugs that interfere with HIV activity, and identify some unique problems associated with AIDS therapy.

Objectives of Therapeutic Drugs

To be effective against a pathogen, a therapeutic drug must either kill the pathogen or prevent it from multiplying in the body. Note, however, that an effective therapeutic agent need not rid the body of all traces of the pathogen. By preventing the pathogen from multiplying, a drug can slow or halt the progress of disease. For example, people with tuberculosis have been able to lead fairly normal lives by taking therapeutic drugs to prevent the tubercle bacilli from proliferating. Unable to multiply, the bacilli do not cause symptoms or pass in significant numbers to the next individual.

It may be impossible to rid the body of HIV because this retrovirus exists in infected cells as a provirus (Chapter 2). Killing all the cells infected by HIV (e.g., helper T-lymphocytes, macrophages, cells of the nervous system) would probably kill the patient. But holding HIV in check could allow infected individuals to lead almost normal lives.

To kill a pathogen or inhibit its multiplication, a therapeutic agent generally interferes with a sequence of biochemical reactions unique to that organism. Such interference is possible in bacteria because they are so different from humans; thus, interfering with bacterial biochemistry does not affect human biochemistry. Penicillin, for instance, interferes with the construction of the bacterial cell wall and prevents bacteria from proliferating (Figure 8.1). Because human cells have no cell walls, penicillin does not interfere with their normal activity. Viruses, by comparison, do not carry out independent biochemical reactions on which a drug can act, and so antibiotics do not affect viruses. However, drugs may interfere with viral replication, a biochemical process of high complexity.

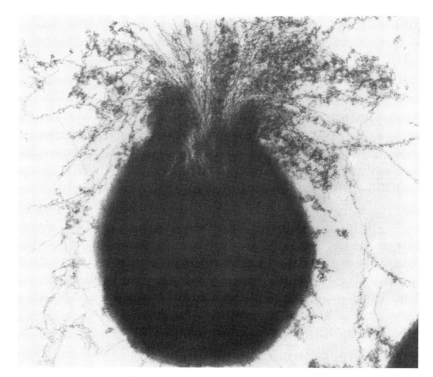

FIGURE 8.1

A photomicrograph of a bacterium exploding on exposure to penicillin (×50,000). The penicillin has interfered with cell wall synthesis in the bacterium and left it with only a surrounding cell membrane. Internal pressures have led to membrane disruption. Penicillin is useful against bacteria but not viruses, because the latter do not synthesize a cell wall.

To be effective, a therapeutic drug must do no damage or only minimal damage to the body. However, years of research and observation have made it clear that taking any therapeutic drug carries risk. Even penicillin, generally regarded as a "safe" drug, can induce severe and sometimes fatal allergic reactions. For many diseases, the risk associated with a drug treatment must be balanced against the benefit. When one has influenza, for instance, it may not be necessary to risk potentially toxic drugs because the disease is usually mild; when one has AIDS, by contrast, the illness is life-threatening, and the risk of taking a potentially toxic drug may be warranted.

There is also the dilemma of when to institute AIDS therapy. Early intervention allows simpler therapeutic management in the long term because patients experience fewer side effects. Early intervention also provides the best chance for minimizing the development of opportunistic infections and reduces the possibility of immune system damage, especially in children where the large size of the thymus encourages a dramatic immune reconstitution. Those opposed to early therapy point up the reduced quality of life for patients who have no symptoms, the possible development of resistant HIV strains if patients do not adhere to the regimen of drugs, and the possible reduction in the useful lifespan of a drug if resistant strains of HIV arise. Ultimately, the treatment decision is made by the patient and his or her physician.

Approaches to Drug Therapy

Against this background, we can begin to appreciate some of the problems that must be considered in developing AIDS treatments. High among these problems is combating HIV in the body without damaging the body. To find HIV's "weak spot," researchers attempt to locate a step in viral replication that is dissimilar to events in the life of a normal host human cell. Locating and interfering with several steps, rather than one step, is clearly more advantageous, which is why a combination of drugs may be better than a single drug.

One approach to drug therapy might be to block the binding of HIV to its host cells by altering the gp120 molecules in the envelope spikes of HIV (Chapter 2). Binding may also be inhibited by blocking the CD4 molecules on the surface of helper T-lymphocytes (Figure 8.2). Another possibility might be to keep viral RNA and reverse transcriptase from escaping their protein coat once HIV has penetrated the cytoplasm. Preventing RNA-to-DNA synthesis via reverse transcriptase (the function performed by AZT) is also a desirable approach. Interference with reverse transcriptase activity is particularly attractive because the enzyme exists only in cells infected with retroviruses such as HIV.

Other opportunities to interfere with viral reproduction exist when the provirus encodes new HIV particles. For instance, if the viral transactivator gene (*tat*) can be inactivated, the provirus will continue to lie dormant. The translation of the genetic message to messenger RNA (mRNA) molecules presents another possibility for interference because synthetic mRNA molecules could be manufactured to bind with and inactivate the natural mRNA molecules. Viral proteins must be modified before assembly with RNA to form new HIV particles, and here lies another opportunity for possible drug action (this is where the protease inhibitors work). Finally, the budding of HIV from infected cells could conceivably be prevented.

Although there appear to be many places where HIV seems vulnerable, there are also many unique features of HIV that require attention. As noted previously, HIV presents an elusive target because it can reside in cells as a provirus. Moreover, HIV infects a variety of cells, so any drug devised must take into account the possible toxic effect on different types of cells. A particularly difficult problem arises with HIV infection of brain cells: Brain cells are separated from the remainder of the body by the blood-brain barrier, a series of membranes that prevent substances from moving out of the blood into the brain cells. To be effective, a drug must cross this barrier. In addition, there is the problem of possible brain cell damage by the drug. Because adult brain cells are among the body cells least able to regenerate themselves, it may be impossible to reverse such brain damage.

Treating children with AIDS presents special challenges for physicians because HIV tends to behave more aggressively in children than in adults (indeed, children progress to AIDS much more rapidly than adults). Moreover, physicians have a relatively small body of research to consult when prescribing anti-HIV medications for children, and fewer drugs are available in acceptable formulations to treat young patients (swallowing pills, for example, can be difficult for young patients).

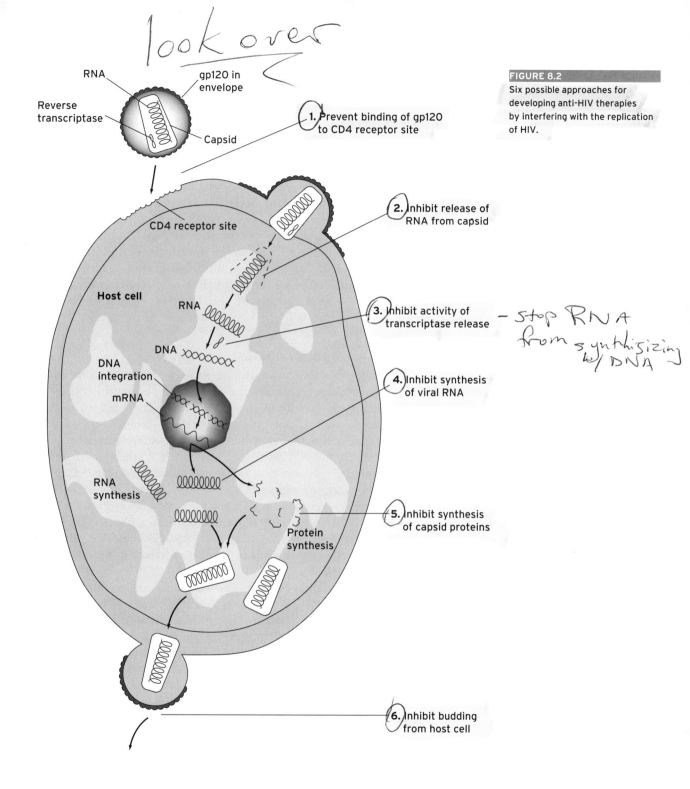

look over

RNA

gp120 in envelope

Reverse transcriptase

Capsid

1. Prevent binding of gp120 to CD4 receptor site

FIGURE 8.2

Six possible approaches for developing anti-HIV therapies by interfering with the replication of HIV.

CD4 receptor site

2. Inhibit release of RNA from capsid

Host cell

RNA

3. Inhibit activity of transcriptase release

— stop RNA from synthisizing w/ DNA

DNA

DNA integration

mRNA

4. Inhibit synthesis of viral RNA

RNA synthesis

5. Inhibit synthesis of capsid proteins

Protein synthesis

6. Inhibit budding from host cell

In addition, treating children has greater urgency because HIV invades the brain early in the disease and the infection retards intellectual development, while impairing motor coordination and stifling physical growth. Families can also experience difficulty in following intensive and strict drug regimens (for instance, when a child is at day care). Despite these difficulties, great strides have been made in reducing the incidence of AIDS in children.

Treating Kaposi's sarcoma and opportunistic diseases while concurrently attempting to destroy HIV represents another challenge. Most infectious diseases are due to a single microorganism, and the physician can usually marshal available resources against that one pathogen. AIDS, by comparison, is a multifaceted disease, bringing numerous opportunistic diseases in addition to the HIV infection. Drug therapy must therefore be multifaceted, and physicians must battle on many fronts at one time. In addition, drugs may interfere with one another, and a patient may be weakened by drug toxicity. The cumulative stress on the body from several concurrent illnesses may make drug therapy very difficult.

Mutations and Other Considerations

Another key issue concerns HIV mutation and the drug resistance related to mutation. As we note in Chapter 2, mutation results in a permanent change in the HIV genome, a change that results in an altered protein. If the altered protein is a drug-targeted enzyme such as protease or reverse transcriptase, then it will resist binding to the drug and the latter will become useless. For example, nevirapine and related drugs inhibit HIV particles by reacting with their reverse transcriptase molecules, but a single mutation in the enzyme-encoding gene changes the active site where the reaction occurs and binding fails. Scientists estimate that at least one mutation occurs each time an HIV particle undergoes replication, and thus in the approximate 10 billion HIV particles produced daily in a patient's body, a host of mutants are probably present. Moreover, it is possible that a mutant with resistance to an antiviral agent such as nevirapine has developed even though the patient has never taken the drug.

How, then, does a population of nevirapine-resistant viruses emerge in the body? The answer is based on the Darwinian process of selection: Nevirapine will react with all the HIV particles that contain susceptible reverse transcriptase and thereby neutralize 99.99 percent of them. But the few resistant viruses will survive and continue to replicate, and soon they will comprise the dominant population (Figure 8.3). Their replication will result in more mutants, probably with increased resistance to the nevirapine, and soon the drug will become ineffective. As we shall discuss presently, physicians learned the implications of mutation-based resistance in the 1990s, and they switched from single-drug therapy (monotherapy) to combinations of drugs (multidrug therapy) to reduce the likelihood of encountering drug-resistant viruses in the body or encouraging the development of resistance.

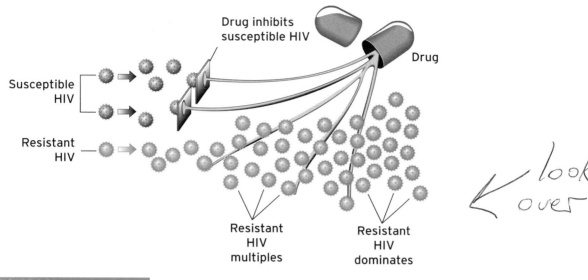

Susceptible
HIV

Resistant
HIV

Drug inhibits
susceptible HIV

Drug

Resistant
HIV
multiples

Resistant
HIV
dominates

look over

FIGURE 8.3

How drug resistance emerges in a population of HIV particles. An anti-HIV drug such as nevirapine reacts with susceptible HIV particles and neutralizes them. In the population, however, some resistant HIV particles exist, as a result of mutation, and these resistant particles soon multiply and become the dominant members of the viral population. The nevirapine is no longer useful.

Because drug resistance is a widespread problem in anti-HIV drug therapy, methods of assessing the resistance are a focus of research efforts. In general terms, the presence of HIV in the blood four to six months after therapy has begun is a signature of HIV replication and potential drug resistance. A test approved by the FDA in 2001 can verify that resistance is occurring. The test, called Trugene, examines the genetic composition of the patient's HIV and checks for mutations, using a software program to compare the genome of the patient's HIV to a list of more than 70 mutations linked to resistance to specific drugs. This is a so-called genotypic test. A phenotypic test, by comparison, checks for resistance by measuring the ability of a specific drug to decrease replication of the patient's HIV by 50 percent under laboratory conditions. If resistance to several drugs is encountered, regaining control of viral multiplication requires salvage therapy. This therapy employs a fresh set of drugs, preferably new to the marketplace; a lower reduction in viral load is anticipated at the outset of the therapy.

The problem of general inexperience in treating viral diseases is also worthy of note. Through the 1980s, most pharmaceutical companies concentrated on drugs that target bacterial diseases. Past efforts had turned up few antiviral drugs, and most viral diseases were not viewed as life-threatening (except, for example, rabies, smallpox, and polio). In addition, viral vaccines were effective in halting epidemics and preventing new ones. Pharmaceutical companies, therefore, were not inclined to conduct exhaustive searches for antiviral drugs; this meant that little experience in the development of such drugs was acquired. This inexperience may be the most significant problem that needs to be resolved if a successful therapeutic agent for HIV infection and AIDS is to be located (Table 8.1).

On the positive side of the ledger, a substantial effort is under way to develop effective therapies for HIV infection and AIDS. As early as 1989, a features reporter for the *American Society for Microbiology News* wrote that endeavors "to develop drugs for combating acquired immune deficiency syndrome (AIDS) make the U.S. 'War on Cancer' seem like a mere skirmish." And in the next paragraph, the reporter wrote, "Unquestionably, a massive AIDS drug development campaign is under way in the United States." To be sure, the search for treatments for HIV infection and AIDS is one of the most intensive research efforts of our time. Led by the National Institutes of Health (NIH), the search consumes hundreds of millions of dollars in federal funds annually. In many quarters, this commitment is viewed as a cause for optimism. In the following sections, we shall examine some of the fruits of the search.

Reverse Transcriptase Inhibitors

Reverse transcriptase is the enzyme that catalyzes the synthesis of DNA using the RNA in the genome of HIV. This synthesis occurs after the HIV particle has penetrated a host cell, a T-lymphocyte (Chapter 2). Reverse transcriptase is a valuable target for anti-HIV drugs because it does not occur in human cells (and thus the drug will not interfere with T-lymphocyte metabolism), and because the gene that encodes reverse transcriptase is an essential element in viral replication. For

TABLE 8.1	Problems Associated with Development of Drugs for HIV Infection and AIDS

- Combating HIV without damaging body cells
- Locating a biochemical point where HIV is vulnerable
- Dealing with the provirus in infected cells
- Crossing the blood-brain barrier
- Damage to nonregenerative brain cells
- Treating opportunistic diseases apart from HIV infection
- Relieving cumulative stresses on the body
- General inexperience in treating viral diseases

these reasons, various reverse transcriptase inhibitors have been developed, as we explore next.

Azidothymidine (AZT)

In 1964, Jerome P. Horwitz, an organic chemist at the Michigan Cancer Foundation, in Detroit, synthesized a new drug for treating cancer. The drug was similar to a building block of DNA but was counterfeit; that is, it was designed to confuse the cancer cells' genetic machinery and stop a tumor's growth. Unfortunately, when Horwitz and his colleagues injected the drug into mice with leukemia, the drug had little effect on the cancer. The drug was azidothymidine, or AZT. AZT would sit on the shelf, with other failed anticancer drugs, for 20 years.

During the 1970s, interest mounted in retroviruses, and a number of investigators tested AZT and similar drugs for activity against mouse retroviruses. The drugs were somewhat effective, but because there were no known retroviruses of humans, a practical benefit from the research was lacking. The drugs therefore remained in relative obscurity.

Then the AIDS epidemic broke out, and researchers began an active search for therapeutic drugs. Two of the researchers were Hiroaki Mitsuya and Samuel Broder of the NIH. In the summer of 1984, Mitsuya and Broder obtained from Robert Gallo a sample of HIV (then known as HTLV-III), and they began testing various drugs against the virus. They took more than 300 drugs "off the shelf" and evaluated them. Fifteen of the drugs interfered with HIV replication in test tubes. One was AZT.

Broder and Mitsuya began an intensive effort to develop AZT as a therapy for AIDS patients. Working with the Burroughs Wellcome Company and researchers at Duke University, they found AZT to be a potent inhibitor of HIV in cultures of T-lymphocytes, and they worked out a concentration at which the toxic effects in human cells would be minimal. The first patients received AZT in July 1985.

A year later, Broder and Mitsuya announced the results of clinical trials conducted at twelve medical centers. Doctors gave the drug to 145 AIDS patients and an inert placebo to 137 AIDS patients. In the test group receiving AZT, the helper T-lymphocyte count rose, the immune response improved, resistance to *Pneumocystis carinii* pneumonia was enhanced, and the patients' lifespans increased over what was expected. In the spring of 1987, the Food and Drug Administration (FDA) licensed AZT as a therapy for AIDS patients in the United States. In 1988, Burroughs Wellcome changed the drug's name from azidothymidine to zidovudine and sold it by the trade name Retrovir. However, since most people know the drug as AZT, we shall continue to use that name.

Mode of Action of AZT Since its introduction to general use in 1987, AZT has been a mainstay for treating AIDS. The chemical name of the drug is azido-2′,3′-deoxythymidine; it is a compound closely related to deoxythymidine (Figure 8.4). Deoxythymidine is an essential component of DNA. AZT acts by replacing deoxythymidine in the synthesis of DNA, a synthesis catalyzed by reverse transcriptase.

FIGURE 8.4

The mode of action of azidothymidine (AZT). (a) The normal DNA molecule consists of a series of nucleosides linked to one another by phosphate (PO_3) molecules. Four types of nucleosides are involved, each having a different nitrogenous base: A stands for adenine, C for cytosine, T for thymine, and G for guanine. Each nucleoside contains the carbohydrate deoxyribose (D). Note that the phosphate molecule links at the 3′ position of the deoxyribose. (b) AZT has a chemical structure similar to that of the nucleoside containing thymine. Thus, when AZT is present, it is erroneously taken up in place of the thymine-containing nucleoside as DNA is being formed. However, the 3′ position of AZT contains an $-N_3$ group, and a phosphate molecule cannot link here. Thus, DNA chain formation comes to an end with AZT's incorporation. In the absence of DNA, HIV replication comes to a halt because proviruses cannot form.

W/ the stopping Using reverse transcriptase.

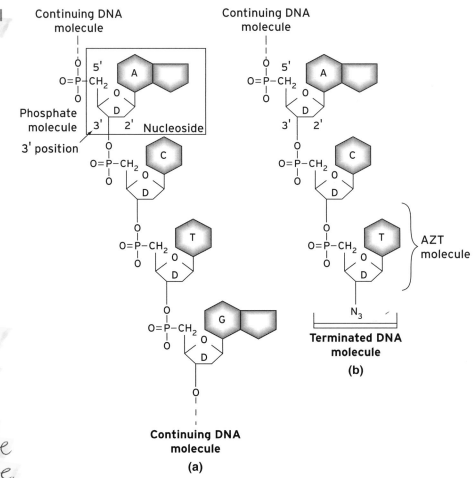

(a)

(b)

The key to AZT's activity lies in its similarity to deoxythymidine (Figure 8.4). Deoxythymidine is a nucleoside consisting of deoxyribose (the carbohydrate in DNA) and thymine (one of the four nitrogenous bases in DNA). In building a DNA molecule, molecules of deoxythymidine are linked by reverse transcriptase to other nucleoside building blocks via phosphate molecules. To form the link at the 3′ (pronounced "3-prime") position, reverse transcriptase removes the –OH group from the deoxythymidine and attaches a phosphate molecule. The phosphate molecule then acts as a bridge to link the deoxythymidine to the next nucleoside in the DNA chain. The next nucleoside can be deoxycytidine, deoxyadenosine, deoxyguanosine, or another deoxythymidine molecule. The phosphate molecule is thus a linkage between the DNA building blocks, a "bridge" that joins the nucleosides together.

This is where AZT enters the picture. Because of its abundance in the cellular cytoplasm (the patient has taken a therapeutic dose) and its resemblance to deoxythymidine, AZT is taken up by reverse transcriptase and is slotted into the position where deoxythymidine should be placed. But AZT lacks the –OH group at the 3′ position; it has a nitrogen group there instead. Reverse transcriptase cannot remove this nitrogen group to attach a phosphate molecule, and without the phosphate "bridge," a link cannot be forged to the next nucleoside. The effect is to abruptly halt the elongation of the building DNA chain. This mechanism, known as chain termination, thus prevents the production of proviral DNA. Essentially, it interrupts the replication cycle of the virus.

AZT can also operate via a second mechanism. Once again, the key is the chemical similarity between AZT and deoxythymidine. Reverse transcriptase normally binds to deoxythymidine to incorporate it into the growing DNA chain, but when AZT molecules are abundant, the enzyme mistakenly binds to the AZT. This binding is irreversible. Reverse transcriptase becomes nonfunctional because it is unable to free itself from the AZT molecule. In effect, the AZT has successfully competed with the nucleoside for the active site on the enzyme molecule; in so doing, AZT has inhibited the enzyme. This mechanism is thus called competitive inhibition.

Theoretically, what AZT accomplishes could be carried out by other nucleoside substitutes, but this does not necessarily occur. A drug molecule, for example, must be able to enter affected cells, and not all nucleosidelike compounds can do so. Furthermore, a drug molecule must hook easily to phosphate at the "upper" end of the molecule (the 5′ position), an ability not possessed by most nucleoside substitute. The question of enzyme preference also arises: Reverse transcriptase prefers AZT to deoxythymidine, whereas host cell enzymes prefer deoxythymidine to AZT for DNA synthesis. The result is that AZT can inhibit reverse transcriptase without affecting other cellular enzymes. Other compounds might not be preferred in this way. In addition, there may be the problem of decomposition: AZT escapes decomposition by cellular enzymes, but a substitute molecule might easily be broken down. A substitute molecule may be a potent inhibitor of HIV replication, but it will have little value if it is rapidly destroyed in cells.

Benefits and Uses of AZT For persons with HIV infection or AIDS, AZT has been found beneficial for a number of reasons: It slows the spread of infection among the T-lymphocytes, and as the T-lymphocytes regenerate themselves, the immune system functions are partially restored (the count of helper T-lymphocytes, or CD4 cells, doubles or better in some patients); patients experience a gain of weight; for many patients, the chronic fever leaves; and in some patients, the fungal infection due to Candida albicans lessens or disappears. Perhaps the most significant benefit of AZT therapy is that the level of HIV declines demonstrably in the infected patient (Healthline 8.1).

There are several factors that add to the value of AZT: It can be given orally because it is absorbed through the intestine; levels of the drug that inhibit viral replication in the laboratory can be achieved in the patient; most of the drug remains active for at least an hour before being converted to an inactive compound by liver enzymes and excreted through the kidneys (the drug must be taken at regular intervals because of this elimination); and the drug can apparently penetrate

1

Q My HIV test came back positive, and the doctor advised me to take AZT. Exactly what is AZT?

A AZT stands for azidothymidine. It is a chemical compound that interferes with the replication of HIV and, in doing so, slows the deterioration of the immune system and/or brain. Approved by the FDA in 1987, AZT can slow the progression to AIDS in persons who are infected with HIV. AZT is a generic (chemical) name of the drug, while Retrovir is the trade (commercial) name of the same substance. The drug is also known by the generic name zidovudine.

2

Q Does AZT have any side effects?

A Unfortunately, AZT has substantial side effects, the most prominent of which is anemia. Patients feel very tired and rather weak, and they tend to have nausea and headaches. The blood-clotting mechanism may also be impaired, and wounds may take unusually long to heal.

3

Q Are ddI and ddC similar to AZT?

A Yes, they are. Both are other drugs approved by the FDA for use against HIV. Both work in the same way as AZT; that is, they are inhibitors of reverse transcriptase. Combinations of either drug with AZT have been shown effective in reducing the amount of HIV in the body because they interfere with different strains of HIV that may emerge.

the blood-brain barrier, enter the cerebrospinal fluid, and reach infected brain cells. Unfortunately, the toxicity of AZT somewhat tempers these positive factors, as we shall see presently.

In 1988, researchers at the National Cancer Institute first reported that AZT could also alter the course of disease in children displaying the neurological symptoms of AIDS. Twenty-one children ranging in age from 1 to 12 were given the drug by continuous intravenous infusion, and all showed improvement. In many children, the intelligence quotient (IQ) rose a significant number of points; in some cases, the youngsters' intelligence level returned to the level at which it was before they became ill. Scans of brain tissue showed that in some cases, shrunken tissue returned to its normal condition after treatment; younger children regained the ability to walk or talk or exhibited other developmental. Because children appear to suffer more brain damage from HIV infection than adults do, the study was particularly encouraging (Figure 8.5).

One of the more remarkable success stories associated with AZT is its use in pregnant women to reduce the risk of HIV transmission to their unborn offspring. Dramatic results reported in 1994 summarized the effects of AZT in 748 HIV-infected women: 25 percent of children born to women administered placebos had HIV infection, while only 8 percent of children born to AZT-treated women were infected with HIV. In the years thereafter, the number of babies who were infected with HIV from their mothers declined substantially, largely due to AZT therapy. For example, in 1992, in the United States the number of newborns who developed pediatric AIDS was 907, while in 1997, the number was 297, a 67 percent decline. And some health officials were postulating that prenatal AZT treatment could reduce the risk of acquiring HIV to 3 percent (that is, only 3 percent of HIV-infected women would give birth to infected babies).

Even limited AZT treatment in pregnant women is of significant value. In 1999, for example, researchers reported that administering AZT and another drug called 3TC during the last few weeks of pregnancy reduces transmission of HIV to the fetus by 50 percent. Furthermore, treating a woman intravenously with AZT at the beginning of labor and administering AZT to babies just after birth reduces HIV transmission by 37 percent (Table 8.2). An important implication of this finding is that the drug intervention is less costly than the standard treatment ($80 vs. $800 per pregnancy), and thus, it is within reach of developing countries where the spread of AIDS has outstripped the nation's health resources. Studies show that the risk of HIV transmission can be further reduced if a woman is treated with AZT and gives birth by cesarean delivery, since the infant has no oppor-

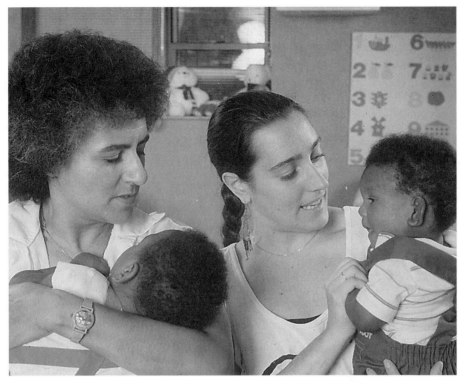

FIGURE 8.5

Studies using azidothymidine (AZT) in young children infected with HIV have shown that the drug can stem the progression to AIDS and can reverse some of the brain damage that often occurs in children. These babies being held by health care workers at the Birk Childcare Center in Brooklyn may be candidates for AZT therapy.

TABLE

8.2 Effectiveness in Newborns of Treating HIV-Positive Pregnant Women with AZT and 3TC

Treatment	Number of Babies Tested	Number of Babies HIV+	Percentage Infected	Percentage Reduction in Risk
From 36 weeks to 1 week postpartum baby treated for 1 week	359	31	8.6	50
From onset of labor to 1 week postpartum; baby treated for 1 week	343	37	10.8	37
From onset of labor to delivery; no treatment of baby	351	62	17.7	0
Placebo	273	47	17.2	0

Source: Science, 1999, Vol. 283, p. 916.

tunity to swallow blood or other fluid from the mother, nor can any of the mother's fluids contact the infant's mucous membranes or abrasions on its skin. And finally, long-term studies indicate that AZT therapy poses no unusual risk for the newborn.

By the start of the twenty-first century, it was clear that AZT, when used in a combination of drugs, slows the progression to AIDS in persons who have HIV infection (as we discuss below). The effects were far-reaching: Many physicians and health officials who had opposed HIV testing because little could be done for those testing positive changed their minds and urged people with a history of high-risk behaviors to take the test. Their recommendations also dramatically increased the pool of potential AZT users to several hundred thousand (the increase lowered the cost of AZT treatment to about $5000 annually). Scientists also found that a lower dose of AZT might be adequate for delaying the symptoms of AIDS. This was good news for two reasons: Lower doses would effectively reduce the cost of therapy and save the patient thousands of dollars annually, and lower doses would lessen side effects, as we discuss next.

Obstacles to AZT Use No drug for microbial disease is taken without risk. Penicillin, for example, can lead to severe and sometimes fatal allergic reactions. Other drugs upset the microbial population of the intestine and permit fungal diseases such as candidiasis ("yeast disease") to emerge. Still others cause liver or kidney damage. In terms of risk, AZT is no different from such other drugs (Table 8.3). As long ago as 1985, the toxic side effects of AZT were known, and bone marrow suppression was a notable problem. The chief effect of this suppression is anemia, often so severe that a choice has to be made between continued use of AZT and the debilitating effects of anemia. Blood transfusions may be necessary to compensate for the anemia's effects.

Another side effect in many individuals who take AZT is thrombocytopenia. This condition develops when the body's blood platelets are progressively destroyed

TABLE 8.3	Benefits and Obstacles to Use of AZT	
Benefits	**Obstacles**
Increases patient life span	Suppresses activity in bone marrow
Interrupts viral replication	Induces anemia
Prevents progression to AIDS	Affects platelets and blood clotting
Penetrates into infected cells	Possible cause of cancer in animals
Remains active for 1 hour	Leads to drug resistance in viruses
Passes blood-brain barrier	May cause headache, nausea
Preferred by reverse transcriptase	Dose reduction causes symptom rise
Can be given orally	High cost

("thrombocytes" are blood platelets; "penia" refers to reduction). Because platelets are required for blood clot formation, their reduction means that the blood fails to clot easily. Increased hemorrhaging, longer clotting times, and greater susceptibility to injury may result. Other side effects of AZT use include headaches, nausea, vomiting, seizures, and confusion. Symptoms such as these vary with individuals, with dosage, and with extent of the HIV infection or AIDS.

Another troublesome problem is the so-called rebound effect. Physicians have reported that when they recommend a lower dose of AZT to minimize anemia and other side effects, the dose reduction incites a dangerous and unexpected flare-up of symptoms. Neurological problems were noted as a characteristic sign in one report, and a sharp increase in the level of bloodborne HIV was pointed out in a second report. Researchers speculated that AZT keeps the virus in check, but viral replication may occur at an increased rate when the drug is withdrawn.

Another problem is drug resistance. Drug resistance can develop when a drug destroys sensitive strains of a microorganism but allows more resistant mutants in the population to survive. As early as 1989, it became obvious that resistant strains of HIV were emerging in persons taking AZT. Of particular concern were people whose immune systems were so severely compromised that heavy doses of AZT were required to keep the HIV in check. In advanced cases of AIDS, increased viral multiplication yields increased possibilities for a strain with resistant traits. In a study at Canada's McGill University, for example, physicians gave AZT to 72 AIDS patients for 36 weeks and found that 20 percent of the patients harbored viruses with AZT resistance at the end of the study. Findings such as these also influence the use of AZT in HIV-infected patients in whom AIDS has not developed, because treating people early and for long periods of time might encourage resistant strains of HIV to emerge and eventually make AZT useless.

Other Dideoxynucleosides

AZT belongs to a group of compounds known as dideoxynucleosides, that is, nucleosides missing oxygen groups at two positions, position 2′ and position 3′ ("dideoxy-"). Two other dideoxynucleosides that show anti-HIV value are dideoxycytidine (ddC) and dideoxyinosine (ddI). Both are inhibitors of the enzyme reverse transcriptase, working as chain terminators in a manner similar to AZT. Their side effects are less severe, however, and include skin rashes as well as peripheral neuropathy, such as headache, pain, and decreased touch, pinprick, temperature, and vibratory sensations. The drugs are often referred to in the technical literature as nucleoside reverse transcriptase inhibitors (NRTIs).

When ddI first became available in 1989, the FDA announced that it would allow wide distribution at the same time as tests were continuing to determine the effectiveness of the drug. This unusual landmark step was taken because the toxicity of AZT was too high for some AIDS patients and because ddI works in essentially the same way and could be expected to show benefits similar to those of AZT. Marketed as Videx, the drug could be used in rotation with AZT to minimize the respective toxicities of the drugs while maximizing their potency. In

1991, the FDA licensed ddI for use against HIV infection and AIDS. The drug is also known as didanosine.

The second dideoxynucleoside, ddC, was FDA-approved in 1992. It was the first drug to be licensed through the Accelerated Approval Program established by the FDA. Another name for ddC is zalcitabine, and the trade name is Hivid. Like AZT and ddI, the drug is an inhibitor of reverse transcriptase, but it is thought to act at a different site. Varying combinations with AZT and ddI are currently recommended for patients. Another compound in the same class of dideoxynucleosides is d4T, which is also known as stavudine (Zerit).

Another dideoxynucleoside is a sulfur-containing derivative of deoxycytidine known as 2′-deoxy-3-thiocytidine, or 3TC (also known as lamivudine or Epivir). In 1996, this drug became the first *initial* therapy drug approved to treat AIDS since AZT was approved nine years previously. Since then, 3TC has also been prescribed in combination with AZT and a protease inhibitor to constitute the three-drug regimen that has significantly reduced the viral load in AIDS patients. As we shall discuss presently, the three-drug therapy has played a major role in the developing view that AIDS may one day be considered a chronic disease that can be maintained and controlled, rather than an acute disease bringing certainty of death (Figure 8.6).

FIGURE 8.6
A patient who has had AIDS since 1990 shows the "cocktail" of drugs he takes daily.

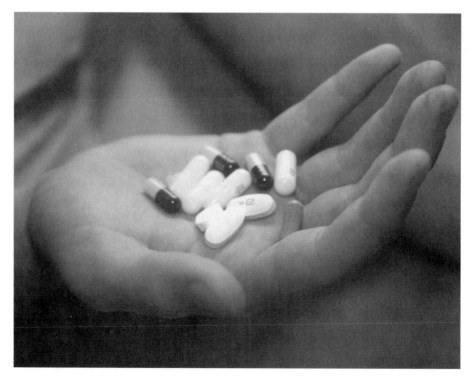

In 1999, the FDA approved an AZT-like drug called abacavir (Ziagen). When used in combination with AZT and 3TC, this drug is significantly more effective in reducing the viral load in patients to "undetectable" levels (i.e., 400 or fewer HIV RNA copies per mL) than AZT and 3TC used together. The drug is particularly useful for treating children and young patients because it is formulated as a palatable liquid that is not bitter (most pills are difficult to swallow and are bitter).

The newest dideoxynucleoside is tenofovir (Viread), which achieved FDA approval in 2001. Tenofovir is called a nucleo*tide* reverse transcriptase inhibitor because it contains an extra phosphate group. This extra group makes the drug a more active chain terminator. Taken once a day, tenofovir appears to circumvent HIV mutations that confer resistance to other drugs. Mild to moderate gastrointestinal disturbances are the only known side effects.

Nonnucleoside Analogs

Although the dideoxynucleoside drugs have achieved a measure of success, some patients cannot tolerate the side effects or are infected with HIV particles resistant to the drugs. For these individuals, nonnucleoside analogs offer a viable option. The drugs target reverse transcriptase and react directly with it (in contrast to the dideoxynucleosides, which trick reverse transcriptase into producing faulty DNA). Some researchers recommend that physicians prescribe nucleoside analogs in combination with the dideoxynucleosides, while others recommend them when the three-drug combination involving a protease inhibitor fails. In the technical literature, the drugs are called nonnucleoside reverse transcriptase inhibitors (NNRTIs).

The three most prominent nonnucleoside analogs are nevirapine, delavirdine, and efavirenz. Nevirapine (Viramune) and delavirdine (Rescriptor) elicit HIV resistance rapidly, so they have received FDA approval for use only with a dideoxynucleoside such as AZT or ddI. Such combinations are more effective than either drug used alone, as a result of the so-called synergistic effect. Presumably this is because reverse transcriptase is being inhibited by two different mechanisms at the same time. In 1999, researchers reported that, like AZT, nevirapine can significantly reduce the possibility of HIV transfer from HIV-infected pregnant women to their newborns. The substantially lower cost of nevirapine adds an economic advantage to its use, especially in developing countries. However, damage to the liver (hepatotoxicity) and skin reactions have been reported in patients taking the drug, and appropriate precautions have been issued.

Efavirenz (Sustiva) received FDA approval in 1998. This drug is taken once a day with normal doses of AZT and 3TC in a three-drug combination therapy. In one study, efavirenz used with ddI and an AZT-like drug called emtricitabine (FTC or Coviricil) reduced viral loads substantially in 98 percent of patients followed over a three-year period. Dizziness, insomnia, impaired concentration, and drowsiness are notable side effects of the drug. And women are strongly advised not to use the drug, as it could cause birth defects.

Other Therapeutic Agents

Since AZT was approved for use in 1987, physicians have shown that the drug is capable of increasing helper T-lymphocyte counts, enhancing survival rates of AIDS patients, and adding to the quality of life for those infected with HIV. In addition, use of AZT has relieved some of the hopelessness that pervaded the early years of the AIDS epidemic, while providing impetus for additional efforts to develop treatments and therapies for AIDS. The work with other compounds has also been significant because it shows that scientists can utilize their understanding of the biochemistry of HIV to synthesize other specific drugs.

But AZT and its related compounds are only a few of the multitude of drugs currently in various stages of experimentation and testing. In this section, we survey some of the other drugs that are in use or hold promise for use against HIV.

Protease Inhibitors

Protease inhibitors first made headlines in 1989. Development of these drugs resulted from determination of the three-dimensional structure of an HIV enzyme known as protease. The chemical determination was so detailed that it specified the arrangement of the enzyme's individual atoms. Protease is essential to the last stages of HIV replication; it trims bulky, unprocessed viral proteins down to working size before they are assembled as protein coats for the new viruses.

Once the exact structure of protease was known, researchers designed drugs to fit precisely into the enzyme's griplike active site and jam its action. They were encouraged by the observation that a form of HIV with an altered protease enzyme could not trim proteins and assemble them to make protein coats. By 1995, twelve pharmaceutical companies were working on the development of an entire series of protease inhibitors that yielded lower levels of HIV in the bloodstream as well as higher counts of T-lymphocytes. The drugs were used alone and in combination with other drugs, and because they affected a relatively small enzyme, the emergence of resistant viruses was rare.

By 1996, the protease inhibitors had assumed their place in medicine as accepted therapies for HIV infection and AIDS. That year, three drugs received FDA approval: saquinavir (Invirase), indinavir (Crixivan), and ritonavir (Norvir). In clinical trials conducted in several parts of the world, all three drugs were shown to decrease viral concentrations in patients' blood and slow disease progression by up to 50 percent in late-stage patients. Side effects were apparently limited to mild nausea, vomiting, and diarrhea as well as fat buildup on the torso and face (i.e., lipid-dystrophy). Soon, researchers were recommending a three-drug combination (a "cocktail" of drugs) consisting of AZT, 3TC, and one of the protease inhibitors. The cocktail therapy came to be known as highly active antiretroviral therapy, or HAART.

The impact of HAART on the AIDS epidemic was immediate; for example, in the first half of 1996, there were 21,460 AIDS-related deaths in the United States, but in the first half of 1997, the number dropped to 12,040 and continued to drop thereafter (Table 8.4). Physicians described in glowing terms how ill

TABLE 8.4 Deaths of AIDS Patients in the United States Between 1993 and 1999

Male adult/adolescent Exposure category	Year of death							
	1993	1994	1995	1996	1997	1998	1999	2000
Men who have sex with men	23,956	25,534	25,044	16,854	8,666	7,048	6,230	5,439
Injection drug users	9,325	10,454	10,844	8,551	5,346	4,476	4,119	3,551
Men who have sex with men and inject drugs	3,188	3,528	3,467	2,591	1,447	1,262	1,182	1,120
Hemophilia/coagulation disorder	357	346	330	246	136	117	100	*
Heterosexual contact	1,600	2,013	2,389	2,111	1,464	1,227	1,257	1,218
Receipt of blood transfusion, blood components, or tissue	314	304	259	217	108	83	73	*
Risk not reported or identified	168	143	102	66	44	28	29	187
Male subtotal	**38,908**	**42,322**	**42,434**	**30,636**	**17,212**	**14,241**	**12,991**	**11,514**
Female adult/adolescent exposure category								
Injection drug users	3,152	3,713	3,824	3,289	2,137	1,900	1,920	1,662
Hemophilia/coagulation disorder	17	28	31	30	20	14	17	*
Heterosexual contact	2,662	3,489	3,999	3,439	2,297	2,029	2,032	1,899
Receipt of blood transfusion, blood components, or tissue	238	224	235	170	93	75	75	*
Risk not reported or identified	77	56	56	32	20	15	19	95
Female subtotal	**6,146**	**7,510**	**8,144**	**6,960**	**4,567**	**4,033**	**4,063**	**3,656**
Pediatric (<13 years old) exposure category	544	586	539	429	221	123	118	74
Total[1]	**45,598**	**50,418**	**51,117**	**38,025**	**21,999**	**18,397**	**17,172**	**15,245**

* = data not available.

[1] Because column totals were calculated independently of the values for the subpopulations, the values in each column may not sum to the column total.

Source: HIV/AIDS Surveillance Report, Vol. 13(1), June, 2001.

patients responded to the therapy, and with the introduction of the viral load test, researchers could chart the disappearance of HIV from the blood, lymph nodes, and other tissues. Some scientists were so excited about the paradigm shift created by HAART (the $10,000 cost per year notwithstanding) that they forecast the imminent eradication of HIV from the population. It was not uncommon to hear the words "AIDS" and "hope" in the same sentence. And *Science* magazine, the preeminent journal of science in the United States declared protease inhibitors to be the 1996 Breakthrough of the Year.

The success of HAART led to numerous other studies involving drug cocktails. In one study, for instance, a combination of two protease inhibitors (ritonavir and saquinavir) showed a reduction in viral load to less than 400 copies per mL (considered undetectable) in 88 percent of patients. Other studies including or excluding protease inhibitors combined delavirdine, AZT, and 3TC; or efavirenz and indinavir; or nevirapine, AZT, and ddI. HAART's success also led to the view that maximum suppression of the virus would minimize damage to the immune system and possibly avert opportunistic diseases. This so-called "hit it early, hit it hard" approach was spearheaded by David Ho of New York's Aaron Diamond AIDS Research Center (Figure 8.7). Ho was among the first to show the efficacy of the protease inhibitors in three-drug combinations and to raise hope for new treatments. Ho was honored in 1996 as *Time* magazine's Man of the Year.

Unfortunately, by 1997, reality was setting in, and HAART drugs were being seen as far from perfect. Many patients had already chosen to stop taking the drugs, complaining of difficulty in adhering to the drug regimen, a complicated

FIGURE 8.7

Former *Time* Man-of-the-Year David Ho, pathologist and AIDS researcher, at an AIDS conference.

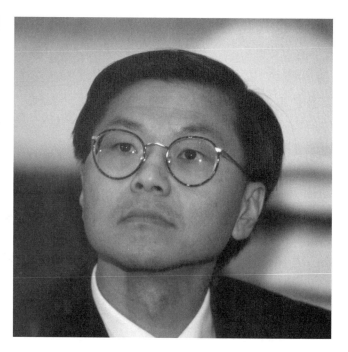

Treating HIV Infection and AIDS

affair that involved taking up to 15 pills a day—some alone and others in tandem, some on a full stomach and others on an empty one (in one study, only 60 percent of patients said that they adhered to the regimen). Others complained of the side effects of the drugs (Table 8.5), and still others expressed the feeling that the drugs were failing to work. That year, the FDA, in an unusual step, sent thousands of letters to physicians advising them that the protease inhibitors were linked to high blood pressure (related to raised cholesterol levels) and new or worsened cases of diabetes. Scientists also noted the emergence of multidrug-resistant HIV strains, often the result of patients' continual switching among the many available drugs.

By 2002, the newer policy advanced by many medical professionals was to back off the "hit it early, hit it hard" approach and consider deferring treatment until the patient showed signs that the immune system was weakening. Moreover, *Guidelines for the Use of Antiretroviral Agents* developed by the United States Department of Health and Human Services had been in place for a year. Among other things, the guidelines recommended beginning HAART drugs when the infected individual's T-lymphocyte count dropped below 350 cells per microliter (as compared to the previous recommendation of 500 cells per microliter). The guidelines are available for downloading at the HIV/AIDS Treatment Information Service website at http://www.hivatis.org.

Researchers have also discovered that as soon as patients stop taking their HAART drugs, HIV rebounds in the body and rises to high levels, possibly due to the influence of chemokines (cytokines) that stimulate the lymphoid cells to produce HIV particles; soon thereafter, the classic opportunistic diseases surface. Scientists once believed that if viral replication could be suppressed for a few years, all the pools of HIV in the body would be exhausted. However, it now appears that HIV is able to find sanctuary in long-lived dormant ("resting") cells of the immune system, lurking in a latent state for many years. This reservoir of latent infection is apparently what prevents HAART from curing patients; instead, it puts patients into remission. The level of HIV is pushed way down, but it fails to hit zero (Figure 8.8).

Still, the reduction of the viral load is apparently very beneficial. In 2000, for example, European investigators reported that with HAART and other new drug therapies, about 80 percent of AIDS patients lived at least 10 years after becoming infected with HIV; before the advent of such drugs, only 55 percent lived 10 years or more. As a writer in *Science* magazine explained, "AIDS research ricochets from breathtaking optimism to stomach-wrenching disappointment and back again."

Fusion Inhibitors

A new class of drugs called fusion inhibitors represents an alternative approach to treating HIV infection and AIDS. Like protease inhibitors, the fusion inhibitors were derived from an understanding of the basic science of HIV, in this case, the method by which HIV fuses with its host T-lymphocyte (Chapter 2). The drugs are designed to interfere with steps taking place before reverse transcriptase and protease act in the host cells.

TABLE 8.5 Some Side Effects Associated with Antiretroviral Drugs

Antiretroviral Class/Agent	Primary Side Effects and Toxicities
Nucleoside reverse transcriptase inhibitors (NRTIs)	
Zidovudine (Retrovir; ZDV; AZT)	Anemia, neutropenia, nausea, headache, insomnia, muscle pain, and weakness
Lamivudine (Epivir; 3TC)	Abdominal pain, nausea, diarrhea, rash, and pancreatitis
Stavudine (Zerit; d4T)	Peripheral neuropathy, headache, diarrhea, nausea, insomnia, anorexia, pancreatitis, increased liver function tests (LFTs), anemia, and neutropenia
Didanosine (Videx; ddI)	Pancreatitis, lactic acidosis, neuropathy, diarrhea, abdominal pain, and nausea
Abacavir (Ziagen; ABC)	Nausea, diarrhea, anorexia, abdominal pain, fatigue, headache, insomnia, and hypersensitivity reactions
Nonnucleoside reverse transcriptase inhibitors (NNRTIs)	
Nevirapine (Viramune; NVP)	Rash (including cases of Stevens-Johnson syndrome), fever, nausea, headache, hepatitis, and increased LFTs
Delavirdine (Rescriptor; DLV)	Rash (including cases of Stevens-Johnson syndrome), nausea, diarrhea, headache, fatigue, and increased LFTs
Efavirenz (Sustiva; EFV)	Rash (including cases of Stevens-Johnson syndrome), insomnia, somnolence, dizziness, trouble concentrating, and abnormal dreaming
Protease inhibitors (PIs)	
Indinavir (Crixivan; IDV)	Nausea, abdominal pain, nephrolithiasis, and indirect hyperbilirubinemia
Nelfinavir (Viracept; NFV)	Diarrhea, nausea, abdominal pain, weakness, and rash
Ritonavir (Norvir; RTV)	Weakness, diarrhea, nausea, circumoral paresthesia, taste alteration, and increased cholesterol and triglycerides
Saquinavir (Fortovase; SQV)	Diarrhea, abdominal pain, nausea, hyperglycemia, and increased LFTs
Lopinavir/Ritonavir (Kaletra)	Diarrhea, fatigue, headache, nausea, and increased cholesterol and triglycerides

Source: MMWR (RR), Vol. 50, June 29, 2001, p. 13.

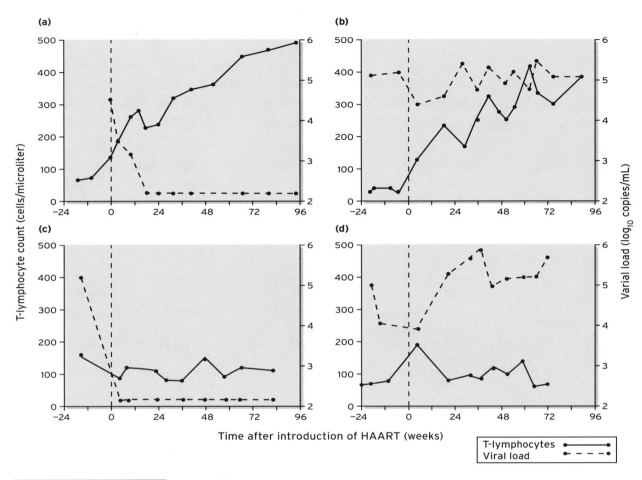

FIGURE 8.8

Four possible results of the anti-HIV therapy HAART and their interpretations. (a) Complete success is recognized as the viral load is suppressed and the T-lymphocyte count rises. In (b) and (c), the treatment is deemed partially successful, while in (d), it is deemed a failure. *Source:* Science, *1988, 80:1872.*

One fusion inhibitor now being tested is a drug tentatively called T-20 (Enfuvirtide). This is a synthetic peptide containing 36 amino acids. The peptide mirrors a key part of the gp41 molecule, the HIV glycoprotein that anchors the gp120 molecule after the latter has contacted the cell membrane of the T-lymphocyte, as we explored in depth in Chapter 3. When T-20 binds to the gp41 molecule, the gp120 molecule cannot contact the T-lymphocyte, and fusion is interrupted. At this writing, T-20 has been shown effective for reducing the viral loads in patients for whom HAART therapy fails, and large-scale clinical trials involving over 1000 patients are under way. But because T-20 is a large molecule that must be injected, researchers are already studying smaller peptides that can be taken orally and will survive the intense acidity of the stomach environment. These smaller molecules target a pocket on the gp41 molecule that is exposed when that molecule unites with the host T-lymphocyte. The research illustrates how the science of structural biology has application in the development of a possible new therapy.

Another group of innovative researchers are developing a fusion inhibitor using genetic engineering technology. They begin with the CD4 receptor molecules at the surface of the T-lymphocytes and determine the chemical structure of these protein molecules. Working backward, they deduce the genetic code for the protein and formulate an artificial gene. When this gene is placed into a producer organism such as a bacterium, the organism synthesizes industrial quantities of soluble CD4 (Receptin) molecules. Injected into patients, soluble CD4 bind molecules to HIV particles and enhance the effects of other drugs such as AZT, as Figure 8.9 displays.

One of the disadvantages of using soluble CD4 molecules is their short half-life in the bloodstream (the half-life is the time for half of the drug to be metabolized by the body and, thus, disappear). Researchers have partly resolved this problem by linking the CD4 molecules to the stem sections of anti-HIV antibodies to produce immunoadhesions. The immunoadhesions remain active in the bloodstream longer than CD4 molecules, and they bind more efficiently to HIV particles, thereby blocking fusion and inactivating the virus at the same time. The preparation called PRO542 has been shown to enhance the activity of T-20, and vice versa.

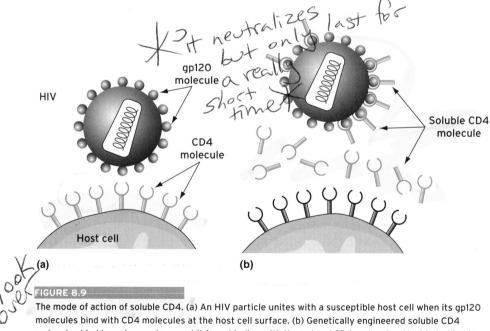

FIGURE 8.9

The mode of action of soluble CD4. (a) An HIV particle unites with a susceptible host cell when its gp120 molecules bind with CD4 molecules at the host cell surface. (b) Genetically engineered soluble CD4 molecules bind to a virus and prevent it from binding with the natural CD4 molecules. Unable to bind to the host cell, the virus is rendered harmless.

Before we leave the fusion inhibitors, we should note recent investigations of the zinc fingers in the capsid of HIV. Zinc fingers are sections of capsid proteins that contain large amounts of the amino acids cysteine and histidine combined with atoms of zinc in arrangements that extend out from the surface. A drug being developed by biochemists at the National Cancer Institute attacks the sulfur atoms in cysteine molecules; this attack leads to ejection of the zinc atoms and incapacitation of the capsid protein. The effect is to limit the ability of HIV to fuse with its host cell and to synthesize the protein it later needs for capsid formation. Because the zinc fingers resist mutation (i.e., they are "mutationally intolerant"), the drug is an attractive anti-HIV therapy (Healthline 8.2).

Entry Inhibitors

Elucidation of the central role played by chemokines and chemokine receptors in HIV's attachment to T-lymphocytes has kindled hopes for therapeutic molecules that will block HIV infection. As Chapter 2 discusses, HIV slips into T-lymphocytes by commandeering CXCR4 and other coreceptor molecules on the cells' surface that normally bind to chemokines. (Chemokines are a set of proteins that act as chemical messengers when produced by cells of the immune system.) This discovery, made in 1996, encouraged scientists to develop treatments that would exploit the HIV/chemokine nexus. One research group developed a synthetic chemokine that works within the cytoplasm of the T-lymphocyte to inactivate the CXCR4 proteins as they are synthesized and before they can be dispatched to the cell surface, where they will provide docking sites for HIV (Chapter 2). The synthetic chemokine has been called an intrakine because it works within the cell, rather than at its surface. In laboratory tests, this intrakine effectively blocked expression of the surface CXCR4 protein and thereby prevented formation of the CXCR4 coreceptor site. Essentially, the HIV particle found itself unable to enter its host cell.

Despite the encouraging results, researchers were quick to point out that the intrakine is not a new therapeutic agent because the gap between basic research and applied technology is usually vast and talk of bridging it is often premature. Nevertheless, the research has opened new possibilities for therapies. Indeed, in 1999, another group found that gene mutation causes some individuals to overproduce a chemokine identified as SDF-1. Individuals with this mutated gene apparently progress more slowly to AIDS than expected, and since SDF-1 molecules normally bind to the CXCR4 coreceptor sites, it is conceivable that these abundant molecules occupy the sites otherwise used by HIV particles. This finding correlates with the 1996 discovery that individuals lacking the CXCR4 coreceptors are able to resist HIV infection (Chapter 2).

Healthline 8.2

1 Q I have read newspaper reports about HAART. What does that mean?

A HAART stands for "highly active antiretroviral therapy." It is an approach to AIDS therapy that employs a three-drug combination. One drug in the combination is usually AZT; another is usually 3TC. The third drug in the combination is a protease inhibitor, either saquinavir, indinavir, or ritonavir. Such a three-drug combination, often called a "drug cocktail," has been shown to considerably delay the progression to AIDS and make HIV infection a disease that can be managed.

2 Q What's a protease inhibitor?

A A protease inhibitor is a chemical compound that interferes with the construction of the HIV particle at the conclusion of its replication cycle. The compound neutralizes the enzyme that is normally used to process the protein used in the viral capsid.

3 Q Can any other drugs be used in HAART?

A Yes. A physician has a choice of numerous drugs approved by the FDA for HAART. Recommendations are constantly changing as a result of new research findings, and physicians are free to use whichever combination they believe will most benefit the patient.

The promising discoveries relating to chemokine receptors are counterbalanced by the possible unanticipated developments. For example, using chemokines or chemokine analogs to block an entry site might encourage HIV to develop a preference for an alternate site such as the CCR5 coreceptor. Nevertheless, researchers are encouraged to continue their work with chemokines since they have already developed profitable drugs that target receptors involved in rheumatoid arthritis, psoriasis, and other inflammatory conditions.

Using an innovative approach described as "set a thief to catch a thief," scientists have formulated a recombined virus to attack HIV particles. Investigators at Yale University began with a well-researched virus called the vesicular stomatitis virus (VSV), which infects cattle and other livestock and causes ulcers on their hooves and tongue. The researchers biochemically removed the genes that encode the capsid proteins of the VSV and inserted in its genome the genes that encode the CD4 and CXCR4 receptors of a T-lymphocyte. When the VSV replicated in cells, its new genome encoded a strain of the virus with CD4 and CXCR4 proteins on the surface instead of the usual capsid proteins. In laboratory tests, this virus bound itself to gp120 and gp41 molecules in the spikes of HIV, thereby neutralizing the HIV. It also united with and eliminated infected T-lymphocytes, since these cells are studded with gp120 and gp41 molecules on their surfaces (the molecules are later incorporated in new HIV particles during budding). The Trojan horse virus, as the recombined VSV came to be called, demonstrates that it is possible to use HIV's so-called grappling hooks (i.e., its gp120 and gp41 molecules) as a target for drug therapy.

Interleukin-2

The finding that HIV rapidly rebounds when HAART is stopped has prompted the conclusion that long-term control of HIV will likely require immune-based therapies to enhance the immune system's ability to combat HIV as well as the agents of opportunistic diseases. Among the well-studied immune-based therapies is interleukin-2 (IL-2), a chemokine (or cytokine) that spurs the development of helper T-lymphocytes and acts as a growth-enhancing factor for cytotoxic T-lymphocytes (Chapter 3). Currently FDA-approved for use against certain kinds of cancer, IL-2 is produced synthetically by recombinant DNA technology and is available as aldesleukin (Proleukin). In recent years, the drug has been used in small-scale studies as a supplemental (adjunctive) therapy to boost the number of helper T-lymphocytes in HIV patients. Two major trials using HAART plus IL-2 are currently under way in 4000 patients in 18 countries. The trials have been established to determine the effect of IL-2 on the clinical progression from HIV infection to AIDS.

Part of the value of IL-2 is its ability to wrest from their quiescent state the reservoir of "safe haven" dormant T-lymphocytes that are infected with inactive HIV. This inactive HIV is invisible to anti-HIV drugs, and it is largely from this cohort of cells that HIV rebounds after HAART is stopped (as we noted previously). Researchers have found that IL-2 can activate the cells and make their indwelling HIV vulnerable to destruction by HAART. Experiments performed in 1998 pointed to the practical benefits of this approach when researchers isolated from patients resting T-lymphocytes purged of HIV. However, before a person can be declared "cured" of HIV infection, it must be shown that no traces of HIV remain in macrophages, brain cells, or any other infected cells. There is also the possibility that the treatment may backfire if the aroused cells become high-rate producers of HIV.

Work on another chemokine called interleukin-16 (IL-16) is also ongoing. As early as 1995, this chemokine was isolated from T-lymphocytes (CD8 cells), which target body cells when they are infected. When administered to patients, IL-16 appeared to interrupt HIV replication by repressing transcription.

Antisense Molecules

The AIDS virus infects a host cell by inserting itself as a provirus into the cell's DNA. To produce new viruses, the provirus then encodes molecules of RNA and sends these as chemical messengers into the host cell's cytoplasm to use the cell's resources and building blocks to form new viruses.

The molecules of RNA so encoded are known as messenger RNA (mRNA) molecules. They are essential components of the process of protein synthesis studied in most basic biology courses. These mRNA molecules are used to produce viral RNA for the genome and direct the synthesis of viral protein for the capsid. To interrupt the production of new viral parts, biochemists have designed a genetic projectile, a synthetic RNA molecule that attacks and neutralizes the mRNA molecule. The synthetic RNA carries a molecular code complementary to that of mRNA. Thus, the synthetic molecule combines specifically with the mRNA, much like bringing a pair of right and left hands together (Figure 8.10). In biochemical jargon, the mRNA molecule formed by an infected cell has a molecular message that makes "sense." The synthetic RNA has a message that is "antisense."

Early in the 1900s, the Nobel laureate Paul Ehrlich introduced the term "magic bullet" to describe a seemingly impossible drug that would attack a microbe without causing dangerous side effects to the body. Antisense molecules could be such a magic bullet because they are directed at targets within the cells, rather than at the cells themselves. Such targets are not essential for normal cell function and are not present in healthy cells. One group of researchers at the National Cancer Institute is testing an antisense molecule aimed at the *rev* gene of HIV. To switch on this gene, a regulatory protein must first bind to it. But to make the protein, an mRNA molecule must provide the code for joining the necessary amino acids in proper sequence. The antisense molecule devised by the researchers is directed at this mRNA.

Antisense molecules have been successfully tested in the laboratory, using infected T-lymphocytes and animals. As of 1995, one antisense molecule directed against HIV, a substance known as Gem 91, was being tested in human volunteers in the United States and France. Another antisense molecule, Fomivirsen,

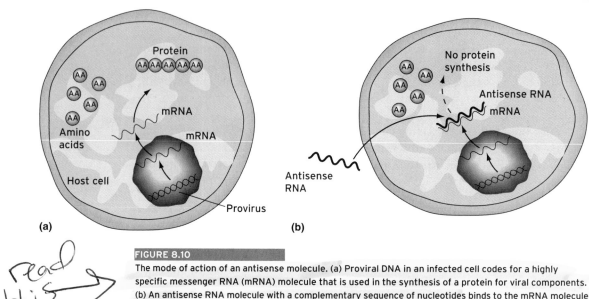

(a) **(b)**

Read this →

FIGURE 8.10

The mode of action of an antisense molecule. (a) Proviral DNA in an infected cell codes for a highly specific messenger RNA (mRNA) molecule that is used in the synthesis of a protein for viral components. (b) An antisense RNA molecule with a complementary sequence of nucleotides binds to the mRNA molecule (the sense molecule) and prevents that mRNA molecule from functioning.

directed against cytomegalovirus was also in the trials stage. In July of 1997, however, the test were halted because of platelet depletion in trial patients.

Miscellaneous Therapeutic Agents

Certain other therapeutic agents merit attention either because they have shown promise in the past or because they are in various stages of development and study. In some cases, the drugs have displayed toxic side effects and are therefore used under limited circumstances.

Interferon is a naturally occurring antiviral substance produced by human cells when they are stimulated by viruses. The interferon does not protect the cell that produced it, but it passes into neighboring cells and induces them to produce proteins, which block the entry of viruses as well as their budding from the host cell cytoplasm (Figure 8.11). Two major American pharmaceutical companies have used genetic engineering to produce a form of interferon called alpha interferon. Alpha interferon is commercially available from the two companies as Roferon and Intron-A. It has been approved by the FDA for use against Kaposi's sarcoma because it was shown to diminish and, in some cases, eliminate the purplish skin tumors that accompany the disease.

After successfully developing therapies based on two HIV enzymes—reverse transcriptase and protease—researchers are zeroing in on the third enzyme, integrase. Integrase incorporates proviral DNA into the DNA of the host T-lymphocyte (Chapter 2). Scientists at Merck Research Laboratories have tested tens of thousands of chemical substances in the company's repository, and in 2000, they reported two diketoacids with anti-integrase activity. Fur-

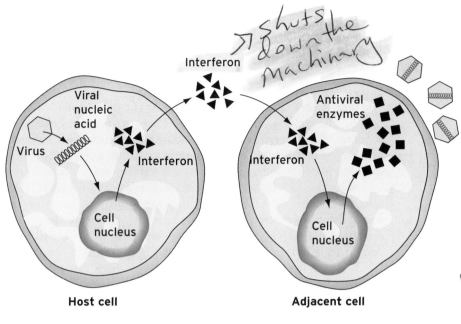

shuts the down the Machinery →

FIGURE 8.11
The mode of action of interferon. When a virus enters a host cell, its nucleic acid stimulates the cell nucleus to set into motion the production of interferon. Interferon passes out of the cell into an adjacent cell, where it stimulates the cell nucleus to code for the production of antiviral enzymes that protect the cell against viral invasion.

read over

thermore, University of California biochemists have developed a chemical model of the integrase molecule, and they have used it to screen a library of compounds to locate inhibitors that might bind to the enzyme's active site. It is hoped that this approach, used successfully years before with protease, will yield equally successful results.

Compound Q made headlines in 1989 as a possible drug for AIDS. Obtained from the root of the Chinese cucumber, compound Q displayed an unusual ability to destroy HIV-infected macrophages taken from AIDS patients and cultivated in the laboratory. In volunteers, however, the extract displayed a less than spectacular ability to improve immune system performance, and in some individuals, it induced confusion, seizures, and coma (Healthline 8.3).

Two compounds under investigation for use as binding inhibitors are AL 721 and peptide T. AL 721 is a composite of several lipids normally manufactured in the body during the metabolism of fats. The compound is thought to act on HIV by dissolving its envelope, thereby interfering with viral attachment to host T-lymphocytes. Peptide T is a series of eight amino acids (an octapeptide), synthesized to resemble a region of HIV's gp120 protein molecule. Investigators envision that the octapeptide will bind to the CD4 receptor site of host cells and thereby block binding of HIV. However, there is concern that peptide T will react with uninfected immune system cells that also carry the CD4 receptor and cause immunosuppression, thereby further endangering AIDS patients.

For more than 20 years, dextran sulfate has been used in Japan as a nonprescription anticoagulant and cholesterol-lowering agent. Though the drug is not approved in the United States, the FDA has permitted its importation for "personal use," and many AIDS patients began purchasing it after learning of its ability to protect cultured T-lymphocytes from HIV infection. Immunologists have

1 **Q** I get severe reactions from AZT and would like to take a different drug for AIDS. Are all the available drugs approved by the FDA?

A There are two general types of drugs available for use by AIDS patients: those that carry the weight of FDA approval and those that are not yet approved by the FDA. Approved drugs can be prescribed by physicians. Unapproved drugs must be obtained elsewhere, sometimes in foreign countries where they have been approved. Another possibility is experimental drugs. These can be obtained by participating in a clinical trial.

2 **Q** Can I get unapproved drugs for personal use?

A Yes, even though the FDA may not give its approval for a drug to be sold commercially in the United States, it may permit importation from foreign countries so long as the drug is for "personal use." This approval implies that the drug is not for sale to others.

3 **Q** Suppose I choose to take an unapproved drug. Can I get a physician to help me?

A Physicians will generally not recommend that you take unapproved drugs, but there is no law that prevents a physician from helping you obtain and use an unapproved drug. A physician may also help you gain entry to a clinical trial where you can benefit from an experimental drug.

shown that dextran sulfate can block the binding of HIV to helper T-lymphocytes and prevent syncytium formation. Dextran sulfate is also a relatively inexpensive drug.

One drug that attracted publicity in the mid-1980s was heteropolyanion 23, or HPA 23. HPA 23 acts to inhibit reverse transcriptase in certain retroviruses, including HIV. Its activity in patients, however, is very limited, and its side effects include a severe reduction of blood platelets and a lowering of the white blood cell count.

Since the 1980s, herpes simplex and cytomegalovirus (CMV) infections have been treated with phosphonoformate (known commercially as Foscarnet). Researchers have also shown the drug to be effective against viruses possessing reverse transcriptase and have demonstrated that it crosses the blood-brain barrier. Activity against CMV makes the drug attractive because this virus causes a major opportunistic disease in AIDS patients. Kidney damage is an important side effect associated with phosphonoformate.

In the 1950s and early 1960s, millions of people worldwide took the drug thalidomide as a sedative. For most, there were no ill effects, but at least 10,000 pregnant women gave birth to babies with missing or stunted limbs. Use of the drug as a sedative in the United States was banned, but it continued to be available for skin lesions in the interim decades. Then, in 1989 was banned, researchers at Rockefeller University found that thalidomide could inhibit production of an immune system substance known as tumor necrosis factor alpha (TNF) by acting at the level of messenger RNA. The researchers raised the possibility that thalidomide might be used as an antiviral agent, since TNF is known to boost replication of HIV. In 1997, a federally sponsored study showed that thalidomide is effective for healing the painful oral and esophageal ulcers associated with AIDS and for retarding the wasting syndrome that often accompanies the ulcers in AIDS patients. An elevation of the TNF levels in patients was an unanticipated finding in view of the earlier research. A troublesome and unexplained increase in the viral load accompanied the TNF rise.

Though not approved for AIDS therapy by the FDA, the anticancer drug hydroxyurea has been used by some physicians because it apparently interferes with the uptake of nucleotides needed by HIV in its replication. Anecdotal reports indicate that when hydroxyurea is used with a protease inhibitor and an AZT analog, there is no rebound of HIV when the therapy is withdrawn. These reports have stimulated further study of the compound.

Work is also continuing on using fullerenes as protease inhibitors. Fullerenes are molecules containing 60 carbon atoms arranged in a structure resembling a soccer ball (and named for Buckminster Fuller, the architect who designed the geodesic dome, which the molecule also resembles). Researchers at the University of California have shown that fullerenes (also called "buckyballs") fit snugly into the cylinderlike binding site of HIV protease. With modifications, they believe that fullerenes can bind there selectively and inhibit the enzyme.

A plant derivative that appears to inhibit syncytium formation by infected T-lymphocytes is castanospermine. Evidence indicates that castanospermine alters the glycoproteins in the HIV envelope and on the surfaces of infected T-lymphocytes, thereby preventing the cross-linking of the cells. Few studies of the drug have been performed in humans, so its effectiveness against HIV and its toxicity remain unknown.

Late in the 1980s, a drug named hypericin was isolated from the herb St. John's wort and shown to have antiviral effects in animals. A decade later, researchers were postulating that hypericin holds the capsid proteins together after HIV enters its host cell, thereby preventing the uncoating stage and the release of viral RNA. The drug shows an unusual propensity to act only when it is exposed to light. Scientists also believe that the drug attaches to the cell membrane of host cells and prevents viral binding. Syncytium formation may also be inhibited.

The final drug we shall consider briefly is Ampligen. Ampligen is so named because it appears to amplify immune system activity, possibly by stimulating interferon production and macrophage activity to hasten the destruction of HIV. The drug consists of a double-stranded RNA molecule. It is believed that this molecule interacts somehow with cellular enzymes to increase immune systems functioning. Tests to determine the usefulness of this drug and other we have surveyed are presently under way. As of July, 2002, Ampligen as an adjunct to HAART has been shown to decrease HIV RNA levels after 4.5 months of treatment.

Postexposure Prophylaxis

Before leaving the therapeutic agents, we should note that none of these drugs is intended for use as a "morning after" pill; that is, none of the drugs is FDA-approved for use in those who fear they may have been exposed to HIV and wish to receive so-called postexposure prophylaxis. Unofficially, however, some health clinics and practitioners offer anti-HIV drugs to high-risk patients, such as those who may have been exposed to HIV during a sexual assault. And studies are ongoing to determine the feasibility of such treatment. Part of the reluctance to prescribe drugs is their often serious side effects and the long duration of the drug regimen.

The situation is somewhat different for health care workers who may have been exposed to HIV through a needlestick or other accident during the course of their work. Guidelines promulgated by the NIH in 2001 suggest that AZT and 3TC remain the basic recommended postexposure regimen (Table 8.6), but that additional choices are available, including didanosine and stavudine. A third drug in the regimen is a protease inhibitor such as indinavir. Advantages and disadvantages are listed in the guidelines so that the physician can choose the most suitable

TABLE			
8.6 **Recommendations for Use of Prophylaxis Therapy in Health Care Workers, 2000**			
Type of Exposure	**Source Material**	**Antiretroviral Prophylaxis**	**Antiretroviral Regimen**
Percutaneous	Blood		
	Highest risk	Recommend	AZT plus 3TC plus indinavir
	Increased risk	Recommend	AZT plus 3TC, ± indinavir
	No increased risk	Offer	AZT plus 3TC
	Fluid containing visible blood, other potentially infectious fluid, or tissue	Offer	AZT plus 3TC
	Other body fluid (e.g., urine)	Not offer	
Mucous membrane	Blood	Offer	AZT plus 3TC, ± indinavir
	Fluid containing visible blood, other potentially infectious fluid, or tissue	Offer	AZT ± 3TC
	Other body fluid (e.g., urine)	Not offer	
Skin, increased risk	Blood	Offer	AZT plus 3TC, ± indinavir
	Fluid containing visible blood, other potentially infectious fluid, or tissue	Offer	AZT ± 3TC
	Other body fluid (e.g., urine)	Not offer	

Source: NIAID AIDS Agenda, *September, 2000.*

combination for the individual case. The severity of exposure and the HIV status of the individual who is the source of the exposure are examples of factors to be considered (Chapter 6).

One could suggest that the value of postexposure prophylaxis for health care workers argues for its use with the general public. However, conditions are much different when treating patients who are not health care workers. For example, a person may fear HIV infection as a result of having unprotected sex while drunk: In this case, the HIV status of the source individual is uncertain; substantial time may pass before treatment is sought; the costly drugs may not be affordable; the strict drug regimen may be hard to follow without support; and the behavior that led to the exposure may be difficult to change. With a health care worker, by comparison, the source individual is known, treatment is immediate, the cost is borne by the institution, support at work is ongoing, and a risky behavior is not involved. Nevertheless, despite the drawbacks, the use of anti-HIV drugs for "morning after" treatment is being investigated.

Treating Opportunistic Diseases

After two decades of dealing with the AIDS epidemic, it has become clear that AIDS patients do not die of AIDS. Rather, they die of encephalopathy, wasting, or any of a series of opportunistic diseases that infect the tissues after HIV has ravaged the immune system (Chapter 4). The obvious way to deal with AIDS is to eliminate the virus or develop a vaccine against it. As long as neither of these is imminent, a reasonable tactic is to treat the opportunistic diseases that commonly cause death.

Pentamidine Isethionate

Among the most intractable diseases to strike AIDS patients is *Pneumocystis carinii* pneumonia. The responsible protozoan multiplies without control in the lungs, fills up all the air spaces, and induces oxygen suffocation. Over half the patients who die from complications of AIDS die of this type of pneumonia. Indeed, about 70 percent of all AIDS patients suffer at least one bout of the disease.

Even before the AIDS epidemic emerged, *Pneumocystis carinii* pneumonia was a treatable disease. The drug of choice then and now is pentamidine isethionate. Originally, the drug was dispensed only by the CDC, but as HIV spread among the U.S. population, it became available locally. Physicians had to administer it by injection, however, so its use was generally limited to those hospitalized. Then, in 1989, the FDA approved pentamidine isethionate in a much easier to use aerosol form and suggested that it be employed for prevention of *Pneumocystis carinii* pneumonia (Healthline 8.4) as well as treatment. The procedure specifies use of the aerosolized drug in AIDS patients who have had one bout of the pneumonia or whose helper T-lymphocyte count drops below 200 cells per microliter (the threshold at which studies show that patients are at risk of developing the pneumonia).

At this writing, aerosolized pentamidine isethionate is believed to be helping an estimated 250,000 or more individuals in the United States and Europe. Most people infected with HIV visit a clinic monthly to inhale a dose of the drug. However, some physicians are skeptical, believing that the drug may protect the lungs, but it does not lend resistance to other organs that *Pneumocystis carinii* may infect, such as the thyroid gland, kidney, spleen, and liver. These rare infections may require therapy with a different drug. A side effect of the aerosolized treatment is a cough, but there are few other side effects. By contrast, injected pentamidine isethionate often leads to damage to the pancreas, reduced white blood cell counts, and altered blood glucose levels.

Among the other drugs for treating *Pneumocystis carinii* pneumonia are trimetrexate, an anticancer drug. Trimetrexate interferes

Healthline 8.4

1 Q I was recently diagnosed with HIV infection and told I should take pentamidine isethionate. What will it do?

A Pentamidine isethionate is a drug that will help prevent *Pneumocystis carinii* pneumonia from developing. This form of pneumonia is among the most common opportunistic diseases associated with AIDS and a major cause of death in individuals who have AIDS.

2 Q Where can I get pentamidine isethionate?

A The drug is now available in an aerosol mist that the patient breathes into the lungs so that the drug can act at the likely site of infection. A physician has the equipment for administering the aerosol (taken much like an antihistamine mist); a local hospital clinic can also supply the drug to you.

3 Q Is pentamidine the only drug available to prevent *Pneumocystis carinii* pneumonia?

A Several drugs are now in use to prevent this pneumonia. If you experience toxic side effects from pentamidine, there are alternatives, including trimethoprim-sulfamethoxazole (Bactrim or Septra). However, pentamidine is the recommended drug.

with the metabolism of human cells and tends to be toxic, but its toxicity can be reduced by administering leucovorin, a vitaminlike substance that somehow protects cells. Another possible treatment is trimethoprim-sulfamethoxazole, an FDA-approved combination of two drugs commonly used for bacterial infections. (The combination is marketed by one company as Septra and by another company as Bactrim.) The antiprotozoal drug atovaquone has also been approved by the FDA for use in treating mild-to-moderate *P. carinii* infection in humans.

Other Drugs

Two opportunistic viruses, the herpes simplex virus and cytomegalovirus (CMV), can also be held in check with drug treatment (Table 8.7). For herpes simplex, the preferred drug is acyclovir (commercially known as Zovirax). Like AZT, acyclovir is a nucleoside that inhibits replication of the herpes simplex virus by interfering with its production of DNA. Acyclovir is available in injectable, cream, and pill forms. It was approved by the FDA in the mid-1980s. In 1989, the FDA approved ganciclovir for the treatment of CMV-induced retinitis, a condition of the eye that affects 25 percent of AIDS patients and often leads to blindness. Because its side effects include anemia, ganciclovir cannot be taken with AZT, which is also associated with anemia.

Other opportunistic diseases can also be controlled with drugs. For tuberculosis, the drugs of choice include isoniazid and rifampin; for preventing mycobacteriosis due to *Mycobacterium avium-intracellulare* (MAC infection), rifabutin (Mycobutin) has been recommended, and for treating established cases, clarithromycin or azithromycin is suggested; for cryptococcosis, there is amphotericin B or fluconizole; *Candida albicans* infections can be controlled with nystatin (Mycostatin), as well as miconazole, clotrimazole, or ketoconazole; toxoplasmosis is treated with pyrimethamine or atovaquone; and the effects of cryptosporidiosis can be lessened with various drugs, although this disease remains very

TABLE 8.7 A Summary of Drugs Used to Treat Opportunistic Diseases

Opportunistic Disease	Available Drugs	Comment
Pneumocystis carinii pneumonia	Pentamidine isethionate Trimetrexate	Available as aerosol Toxicity reduced with leucovorin
Cytomegalovirus disease	Ganciclovir	Useful for retinitis
Herpes simplex infection	Acyclovir	Available in several forms
Tuberculosis	Isoniazid, rifampin	Long therapy required
Cryptococcosis	Amphotericin B	Toxic side effects
Candidiasis	Nystatin and others	Few side effects
Toxoplasmosis	Pyrimethamine	Kidney damage possible

difficult to treat and patient rehydration by intravenous infusions of fluids is often required.

Anemia remains one of the most worrisome side effects of many drugs used to treat AIDS patients. Physicians have estimated, for example, that half the individuals taking AZT suffer anemia. To lessen the possibility of this disorder, the FDA has approved the clinical use of erythropoietin. Erythropoietin is a protein hormone normally produced by kidney cells. The hormone promotes red blood cell production in the bone marrow. Biotechnologists have deciphered the genetic code for this protein and have synthesized abundant supplies. Physicians recommend it for use in patients taking AZT to lessen the need for blood transfusions.

The reasonably effective arsenal of drugs for fighting opportunistic diseases should encourage persons with the early signs of AIDS to place themselves under the care of a physician. Physicians with long experience in treating AIDS have noted that persons who delay therapy for opportunistic diseases are at greater risk for future bouts because of damage to their tissues. If, however, a person seeks medical help at the first sign of an AIDS-related illness, there is a good possibility that the effects can be lessened.

Drug Development and Testing

To receive the most promising drugs, a person who has HIV infection or AIDS must usually find a way to enter a sophisticated clinical trial at a major medical center. There the individual must meet strict criteria set by researchers and agree to use the test drug or a placebo, usually without knowing which is being administered. The fortunate ones emerge from the trial healthier; the unfortunate ones seek solace in the fact that they have helped develop the knowledge base of science. Essentially, the formal scientific evaluation of unproven therapies is performed more for the benefit of tomorrow's patients than for today's.

But this approach to testing is undergoing a gradual change, stimulated in part by the AIDS epidemic. Driven by the intense need for new drugs, the medical establishment has been relaxing its procedures to bring promising drugs to patients more quickly. Neighborhood clinics are being allowed to conduct clinical trials, and the FDA has changed its traditional rules to put certain drugs on a "fast track" for approval. In some situations, for example, an investigational new drug for treatment (a so-called treatment IND) can be released to physicians, even though the drug is still undergoing trials and awaiting FDA approval (Healthline 8.5). Aerosolized pentamidine isethionate was such a drug. Still another proposal is the

Healthline 8.5

1 **Q** I often hear that "FDA approval" is needed for a drug before it can be sold commercially. What exactly is the FDA?

A FDA stands for Food and Drug Administration. The FDA is an agency of the federal government created by Congress in 1962. Spurred by the 1960s scandals associated with thalidomide, red dye No. 2, and other drugs and food additives, the FDA instituted an elaborate system to test such substances to ensure their safety and effectiveness. Pharmaceutical companies are required to submit potential drugs for FDA approval before offering them for general use.

2 **Q** Will insurance cover drugs that have not been approved by the FDA?

A Most insurance companies will not compensate patients for the cost of drugs unless and until they are approved by the FDA.

3 **Q** Does the FDA have any legal clout to force drug manufacturers to test drugs in certain ways?

A The FDA has no legal basis for requiring drug testing in the manner it has prescribed, but it is generally agreed that federal support for research can be denied if procedures set down by the FDA are not followed. And the FDA can refuse to approve a drug for which testing has been incomplete or otherwise unacceptable.

"parallel-track" procedure that would allow patients not eligible for trials to use a medication along with the trial group.

Drug Trials

A classical clinical trial for a new drug may take more than ten years from laboratory synthesis to FDA approval. In preclinical testing, studies are conducted in laboratory animals to determine whether the drug is safe to use and is biologically active. Two years may be consumed by these studies. Then comes a three-part clinical trial (Figure 8.12). In Phase I, the drug is tested on fewer than 100 paid, healthy human volunteers, with a slow increase in dosage over a period of time to determine any toxic side effects and to see how the drug is handled by the body. This can be a frightening experience for both volunteers and researchers—although animal tests have been performed, animals cannot express such things as dizziness, nausea, or psychiatric symptoms. Serious side effects, not apparent in animals, could also develop in human tissues. Researchers closely monitor the volunteers' blood pressure and temperature, and they carefully scrutinize drug distribution and drug elimination. A Phase I trial usually takes about one to two years.

Phase II trial is next. The drug is given to several hundred patients to pinpoint the conditions under which it will elicit the most effective response. The optimum dose must be established, and the endpoint must be set that is, when can physicians say the drug "works" (for HIV infection, this may mean reduction of the viral load to less than 400 copies of HIV RNA per milliliter of blood, a level currently considered "undetectable"). A control group is used in a Phase II trial, and those participants receive either a placebo or the best therapy available. The control group allows scientists to gauge the effectiveness of the candidate drug in an experimental situation and observe any special side effects related to the drug. Ideally, the test should be double-blind—neither the participants nor the physicians know who is getting the drug and who is in the control group (ensuring that the placebo resembles the drug is helpful in this regard). A two-year period is commonly taken up by a Phase II trial.

In a Phase III trial, the drug is tested in thousands of volunteers over a three-year period or more. Statistics are compiled carefully to determine whether the drug is more effective than the control therapy. A successful trial is often followed by a second, confirmatory trial; or, if the trial results are inconclusive, the data are examined to discover whether a Phase III trial with new parameters is justified. Finally, the results are submitted to either of two agencies for approval: In the United States, the Food and Drug Administration (FDA) can grant or deny approval for sale or request additional information. In Europe, approval is sought from the European Agency for the Evaluation of Medicinal Products.

For every drug approved by this process, an estimated 5000 drugs do not survive the rigorous tests. Supporters of the process suggest that it must be followed if potentially dangerous drugs are to be weeded out. Opponents point out, however, that thousands might die while a useful medication remains in lengthy testing phases. Community-based clinical trials may be a solution to this dilemma. Run

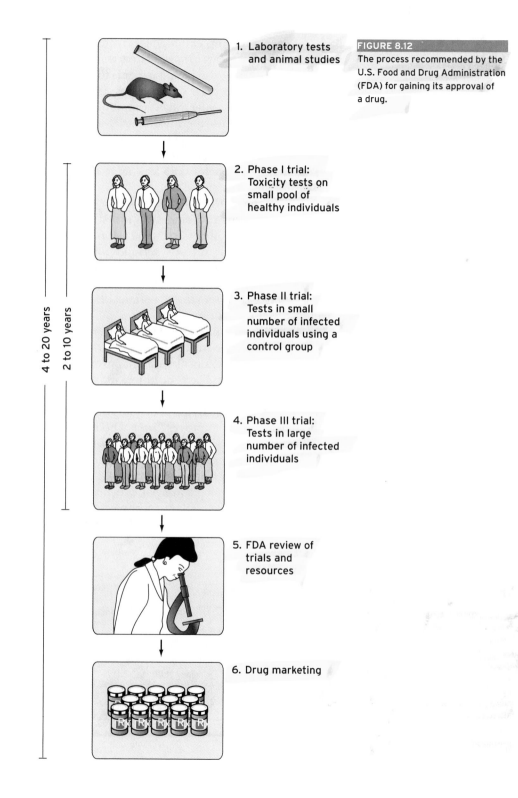

4 to 20 years

2 to 10 years

1. Laboratory tests and animal studies

2. Phase I trial: Toxicity tests on small pool of healthy individuals

3. Phase II trial: Tests in small number of infected individuals using a control group

4. Phase III trial: Tests in large number of infected individuals

5. FDA review of trials and resources

6. Drug marketing

FIGURE 8.12
The process recommended by the U.S. Food and Drug Administration (FDA) for gaining its approval of a drug.

by private organizations employing private doctors and clinics, the community-based trials allow patients to suggest how trials might be operated and to contribute their experience. They also permit patients to receive experimental drugs from their own physicians in a familiar setting, a less stressful situation than they would experience at a university center. Such community trials try to avoid placebos, opting instead to compare the experimental drug with an established drug such as AZT. In the 1990s, community-based groups in San Francisco and New York City were conducting trials on 15 potentially useful AIDS drugs. The San Francisco group was largely responsible for data leading to the approval of aerosolized pentamidine isethionate.

In 1987, the FDA instituted its fast-track procedure to speed up drug approval. Under this procedure, an investigational new drug (IND) for treating "life-threatening" illnesses can be released during its Phase II trial while clinical trials continue. For treating "serious" illnesses, an IND can be released during Phase III trial. No one quarrels with the compassionate motives that underlie this innovation. However, opponents of the fast-track procedure question whether AIDS patients would remain in a clinical trial (where they might be receiving a placebo) if they could leave the trial and purchase the experimental drug or have it prescribed by their physicians. Other issues include the reluctance of uninformed physicians to prescribe treatment with INDs and the refusal of certain insurance companies to cover treatment with unapproved drugs.

For the parallel-track procedure, individuals are enrolled when they are ineligible for controlled clinical trials and in need of experimental drugs (Figure 8.13). Such individuals include those who cannot tolerate a standard treatment or who have failed to improve. Those who live far from an institution-sponsored clinical trial are also eligible. The drugs to be used in this procedure are determined on a case-by-case basis. Opponents of the plan fear that people with AIDS may be diverted away from clinical trials where their participation is needed. The possibility also exists that some patients may stop using a good drug in favor of a poor one. Proponents point out that participants in the parallel-tract procedure will believe they are receiving state-of-the-art and, possibly, better care.

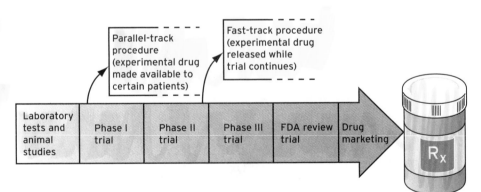

FIGURE 8.13

The parallel- and fast-track procedures for testing an experimental drug. In the parallel-track procedure, experimental drugs are made available to certain patients while Phase I trials are taking place. Under the fast-track procedure, an investigational new drug (IND) is released during Phase II trial while the trial continues. Presence of a life-threatening illness could be the basis for a fast-track release.

Key Questions about Drug Testing

Those who desire to participate in a drug trial may not find it easy because certain criteria must be met. The trial, for example, may be limited to persons in a specific stage of HIV infection. In addition, most trials place limits on other drugs the patient may take (those taking ganciclovir could not take AZT, for example), and such limits may be difficult to enforce. Moreover, a study may be restricted to certain groups, such as injection-drug-using males. The possibility also exists that a participant may receive the placebo, a circumstance that may not be desirable to an infected individual. And a trial may be in a certain phase that is not personally acceptable (a Phase I toxicity trial, for instance, may require confinement to a hospital).

By 2000, approximately 75 antiviral agents and vaccines were undergoing investigation at university and government medical centers. Still unresolved are such questions as whether small manufacturers of drugs will pay for the standard tests preceding approval. Nor is it certain whether insurers will cover the costs of medical care, laboratory tests, and other expenses incurred during broad-based trials. Moreover, it has not yet been determined whether physicians, manufacturers, or the FDA will be held liable should unapproved drugs prove fatal.

There is also the pressing question of whether scientists and doctors should prevent patients from having access to drugs that patients believe will help them. Should a patient be allowed to accept the risk that an experimental drug carries, or should the medical establishment have the final say? Who, essentially, has the ultimate responsibility? And which is the greater good?

Alternative Therapies

Thus far in this chapter, we have discussed AIDS treatment in terms of drugs. This should not be construed to mean that alternative therapies are unavailable. Unfortunately, many such therapies are based on half-truths and false hopes and are potentially lethal because they have little or no scientific basis.

For example, striking one's chest does little to stimulate the thymus gland, as some would believe. Nor do injections of blood cells from fetal calves improve immune functions. And applying dinitrochlorobenzene (DNCB) to the skin lesions of Kaposi's sarcoma does not relieve the symptoms of the disease. Such purported panaceas may be expensive and may tend to divert AIDS patients from recognized treatments.

One alternative therapy being tested is ozone treatment. Ozone is a highly reactive form of oxygen that oxidizes chemical compounds and has been used in Europe against various ailments. Ozone may conceivably change the chemistry of the lipid envelope of HIV if direct exposure takes place. Tests have been performed in which blood from an HIV-infected patient is passed through fine gas-permeable hollow fibers that interface with an ozone-oxygen gas mixture. The gas mixture flows in a direction opposite to the blood flow, and ozone passes through the fibers into the blood. Patients are subjected to one-hour treatments on alternate days over 12 weeks. During each treatment, a volume of 300 cubic centimeters of blood is treated.

Another alternative therapy is centered in boosting the body's immune homeostasis (tendency to maintain a stable state). This therapy, known as immune therapy, can take several forms. For example, therapy with immunoglobulins is performed by intravenously infusing AIDS patients with antibodies using a preparation called HIV hyperimmune globulin (HIVIG). The concentrated antibodies are obtained from healthy HIV-infected individuals, and they render a type of passive immunity. In two studies reported in 1994, HIVIG significantly helped advanced AIDS patients. Researchers were quick to caution, however, that the therapy requires much additional study. One physician referred to HIVIG treatment as having a "quality-of-life effect" rather than a therapeutic effect. The preparation has also been tested for its ability to prevent maternal-fetal transmission of HIV in pregnant women. As of 2002, however, the results are equivocal.

The course of HIV infection is often complicated by malnutrition associated with decreased food intake, abnormalities of metabolism, and high nutrient loss due to malabsorption through the intestinal tract and diarrhea. Nutritional therapy can benefit the patient, especially if instituted at the time of diagnosis. The goals are to maintain body weight, body cell mass, and serum protein levels. Patients are educated on the principles of an adequate diet to prevent weight loss and protein and nutrient depletion. Instruction is provided on safe storage and cooking of food to preclude infection: For example, meat should be cooked well to prevent the transmission of toxoplasmosis; raw eggs should be avoided to preclude salmonellosis; and leftovers should be heated well to avoid food poisoning. Information on nutritional supplements of questionable value is also often provided.

Bone Marrow Transplants

One alternative therapy that may hold promise for the future is the bone marrow transplant. In this procedure bone marrow cells from a donor are transplanted into the bone marrow of the AIDS patient, in the hope that they will restore the immune system cells that have been destroyed. The body normally rejects foreign tissue, so the donor and recipient must be closely matched genetically (the ideal pairing is identical twins, a perfect match).

In the past, researchers have performed bone marrow transplants among sets of identical twins, each set consisting of a healthy twin and a twin with HIV infection or AIDS. Although some partial restoration of the immune system was observed, HIV eventually attacked the incoming cells and destroyed them. More encouraging reports appeared in the 1990s when AZT treatment accompanied the transplant; HIV appeared to be absent in the tissues while the marrow cells were establishing themselves.

Inherent in a bone marrow transplant are several problems that must be circumvented. The process is very dangerous because the remnants of a patient's own bone marrow must be completely destroyed with radiation or toxic chemicals, otherwise patient cells will immediately attack the incoming cells. Finding suitable donors is also difficult, and the transplant procedure is extremely expensive. Though theoretically possible, the prospects remain dim that bone marrow transplants will become a commonplace therapy for treating AIDS.

Gene Therapy

Gene therapy is one of the most innovative and imaginative uses of the DNA technology and genetic engineering that emerged in the 1970s. For gene therapy, cells are taken from the patient, altered in the laboratory by adding genes, then placed back into the patient. It is anticipated that the new genes will provide the genetic codes for certain proteins not normally produced by the cells.

Gene therapy may be used one day to relieve the effects of HIV infection and AIDS. In 1993, the Recombinant Advisory Committee of the U.S. government approved the first clinical test involving patients with HIV infection. The test used a mutant strain of HIV having defective forms of the *rev* and *env* genes. This strain, produced by researchers at the University of California at San Diego, cannot replicate with the mutated genes (*rev* is a regulatory gene and *env* encodes envelope proteins). Researchers removed T-lymphocytes from HIV-infected patients and inserted mutated viruses into the cells. Then they cultivated large numbers of the cells and injected them back into the patient. The virus-containing T-lymphocytes could not produce viruses, but they did stimulate the body to produce cells called killer T-lymphocytes. These killer cells are specifically manufactured to react with HIV-infected cells. Tests with patients are ongoing.

In another form of gene therapy, genes that encode HIV proteins are attached to the DNA of mouse viruses, which are harmless for humans. The reengineered viruses are then injected into HIV-infected individuals, where they enter receptive cells. Researchers hope that the HIV genes will stimulate normal body cells to produce HIV proteins. The proteins will then act as a vaccine and stimulate the immune system to produce anti-HIV antibodies. These antibodies may help prevent HIV expression in the patient.

Still another possible form of gene therapy involves trying to get HIV-infected cells to produce anti-HIV antibodies. DNA technologists at the Dana Farber Cancer Institute in Boston have synthesized the gene for an antibody called F105. This antibody reacts with and inactivates gp120, the envelope spike glycoprotein essential for HIV's binding to host cells. The scientists have refined the gene so that the F105 antibody molecule will be produced at the cell's endoplasmic reticulum (ER), the membranous structure of the cytoplasm where gp120 is also synthesized. And they added a gene segment so that antibody protein will anchor to the ER and not leave the cell (as antibody molecules usually do). The reconstructed gene was attached to a standard plasmid (a loop of bacterial DNA) and inserted into HIV-infected cells derived from a laboratory animal. The cells were soon producing the F105 antibody, an innovative result in which infected cells produce antibodies against the very thing infecting them. The synthesis of gp120 was dramatically reduced in these cells, and the synthesis of HIV particles slowed considerably. Moreover, the cells did not display any toxic effect from the indwelling plasmid.

Experiments such as these illustrate the novel approaches gene engineers are taking to fight HIV. Practical use of these methods remains in the future, but it is comforting to know that alternatives to drug therapy are both possible and feasible.

Thinking Well

The idea that mental states can influence the body's susceptibility to and recovery from disease has a long history. The Greek physician Galen, for example, asserted that cancer struck more frequently in melancholy women than in cheerful women. During the past quarter-century, the concept of mental state and disease has been researched more thoroughly, and several links have been established between the nervous system and the immune system.

One such link occurs between the hypothalamus and the T-lymphocytes. The hypothalamus is a portion of the brain located beneath the cerebrum. It produces a chemical-releasing factor that induces the pituitary gland, positioned just below the hypothalamus, to secrete a hormone (ACTH) that targets the adrenal glands. The adrenal glands, in turn, secrete steroid hormones (glucocorticoids) that influence the activity of T-lymphocytes in the thymus gland.

Another link is established by branches of the autonomic nervous system that extend into the lymph nodes and spleen. The autonomic (or "automatic") nervous system typically operates on its own to regulate the involuntary actions of such organs as the heart, stomach, and lungs through myriad nerve fibers. The anatomical link between the nervous and immune systems permits direct two-way communication.

A third link between the nervous and immune systems involves thymosins, a family of substances originating in the thymus gland. When experimentally injected into brain tissue, thymosins stimulate the pituitary gland via the hypothalamus to release hormones, including the one that stimulates the adrenal glands. Although the precise functions of thymosins are still to be determined, it appears that they serve as specific molecular signals between the thymus and the pituitary gland. A circuit is apparently present that stimulates the brain to adjust immune responses and the immune system to alter nerve cell activity.

The outcome of these discoveries is the emergence of a strong correlation between a patient's mental attitude and the progress of disease (Figure 8.14). Rigorously controlled studies conducted in recent years have shown that the aggressive determination to conquer a disease can increase one's lifespan. Therapies can consist of relaxation techniques as well as the use of mental imagery that HIV is being crushed by the body's stalwart defenses. Behavioral therapies of this nature can amplify the body's response to disease and accelerate the mobilization of its defenses.

Few reputable practitioners of behavioral therapies believe that such therapies should replace drug therapy. However, the psychological devastation associated with AIDS cannot be denied, and it is this intense stress that the "thinking well" movement attempts to address. Very often a person learning of a positive HIV test goes into severe depression, and because depression can adversely affect the immune system, a double dose of immune suppression ensues. Perhaps if the psychological trauma is relieved, the remaining body defenses can adequately handle the virus.

As with any emerging treatment method, behavioral therapies have numerous opponents. Some opponents argue that naive patients might abandon con-

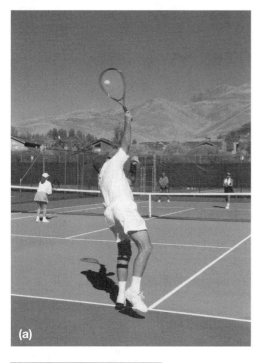

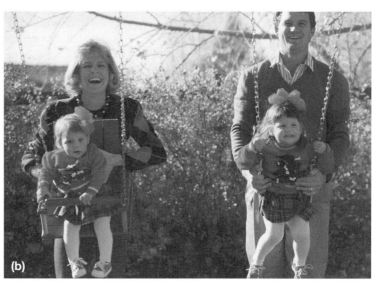

(a)

(b)

FIGURE 8.14

Numerous studies have shown that a person's mental attitude can influence the course of an infectious disease such as AIDS. Such things as exercise (a) and the support of family members (b) can have a positive influence.

ventional therapy; another argument is that therapists might cause enormous guilt to develop in patients whose will to live cannot overcome failing health. Proponents counter with the growing body of evidence showing that AIDS patients with strong commitments and a willingness to face challenges—signs of psychological hardiness—have relatively greater numbers of T-lymphocytes than passive, non-expressive patients. No study has yet proven that mood or personality has a life-prolonging effect on immunity. Still, doctors and patients are generally inspired by the possibility that the mind can be used to help stave off the effects of AIDS. Though unsure of what it is, they generally agree that *something* is going on.

LOOKING BACK

Toward the end of the 1980s, new therapies for AIDS came into use, and with their acceptance, the length and quality of life for AIDS patients have improved. Drugs may not effect a cure, but they can control HIV infection to allow individuals to lead almost normal lives. Among the HIV activities that can be targets for drug inhibition are binding of HIV to host cells, the functioning of reverse transcriptase, and the budding of HIV from host cells. Toxicity, the variety of cells that can be involved in AIDS, and brain cell damage limit the use of drugs.

Azidothymidine (AZT) has been approved by the FDA since 1987 for treating AIDS. The drug replaces deoxythymidine in the synthesis of proviral DNA mediated by reverse transcriptase. Additional nucleosides cannot attach to the DNA chain with AZT in place, and DNA chain development comes to an end. The major side effect is bone marrow suppression leading to anemia.

Other therapeutic agents used for therapy for HIV infection and AIDS include other dideoxynucleosides, which work in the same way as AZT but are less toxic. Examples include ddI, ddC, 3TC, abacovir, and tenofovir. Often one or more of these drugs are used in combination with AZT to overcome HIV resistance. Similar drugs that react directly with reverse transcriptase include nevirapine, delavirdine, and efavirenz. Easier dosage and limited side effects are notable characteristics of these drugs.

The protease inhibitors achieved prominence in 1996 as part of a combination drug therapy known as highly active antiretroviral therapy (HAART). Combined with AZT and another drug (such as 3TC), the protease inhibitor can bring about a significant decline in AIDS-related deaths. The success of this therapy was tempered by its difficult regimens, side effects, and the HIV rebound effect when drug therapy was interrupted.

New classes of anti-HIV agents include the fusion inhibitors and the entry inhibitors. One fusion inhibitor seeks to react with gp41 molecules of the HIV envelope and thus prevent the HIV particle from fusing with its host T-lymphocyte; another uses synthetic CD4 molecules. Entry inhibitors attempt to block HIV entry into host cells by destroying the necessary receptors on the cells' surface.

Other approaches to HIV therapy include using interleukin-2 to spur the development of infected T-lymphocytes so that their indwelling proviruses can be eliminated. Research is also proceeding on antisense molecules that would deactivate the mRNA molecules used by HIV to encode new particles. Alpha interferon, a synthetic version of a naturally occurring antiviral protein is another possible therapeutic agent, along with compound Q, peptide T, dextran sulfate, and HPA 23. None of these, however, has FDA approval. Research has shown that thalidomide, once used as a sedative, is useful for healing the painful oral and esophageal ulcers associated with AIDS. The anticancer drug hydroxyurea and a derivative of St. John's wort called hypericin also show promise for inactivating HIV.

For treating the opportunistic diseases associated with AIDS, aerosolized pentamidine isethionate has been found effective to preclude the development of *Pneumocystis carinii* pneumonia, and ganciclovir is used for cytomegalovirus-induced retinitis. Many other drugs can lessen the effects of *Cryptococcus, Candida, Toxoplasma,* and other opportunistic organisms.

Before drugs are approved by the FDA, they are subjected to a multiyear series of trials, including preclinical trials (in animals), Phase I trial (to determine dose and toxicity in healthy humans), Phase II trial (in small groups of infected humans to determine antimicrobial effects), and Phase III trial (in large groups of volunteers). Parallel-track and fast-track procedures have been used to reduce the time between drug development and FDA approval.

Certain alternative therapies for AIDS do not use drugs. Bone marrow transplants, for example, seek to replace damaged cells in the body, and gene therapy experiments are being attempted to encourage body cells to produce anti-HIV antibodies. Attitudinal and behavioral changes can also affect the outcome of the disease, and physiological and anatomical links have been established between the immune and nervous systems.

REVIEW

Once you have finished this chapter, you should be familiar with the drugs used for therapy in patients with HIV infection and AIDS. To check your knowledge, match the the drug or therapeutic agent on the right with the characteristic listed on the left by placing the appropriate letter in the space (a letter may be used more than once). The correct answers are in Appendix A.

_L_ **1.** Preferred drug for treating herpes simplex infections

_D_ **2.** Combined with sulfamethoxazole for treating *Pneumocystis carinii* pneumonia

_F_ **3.** Approved by FDA in 1987 but causes suppression of bone marrow and anemia

_K_ **4.** Used with AZT; also known as lamivudine

_C_ **5.** Binds to gp120 and gp41 proteins of HIV

_H_ **6.** Inhibits tumor necrosis factor

_D_ **7.** Primary drug for treating *Pneumocystis carinii* pneumonia

_G_ **8.** Acts on reverse transcriptase, but unlike AZT

_F_ **9.** Approved for treating HIV-infected persons to forestall progression to AIDS

_O_ **10.** Possible alternative to AZT with fewer side effects; also called didanosine

A. Alpha interferon

B. Interleukin-2

C. Trojan horse virus

D. Pentamidine isethionate

E. Antisense molecule

F. Azidothymidine (AZT)

G. NRTI

H. Thalidomide

I. Protease inhibitor

J. Ganciclovir

K. 3TC

L. Acyclovir

M. Isoniazid

N. Ritonavir

O. Dideoxyinosine (ddI)

P. T-120

_M_ **11.** Commonly used to treat tuberculosis

_D_ **12.** Aerosolized form used to prevent *Pneumocystis carinii* pneumonia

_B_ **13.** Induces T-lymphocytes to mature

_A_ **14.** Synthetic antiviral substance used against Kaposi's sarcoma

_O_ **15.** Marketed as Videx and used in rotation with AZT; a similar nucleoside

_E_ **16.** Synthetic molecule that combines with HIV-specific mRNA during viral replication

_F_ **17.** Also known as zidovudine and Retrovir

_I_ **18.** Structured to react with a protein-processing enzyme in viral reproduction

_G_ **19.** Has a synergistic effect when used with AZT

_J_ **20.** Recommended for cytomegalovirus-induced retinitis

_N_ **21.** Protease inhibitor; also known as Norvir

_A_ **22.** Commercially available as Roferon and Intron-A

_E_ **23.** Complementary to RNA molecule produced during viral replication

_P_ **24.** Fusion inhibitor

_G_ **25.** Category that includes nevirapine

FOR ADDITIONAL READING

Adler, T. 1994. "The return of thalidomide." *Science News* 146: 424–427.

Bartlett, J. G. and R. D. Moore. 1998. "Improving HIV therapy. *Scientific American*, July.

Bischfberger, N., and R. W. Wagner. 1992. "Antisense approaches to antiviral therapy." *Semin. Virol.* 3: 57–66.

Buchbinder, S. 1998. "Avoiding infection after HIV exposure." *Scientific American*, July.

Centers for Disease Control and Prevention. 1990. "Public health service statement on management of occupational exposure to human immunodeficiency virus, including considerations regarding zidovudine post exposure use." *MMWR* 39(RR-1): 1–14.

Chicurel, M. 2000. "Probing HIV's elusive activities with the host cell." *Science* 290: 1876–1880.

Christensen, D. 2000. "Taking a break: Can interrupting their treatment benefit HIV-infected people?" *Science News* 157: 248–250.

Cohen, J. 1993. "Early AZT takes a pounding in French-British 'Concorde' trial." *Science* 260: 157–158.

Cohen, J. S. 1994. "The new genetic medicines. *Scientific American*, December.

Cohn, J. 1998. "Failure isn't what it used to be . . . but neither is success," *Science,* 279: 1133–1134.

Fischl, M. A., et al. 1993. "Zalcitabine compared with zidovudine in patients with advanced HIV-1 infection who received previous zidovudine therapy." *Ann. Intern. Med.* 118: 762–769.

Hall, N. R., and A. L. Goldstein. 1986. "Thinking well." *The Sciences,* March/April.

Hart, C. 2001. "Interleukin-2 redux," *Modern Drug Discovery*, July.

Hirsch, M. S., and R. T. D'Aquila. 1993. "Therapy for human immunodeficiency virus infection." *N. Eng. J. Med.* 328: 1686–1695.

Lallemant, M., et al. 2000. "A trial of shortened zidovudine regimens to prevent mother-to-child transmission of HIV-1." *N. Eng. J. Med.* 343: 982–991.

Lange, J. M. A. 1997. "Current problems and the failure of antiretroviral trials." *Science* 276: 548–551.

Pendick, D. A. 1993. "Structure-based rug designers eye HIV protease." *ASM News* 59: 382–387.

Perrin, L., and A. Telenti. 1998. "HIV treatment failure: Testing for HIV resistance in clinical practice. *Science* 2809: 1871–1873.

Smith, K. A. 1993. "Lowest dose interleukin-2 immunotherapy." *Blood* 81: 1414–1423.

Underwood, A. 1994. "A 'bad' drug may turn out to do good." *Newsweek,* September 19.

Zivin, J. A. 2000. "Understanding clinical trials." *Scientific American*, April.

CHAPTER 9

An AIDS Vaccine

LOOKING AHEAD

Developing a vaccine for AIDS is among the highest priorities of today's medical researchers. This chapter surveys many aspects of this search. On completing the chapter, you should be able to . . .

- Identify how vaccines work in the body and understand the various forms a microbial vaccine can take.

- Appreciate the various strategies for developing AIDS vaccines and differentiate between sterilizing and therapeutic immunities.

- Describe the various components that can be used in an AIDS subunit vaccine and delineate the advantages of each.

- Explain the composition of a viable-vector vaccine and specify how it works to elicit immunity to HIV.

- Identify the whole virus vaccines that are being developed and indicate some advantages and disadvantages of each.

- Discuss the various problems associated with development of an AIDS vaccine and describe how some of these may be overcome.

- Describe how clinical trials for AIDS vaccines are conducted and anticipate some of the technical, ethical, and social difficulties that such trials will encounter.

INTRODUCTION

Smallpox has historically been among the worst killers of humanity. In the 1600s and 1700s, for example, smallpox epidemics were so severe in England that one-third of all children died before reaching the age of 3. Many smallpox victims were blinded by the disease, and those who recovered were pockmarked for life.

But for those who survived smallpox, the disease did not strike again. People therefore sought a way to contract the disease during a "mild" year, hoping to acquire immunity. At one point, the custom of "buying the pox" arose. Unfortunately, this method of acquiring immunity was haphazard and quite risky. Thus, excitement surfaced in the late 1700s when the method for immunization was improved considerably by an English country surgeon named Edward Jenner. Jenner observed that people who had suffered from a similar disease, cowpox, were apparently immune to the more deadly smallpox. Although cowpox (technically known as vaccinia) primarily occurs in the udders of cows, it also occurs as a mild skin disease in farmers, herders, and those who tend cows.

Jenner pondered whether intentionally giving cowpox to people would protect them against smallpox. In 1796, he tested his theory, enlisting the help of Sarah Nelmes, a dairy maid who had cowpox, and a young boy named James Phipps (Figure 9.1). Jenner took pus from lesions on Nelmes' arm and injected the boy's skin with the material. Phipps developed a swelling at the inoculation site but little else. Several weeks later, Jenner carefully injected Phipps once again, this time with pus from the lesion of a smallpox patient. Within days, the boy developed an uncomfortable feeling, but he did not develop smallpox. Phipps had been successfully immunized. Prominent physicians confirmed his work, and word of Jenner's method of "vaccination" spread quickly throughout the world. By 1801, an estimated 100,000 people in England had been vaccinated.

A hundred years would pass before scientists understood that the cowpox virus stimulates the immune system to produce antibodies, which neutralize the deadly smallpox viruses as well as the mild cowpox viruses. Hailed as one of the great medical-social advances in history, Jenner's immunization method was among the first attempts to control disease on a national scale. It was also the first effort to protect the community as a whole, rather than the individual.

Modern vaccines are as effective as Jenner's but more refined. They are composed of weakened or killed microorganisms, or in some cases, they contain molecular fragments of microorganisms or their chemically altered toxins. Such vaccines work by exploiting the immune system's ability to recognize specific antigens and respond with antibodies and other defenses that later attack and destroy invading microorganisms and their toxins (Chapter 3). A good vaccine prevents infection or disease and protects against different strains of the pathogenic virus. It gives long-lasting protection against both free viruses and cells infected with viruses; and it induces an immune response not only within the blood and tissues, but also at body surfaces, as in the gastrointestinal, respiratory, and urinary tracts.

In this chapter, we first discuss some general principles of immunization, then focus on the intensive effort to develop a vaccine for AIDS. In a sense, AIDS is the smallpox of our era. Indeed, the fear about contracting AIDS rivals the fear people expressed about contracting smallpox in past centuries. And developing an AIDS vaccine carries the priority once given to developing a smallpox vaccine because over 35 million people of the world are currently infected with HIV, and over 1 million will die of AIDS this year (in the United States, AIDS remains the number one killer of individuals in the 25 to 44 age bracket).

FIGURE 9.1

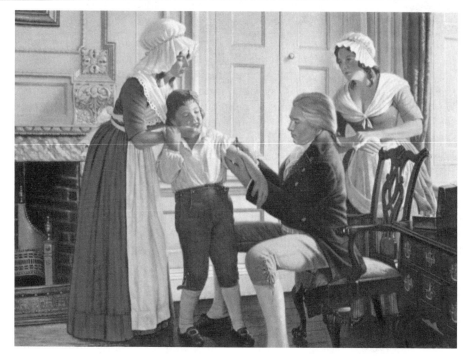

A painting by Robert Thom depicting Edward Jenner vaccinating the young James Phipps. The dairy maid at the right, Sarah Nelmes, is holding the lesion on her wrist where the cowpox material was taken from.

AIDS affects not only those who engage in risky behavior (such as injection drug users), but also the tens of thousands of babies born to infected mothers, the countless numbers of heterosexuals who cannot be reached by educational resources, and the masses of illiterate individuals who simply do not understand that certain behaviors are irresponsible. Preventing AIDS with a vaccine is vital to the economic health of nations because treating an infected individual with drugs costs over $100,000 over his or her lifetime, while immunizing with a vaccine costs only $100 per person. For these reasons and numerous others, the effort to develop an AIDS vaccine is proceeding at full speed in laboratories throughout the world.

General Vaccine Strategies

One of the significant developments of modern medicine was devising a tissue culture technique for the propagation of viruses. Pioneered in the 1930s by Alexis Carrel of Rockefeller Institute in New York City, the tissue culture technique uses bits of living tissue removed from an organism and placed in a sterile growth chamber with nutrients needed for cell growth. In the 1940s, the technique was refined for culturing animal cells by Nobel laureates John Enders, Thomas Weller, and Frederick Robbins. Their technique led to the development of vaccines against polio, measles, mumps, and other diseases because it allowed laboratories to grow sufficient viruses for vaccine production.

Types of Vaccine

By the 1960s, vaccine manufacturers were able to produce two types of vaccines: One contained inactivated viruses, that is, viruses unable to multiply in the body because of chemical or physical treatment; and a second type contained attenuated viruses, that is, viruses able to multiply in the body but at a rate so low that disease does not occur. The Salk injectable polio vaccine typifies a vaccine containing inactivated viruses; the Sabin oral polio vaccine has attenuated viruses. Both are referred to as first-generation vaccines because they contain whole microorganisms (Figure 9.2).

During the 1970s, researchers developed another type of vaccine, the subunit vaccine. Manufacturers found that they could use concentrated suspensions of viral or bacterial fragments known as subunits to mimic whole microbes and stimulate the body's immune system. Such a vaccine is safer than a whole-virus vaccine because subunits cannot possibly infect cells. If the microbe invades the body, antibodies bind with the portion of the microbe corresponding to the subunit and neutralize it.

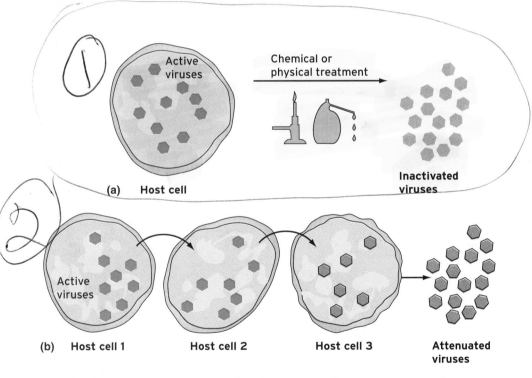

FIGURE 9.2

Methods for producing two types of viral vaccines. (a) Viruses are cultivated in cells in tissue culture and then treated with a chemical or physical agent to yield inactivated viruses. (b) Viruses are transferred from cells in tissue culture to new cells in tissue culture until a variant with reduced virulence emerges. These are attenuated viruses. The Salk polio vaccine contains inactivated viruses, while the Sabin polio vaccine has attenuated viruses.

The vaccine currently used against bacterial pneumonia typifies a subunit vaccine. Licensed in 1983, the vaccine contains polysaccharides obtained from the capsule (outer layer) of the bacterium *Streptococcus pneumoniae*. Specific antibodies form against the polysaccharides and circulate in the blood, binding to the capsule when the bacterium enters the body at a later date. The antibodies cripple the bacterium, preventing its proliferation and aiding its destruction by other cell defenses. Such a vaccine composed of subunits is known as a second-generation vaccine.

Another form of vaccine is composed of synthetic microbial proteins. This is known as a third-generation vaccine. Such a vaccine derives from the sophisticated and practical application of recombinant DNA technology. To produce the vaccine, the immune-stimulating antigen (usually a protein or a protein fragment) and the genes that produce it are identified. Living cells such as harmless bacteria are then modified with the genes to produce the protein, and the size of the protein is increased to promote its uptake and ability to stimulate an immune response. The current vaccine for hepatitis B is an example of a third-generation vaccine. Licensed since 1987 and available as Recombivax, the synthetic vaccine is considered safer than the previous hepatitis B vaccine, which utilized proteins isolated from human blood. The vaccine is a product of more than 18 years of development.

The newest type of vaccine under development is the DNA vaccine. Such a vaccine consists of plasmids modified to carry one or more protein-encoding genes. Plasmids are submicroscopic loops of DNA found in bacterial cells (Figure 9.3). DNA vaccines are safer than vaccines with whole microorganisms because the plasmids are not infectious or able to replicate, nor do they encode any proteins other than those specified by the genes. When injected into muscle tissues, the

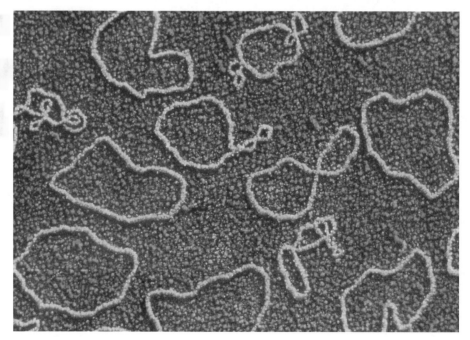

FIGURE 9.3

Plasmids, ultramicroscopic ringlets of double-stranded DNA, exist apart from the chromosome. Plasmids can be spliced with fragments of DNA of unrelated organisms and inserted into host organisms. The host organisms then produce the protein whose genetic message is carried by the foreign DNA.

plasmids enter the muscle cells and stimulate them to synthesize the gene-encoded proteins and place them at the cell surface; here the proteins are recognized as foreign and stimulate an immune response.

One problem with DNA vaccines is that they are difficult to produce because the plasmids must contain various high-technology genes that will ensure their survival and activity in the host cell. Nevertheless, researchers are buoyed by the observation that DNA vaccines appear to stimulate both cell-mediated and antibody-mediated immunity. We shall encounter them and the other types of vaccines in the following pages.

AIDS Vaccine Strategies

Because of the high mortality associated with AIDS, developing a vaccine presents one of the major medical challenges of modern times (Healthline 9.1). In the United States alone, tens of millions would be candidates for the vaccine, among them almost 3 million men at risk because of their homosexual practices with infected partners, and 1 to 2 million men who are bisexual. Also at high risk are several million Americans who regularly inject illicit drugs, as well as their sexual partners. In the medium-risk group are persons likely to come in contact with contaminated blood, such as millions of allied health science professionals. These include doctors, nurses, dental hygienists, pathologists, paramedics, and funeral service employees. Police and correction officers and members of the military are also vaccine candidates, as are highly sexually active, nonmonogamous heterosexuals.

But developing a vaccine for AIDS is far from easy: HIV has an extraordinarily high mutation rate; it is able to weave its genes into host cells and establish latent (silent) infections in those cells; and, like an arsonist attacking a firehouse, it progressively destroys the very T-lymphocytes that the immune system uses to control microbial agents. To develop a vaccine against such a formidable foe, the most simple and direct approach would seemingly be to cultivate mass quantities of the viruses, permanently inactivate them with chemicals, and inject these noninfectious viruses into the body. The body would then produce antibodies and make other specific immune responses to the weakened viruses, thus yielding immunity against future infection by full-strength viruses. Unfortunately, HIV is so dangerous that the effects of a bad batch of vaccine (for example, one containing a few active viruses) would be terrible. For the same safety reason, a vaccine composed of attenuated viruses has also been viewed with skepticism.

Another dilemma is deciding which immune response to trigger. Most viral vaccines work by calling forth a strong antibody

Healthline 9.1

1 Q Why can't an AIDS vaccine be made like a measles or other viral vaccine?

A Most viral vaccines are produced by taking whole viruses, inactivating (killing) them, and using them as vaccines. Using HIV in this way would be very dangerous, because if any HIV particles remained active (alive) in the vaccine, they might cause HIV infection and AIDS. Also, HIV is much more complex than other viruses for which vaccines have been made, so much deeper understanding of its activity is required before it could be used in a vaccine.

2 Q What are the "subunit vaccines" I sometimes read about?

A Though a whole-virus vaccine may be possible, most scientists believe that a vaccine composed of protein fragments of the virus would be safer because there would be virtually no possibility that the fragments could infect a person. The fragments or other chemical components of the virus are called subunits.

3 Q How widely would an AIDS vaccine be used?

A The AIDS vaccine would be recommended for those who may come in contact with HIV-infected blood or semen. Individuals practicing anal intercourse would be candidates for the vaccine, as would injection drug users. Allied health science professionals would also be candidates because they contact blood in the regular course of their work. Anyone for whom the hepatitis B vaccine is currently recommended (such as the individuals just cited) would also be a potential recipient of the AIDS vaccine.

response. The antibodies bind to the virus and prevent it from infecting its host cell. But the other arm of the immune system depends on activity of the cytotoxic T-lymphocytes (Chapter 3). These cells interact with and destroy microbe-infected body cells, such as those with indwelling HIV in its proviral state. Researchers must study how best to exploit the capabilities of both arms of the immune system.

Furthermore, researchers have found that even if pathogenic HIV could be modified to a nonpathogenic variant, retroviruses in general do not elicit sufficient amounts of antibodies to prevent subsequent infection. For example, the retrovirus that causes feline leukemia elicits a low level of protection when used in the inactivated form as a vaccine. Researchers have also reported that nonpathogenic viruses could revert to pathogenic viruses in culture. There is concern, therefore, that an inactivated nonpathogenic variant of HIV could revert to its pathogenic form. It is also possible that gene segments of viruses in a vaccine could integrate into human chromosomes and promote tumor formation, since certain retroviruses are known to be tumor-inducing.

To counter this pessimism, virologists point out that in contrast to the feline leukemia virus, HIV apparently calls forth a strong antibody response when it enters the body. Studies have also shown that HIV antibodies can hold the virus in check for considerable periods of time (months or years). One objective of vaccine research is to locate the part of HIV (e.g., capsid protein, reverse transcriptase, or envelope protein) that elicits the strongest immune response and amplify that part for a possible vaccine. This may be a considerable task because no individuals completely immune to AIDS have yet been found, so no one is really sure about the nature of the immune state. Nevertheless, major interest has focused on various subunits of HIV, as we shall see presently.

Sterilizing and Therapeutic Immunities

Since HIV was first isolated, scientists have been hunting for a vaccine that could prevent it from infecting humans, similar to the vaccines for measles, mumps, rubella, hepatitis B, yellow fever, smallpox, and polio (Figure 9.4). The key word here is "prevent" because the definition of a vaccine implies a preparation that brings about immunologic surveillance and stops microorganisms before they establish themselves in the body. In modern terminology, this form of immunity has been termed sterilizing immunity to distinguish it from a newer concept of immunity known as therapeutic immunity.

In the early days of AIDS vaccine research, the preventive vaccine was the gold standard. Then, in the early 1990s, tests performed on monkeys yielded dispiriting results indicating that a preventive vaccine might be an impossible goal to attain. Some frustrated scientists turned to therapeutic vaccines as a method of preventing "disease" rather than "infection." They accepted the fact that a vaccine could not stop HIV from establishing itself in body cells and turned their efforts to preventing the symptoms of disease from developing. With that assumption, their definition of success changed, and many researchers set modified goals for themselves.

Therapeutic vaccines are used to prolong life, promote a disease-free period, prevent progression of the disease, and possibly, eliminate the virus. In addition,

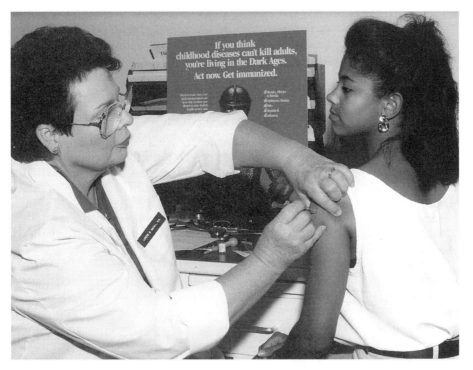

FIGURE 9.4

An adult being immunized against a number of "childhood" diseases.

a therapeutic vaccine could be used to protect the offspring of a pregnant woman who is HIV-positive. For example, a therapeutic vaccine could induce an immune response to reduce the amount of virus present in her bloodstream and reduce the possibility of passage across the placenta to the fetus.

The advantages of therapeutic immunity are numerous: Antibodies induced by the vaccine reduce the viral load in the body and make the patient less likely to spread HIV to the next individual; the delay of symptoms is clearly beneficial to the patient; and the economic pressure on the health care system is reduced. Moreover, as the concept of sterilizing immunity is increasingly rejected and that of therapeutic immunity grows in acceptance, scientists will have a better selection of vaccines for clinical trials; also, reduction of viral load can be used to compare vaccines' efficacies much better than the current approach of determining how many immunized persons fail to contract HIV infection. The current thinking is therefore dualistic: Many researchers still contemplate a preventive vaccine, but others have begun to consider the advantages of a therapeutic vaccine. Both paradigms are represented in the vaccines currently being developed, as the next sections shall survey.

AIDS Subunit Vaccines

Using viral subunits such as proteins or glycoproteins is a viable alternative to using whole-virus vaccines. In the 1990s, technological advances using recombinant DNA made it possible to produce an unlimited supply of subunits employing various types of cells as "factory organisms," or vectors (Figure 9.5). The genes that provide the genetic code for a particular subunit are first identified; then the genes are copied in huge numbers. Next, the researcher selects a vector, an organism such as a bacterium, yeast, or insect cell, and biochemically inserts the genes into the nuclear material of the vector. When the vector's genes express themselves during protein synthesis, the subunit's genes also express themselves, and large quantities of the subunit proteins are synthesized. These proteins can then be isolated and purified from the cellular material.

Among the major subunits being considered for an AIDS vaccine are glycoprotein 120 (gp120) and glycoprotein 41 (gp41). Both glycoproteins exist in the HIV envelope spikes; gp120 juts out and contacts the CD4 receptors and coreceptors, and then gp41 penetrates the membrane and serves as an anchor for gp120 molecules (Chapter 2). Both gp120 and gp41 are essential for the binding of HIV to host T-lymphocytes and brain cells. Antibodies produced against these glycoproteins would presumably unite with the glycoproteins and prevent HIV's interaction with its host cells.

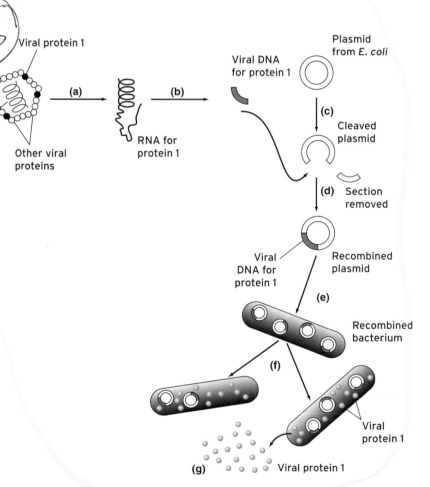

Another avenue of research centers on a third glycoprotein known as gp160. This glycoprotein is a precursor molecule (a forerunner) to both gp120 and gp41. Researchers have shown that gp160 can stimulate antibody production when used in a vaccine.

Still another approach to an AIDS vaccine involves an HIV protein known as p17. This protein is located in the capsid surrounding the HIV genome. The protein is believed to protrude into the envelope of HIV and come near enough to the viral surface to provoke an immune response. Biotechnology companies using recombinant DNA technologies produce the protein in bulk, then chemically cut the molecule into smaller and smaller subunits to determine which subunit most efficiently elicits antibody production by the immune system. The commercial vaccine made by this process is called HGP-30. It contains a 30-amino-acid region of the p17 protein. One distinct advantage to using p17 is that this protein does not display the propensity to mutate shown by envelope proteins such as gp120 and gp41. This is because the *gag* genes for p17 are apparently more stable than the *env* genes for the envelope proteins.

A novel approach to an AIDS vaccine employs antibodies produced against CD4 molecules, the sites where HIV binds to host cells. Scientists produce great quantities of CD4 molecules and use them to produce anti-CD4 antibodies by injecting them into animals. Then they fragment these anti-CD4 antibodies and isolate the key regions at the variable ends, where the antibody molecule binds to the CD4 molecule. Regions such as these are called idiotypes. An idiotype can be visualized as a type of key fitting into the CD4 lock. In the body, idiotypes induce the immune system to produce antibodies that resemble CD4 molecules (the keys have been used to build locks). Such antibodies resemble CD4 molecules and compete for sites on the HIV surface. They "muddy up" the sites and prevent the viruses from uniting with the CD4 receptor sites on the host cell. A comparison can be made with treated CD4 molecules injected into an ill person for a similar purpose (Chapter 8). However, the injection of CD4 molecules is for a therapeutic purpose, while the use of the idiotype vaccine is to induce antibodies for a preventive purpose.

Chemical subunits such as gp120, gp41, p17, and idiotypes generally do not elicit large amounts of antibodies. One reason is that they are not easily engulfed by the body's macrophages or efficiently delivered to the immune system during the immune process (Chapter 3). Subunits are therefore made more attractive to macrophages by chemically binding them to "carrier" particles or to chemical substances referred to as adjuvants. Adjuvants include molecules of aluminum sulfate (alum), globules of peanut or mineral oil, artificial membranes called liposomes, and certain noninfectious viruses, as we discuss presently). A potentially affective adjuvant now in testing stages is granulocyte-macrophage colony-stimulating factor. This chemical substance is often used to boost blood counts in transplant and cancer patients.

Unfortunately, even the best adjuvants are not always able to encourage a strong antibody response. For example, in the early 1990s, optimism was high that a gp120 vaccine might become the weapon of choice against HIV (Figure 9.6). However, two gp120 vaccines formulated independently by two different com-

look over

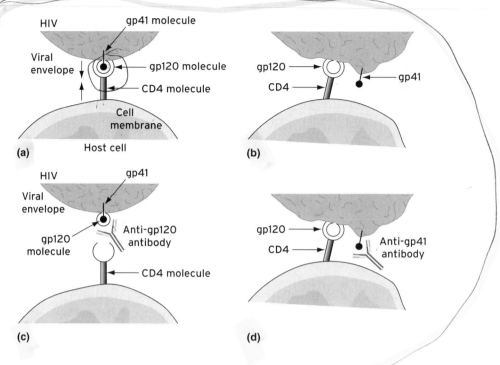

FIGURE 9.6

How antibodies prevent binding of HIV to host cells. (a) When HIV associates with a host cell, its gp120 protein binds to the CD4 receptor site on the host cell. (b) Once the initial binding has taken place, the gp41 protein anchors HIV to the host cell membrane and encourages penetration. (c) Antibodies against gp120 will combine with gp120 and prevent the latter's binding with CD4, and (d) antibodies against gp41 will inhibit gp41's anchorage to the host cell. By interfering with both gp120 and gp41 activity, the attachment of HIV to host cells can be prevented.

panies failed to elicit a strong antibody response to freshly isolated HIV, and in 1994 the National Institutes of Health (NIH) was prompted to abandon human trials using gp120 molecules. The decision dampened enthusiasm for vaccine development for several years.

But the gp120 vaccine was back in the news by the end of the decade. In 1998, VaxGen Inc. of San Francisco was given FDA approval to launch a trial of its newly formulated alum-adjuvant gp120 vaccine called AIDSVAX. The so-called bivalent vaccine contains two types of gp120 molecules, one type from a laboratory strain used in previous vaccines and one from currently circulating HIV. In the United States, about 5000 uninfected gay men volunteered for the trial (two-thirds received the vaccine and one-third a placebo); in Thailand, about 2500 uninfected injection drug users offered their services. Effectiveness of the vaccine was determined by recording how many in each group became infected with HIV and the viral load in those infected. A total of seven inoculations over a 30-month period were administered. Early results generated optimism that the vaccine could induce at least some immunity. The benchmark for effectiveness of the vaccine was that 30 percent of those receiving it should develop cytotoxic T-lymphocytes for protection against HIV. In 2002, plans were drawn up to use the gp120 vaccine in the "boost" phase of the so-called prime-and-boost approach that we discuss below. The canarypox vaccine (explored presently) was used in the "prime" phase.

Another approach seeks to uncover the vulnerable parts of the gp120 molecule (the V3 loops discussed in Chapter 2) that are crucial to infection and that elicit the strongest possible antibody response. These hidden portions of gp120 are not normally available to react with antibodies, but they become exposed when HIV interacts with the host cell's CD4 receptors and coreceptors. Indeed, the camouflaging of these sites may be a reason why they are poor targets for antibodies and why infected individuals mount limited antibody responses.

In 1999, to expose the V3 loops, scientists at the University of Montana added HIV genes to cultured cells and induced the cells to produce gp120 molecules at their surface. Then they engineered neuroblastoma cells to produce CD4 and CCR5 molecules at their surface. Next, they combined the two cell types and just as the cells fused, they added formaldehyde to "freeze" the cells during fusion, a time when critical regions of the gp120 molecules are exposed. Injections of the fused cells into laboratory animals resulted in anti-gp120 antibodies that thwarted HIV infection but did not protect against SIV infection (thus implying that the antibodies were very specific for the structures they neutralized). Practical applications of the idea are still in early testing stages.

And, finally, some vaccine work has been done using the *tat* protein as an immunizing agent. The *tat* gene is one of the nine HIV genes (Chapter 2). It encodes a regulatory protein (*tat*) that appears to enhance the expression of HIV genes, although this observation is not universally accepted. Tests have shown that in humans, some delay in progression to AIDS can be achieved when antibodies that neutralize the *tat* protein are present in the blood. However, working with the *tat* protein is difficult because it occurs in two forms (encoded by two regions of the *tat* gene), and the two forms appear to trigger different actions. Nevertheless, the experiments continue, and in 1999, five of seven primates immunized with *tat* protein and challenged with viruses appeared to resist infection.

Viable-Vector Vaccines

A high priority of vaccine researchers is to complex an HIV subunit with a non-pathogenic microbe. To form this combination, a virus such as the cowpox (vaccinia) virus is genetically engineered to incorporate HIV genes into its genome. In the laboratory, this is accomplished by infecting a culture of lymphocytes with HIV and permitting the RNA of HIV to be transcribed into DNA. Then the DNA is extracted and chemically linked to DNA of the cowpox virus. Next, the virus is allowed to multiply in host cells to produce enough for a vaccine. Animals inoculated with the recombined virus develop antibodies both to the virus and to the HIV subunits whose genes are carried by the virus. The vaccine so produced is known as either a viable-vector vaccine or an infectious recombinant virus vaccine.

One viable-vector vaccine that has entered clinical trials begins with a weakened virus used to immunize canaries and other birds against canarypox. The large genome of the canarypox virus is recombined by adding the HIV *env* gene for surface protein, the HIV *gag* gene for core protein, and the HIV gene for protease, also a protein. The virus does not replicate in human cells, but when it enters them, they package genome-encoded proteins into empty lipid shells called pseudovirions. The latter are not infectious, but they trigger an immune response consisting of antibodies against the three HIV proteins and against the HIV-infected cells. Moreover, the infected cells display gp120 molecules and other HIV proteins on their surfaces, and these marked cells elicit an immune response from cytotoxic T-lymphocytes in cell-mediated immunity. As noted earlier, the vaccine was prepared in 2002 for use in the "prime" phase of the prime-and-boost trials slated to take place in the United States, Canada, the Netherlands, and Thailand. Over 25,000 volunteers were expected to take part in the trial.

One unique feature of the canarypox vaccine is its possible use by application to the mucosal surfaces of the respiratory, urinary, and reproductive tracts. These applications are novel routes of immunization. Laboratory tests are seeking to determine whether the vaccine elicits a special class of antibodies (called IgA) that are known to act at body surfaces and attack free-floating viral particles.

Another viable-vector vaccine being studied consists of cells of the bacterium *Salmonella* engineered with genes for the gp120 glycoprotein (Figure 9.7). The *Salmonella* used in the vaccine has been modified to prevent its reproduction in human tissues and thereby prevent infection. The theory is that macrophages will pick up the bacteria more efficiently than a chemical adjuvant would and transport them to the immune tissues, where antibodies against gp120 molecules will form.

A Whole-Virus Vaccine

Despite the drawbacks cited earlier, some researchers have continued their quest for a whole-virus vaccine in part because a whole virus would present immune-

Scanning electron micrograph of *Salmonella* cells.

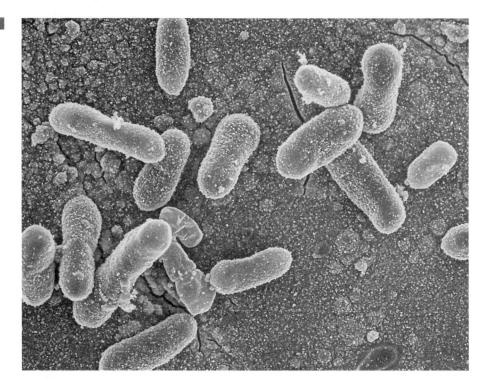

stimulating proteins in their natural form and provide a better target for antibodies. Among the groups seeking such a vaccine is one formerly led by Jonas Salk, developer of the polio vaccine containing inactivated viruses (Salk died in 1995). In 1989, Salk presented evidence that HIV inactivated by chemical treatment and gamma radiation could be safely used as a vaccine. For vaccine production, the envelope of HIV was completely disintegrated by the inactivation treatment, thereby preventing any possible union with host cells. In the late 1990s, plans were under way to test the whole-virus preparation as a therapeutic vaccine in a three-year study involving 3000 people. Proponents pointed out that the vaccine was not intended to provoke an antibody response (since it had no envelope proteins) but rather to enhance cell-mediated immunity centered in cytotoxic T-lymphocytes (Chapter 3). It was hoped that this immune process would keep the viral burden under control while the patient's immune system underwent repair.

Proponents of the whole-virus vaccine are encouraged by a 1995 discovery that an HIV strain lacking most of its *nef* gene apparently discourages the progression from HIV infection to AIDS (the *nef* gene is a regulatory gene discussed in Chapter 2). The discovery culminated a long study in which 7 Australian recipients of HIV-contaminated blood did not progress to AIDS for 14 years (neither did the person who donated the blood). The virus lacking *nef* seemingly infects T-lymphocytes but encodes so few new viruses that the patient's viral load remains within limits that the body can control. Although the *nef* gene was seen as a possible target for drug or vaccine development, the hopes of researchers were dampened by the 1999 report that 2 of the 7 Australian blood recipients had begun the progression to AIDS.

An alternative whole-virus vaccine is one containing simian immunodeficiency virus (SIV), the virus that causes AIDS in monkeys. In 1998, Ronald Desrosiers and his colleagues at Harvard University reported mildly encouraging results three years after vaccinating rhesus monkeys with two forms of SIV, one weakened by excluding three of HIV's nine genes, and the other by excluding the *nef* gene. Some of the monkeys so treated resisted infection when given lethal dose injections of SIV. Moreover, very little SIV could be found in the tissues, and the T-lymphocyte count remained normal in some experimental animals. Since the possibility exists that weakened viruses can mutate to a virulent form or acquire deleted genes, Desrosiers and his colleagues shifted their attention to mutated SIV particles unable to synthesize parts of their gp120 molecules. Work on deleting the so-called V2 region of gp120 was apparently productive, as the group reported in 2001, and the research turned to producing a vaccine with whole, inactivated SIV having the deletion.

Evidence also exists that individuals infected with the milder (but nevertheless infectious) HIV-2 seem to be protected against infection by the more virulent HIV-1. A controversial, decade-long study of 756 African women was concluded in 1995, and researchers found that those initially testing positive for HIV-2 were 70 percent less likely to become infected with HIV-1 than women not previously infected with HIV-2. Studies such as these give hope that alternative milder viruses can protect against virulent viruses in much the same way cowpox viruses protect against smallpox viruses.

Proponents of the whole-virus approach to a vaccine suggest that using the traditional method would reduce the time necessary for vaccine development by several years. They argue that the subunit approach is basically a hit-or-miss technique; that is, it requires the development of costly vaccines that use every part of the virus until the most desirable part is found. Using the whole virus without taking it apart is the sensible approach, the proponents maintain. Opponents continue to point to the safety risks in using whole viruses as they continue to develop subunit vaccines.

In the final analysis, the ideal AIDS vaccine should stimulate two forms of immunity: Cell-mediated immunity (CMI), based on T-lymphocyte activity, would result in cytotoxic T-lymphocytes that attack and destroy HIV-infected cells, thereby ending HIV infection in the body; and antibody-mediate immunity (AMI), a second form that is based on B-lymphocyte activity, would result in antibodies that bind to HIV and prevent it from attaching to host cells. This viewpoint is now gaining favor as well as practical application: The prime-and-boost approach we noted earlier uses a whole-virus vaccine followed by a purified subunit vaccine. The first vaccine stimulates CMI, while the second elicits AMI.

DNA Vaccines

Although enthusiasm for the new DNA vaccines ran high in the 1980s, tests performed in humans in the early 1990s did not yield strong immune responses. Nevertheless, researchers continued their work, and by the end of the century, the future looked more promising. For example, scientists at Chiron Corporation attached DNA molecules to microparticles of a new adjuvant called polylactide coglycolide (which is used in surgical sutures), and they found that the combination boosted both CMI and AMI in laboratory animals.

Another test performed by Harvard researchers was reported in 2000. In this case, rhesus macaque monkeys were immunized with plasmids containing the genes that encode proteins in both HIV and SIV, that is, the SIV *gag* gene and the HIV *env* gene. As an adjuvant, some monkeys were also administered human interleukin-2 (IL-2), a chemokine that encourages the proliferation of cytotoxic T-lymphocytes; alternately, some monkeys received the genes that encode IL-2. The monkeys were then challenged with HSIV, a hybrid virus containing a core of SIV and envelope proteins of HIV. They remained healthy. Although only modest antibody production was noted, there was a substantial increase in the number of cytotoxic T-lymphocytes specifically programmed to lock onto HIV particles. Moreover, the animals displayed suppressed replication of SIV and had low or undetectable viral loads when tested (control animals given no vaccine fared poorly in the test). One researcher suggested that a therapeutic vaccine combined with HAART (Chapter 8) may be a long-range solution to keeping HIV under control in the body.

Between 1986 and 1992, Merck & Company was a leader in AIDS vaccine research, specializing in HIV vaccine components that elicit antibody response. When these vaccines proved questionable, the company changed its focus to vaccines that stimulate CMI. Ten years later, in 2002, Merck was ready to reenter the field with a number of new vaccines, among them three vaccines containing plasmids with the SIV *gag* gene, one with the HIV *gag* gene spliced into the genome of a cowpox virus, and one with the HIV *gag* gene spliced into the genome of a common cold virus known as the adenovirus. Tests with these new vaccines and a number of novel adjuvants are ongoing.

Problems in Vaccine Development

The optimism generated by continuing work on an AIDS vaccine is overshadowed by problems encountered during vaccine development and testing. Among the major problems that confront vaccine researchers are the complexity of the virus and its persistence in the body, the lack of animal models for testing vaccines, the tendency of HIV to mutate, and the nagging possibility that traditional vaccine approaches will not work with HIV. There are other problems to be addressed as well (Table 9.1). A synthetic vaccine, for example, may contain traces of carrier protein (e.g., bacterial, insect cell, mammalian cell), and this protein may induce an allergic response in the recipient. Another challenge is developing improved adjuvants to ensure uptake by macrophages. And as mentioned previously, safety remains a key concern in vaccine development. Problems like these have made vaccine development a herculean task.

Complexity of HIV

High on the list of concerns is the finding that HIV is much more complex than other viruses, such as those causing measles, mumps, rubella, or polio. In these cases, no integration of the viral genome into the host cells' DNA takes place, and antibodies elicited by the vaccines can neutralize the viruses in the extracellular fluids. HIV, by comparison, is an integrating retrovirus that installs its genes as a provirus, and since antibodies do not enter body cells, the virus can escape neutralization by remaining inside cells for months or years. It is therefore unlikely that

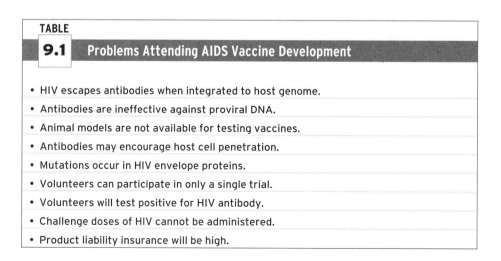

TABLE 9.1	Problems Attending AIDS Vaccine Development

- HIV escapes antibodies when integrated to host genome.
- Antibodies are ineffective against proviral DNA.
- Animal models are not available for testing vaccines.
- Antibodies may encourage host cell penetration.
- Mutations occur in HIV envelope proteins.
- Volunteers can participate in only a single trial.
- Volunteers will test positive for HIV antibody.
- Challenge doses of HIV cannot be administered.
- Product liability insurance will be high.

1 **Q** Could I receive an injection of AIDS vaccine even if I had been previously exposed to HIV?

A The basic principle of a vaccine is to build up the body's immunity so that infection cannot take place at all. However, if infection has already occurred, a vaccine could be used to marshal the body's defenses and keep HIV under control, thereby preventing the development of symptoms. Drugs could be combined with the vaccine to further limit the spread of HIV in the body.

2 **Q** When will a vaccine for AIDS be available?

A By most optimistic estimates, an AIDS vaccine will probably not be available for general use until 2010 or so. Vaccine development is an arduous task, and clinical trials to ensure the usefulness and safety of the vaccine consume a great deal of time.

3 **Q** What is the "human mouse" I sometimes read about?

A Obviously, there is no such thing as a human mouse. However, to help research on AIDS and other diseases, scientists have biologically altered mice so that their immune systems contain human cells rather than mouse cells. Scientists can then study reactions in immune system cells in mice rather than in humans.

antibodies elicited by an AIDS vaccine would be able to locate every viral particle or completely rid the body of HIV. Moreover, antibodies generally react with capsid proteins, and because HIV exists in its proviral form, the antibodies would be ineffective against its DNA (indeed, the viral protein does not even exist at the proviral stage). For these reasons, attention is focusing on prime-and-boost vaccines that stimulate CMI as well as AMI.

But ridding the body of every single viral particle may not be necessary. To be sure, controlling the virus in an infected individual may be a valuable function performed by a whole-virus vaccine such as that developed by Salk's group (Healthline 9.2). The vaccine could be used to boost the level of HIV antibodies in the blood and prevent the viral replication that leads to host cell destruction and development of symptoms. Even if the vaccine contained some active viruses, there would be little effect on the person receiving the vaccine because infection has already occurred. Such a "post-exposure vaccine" has traditionally worked for people infected with rabies viruses (rabies has an incubation period measured in months or years), and the approach could possibly be useful for those previously exposed to HIV.

The ability of HIV to mutate remains a lingering problem in the quest for a vaccine. Like the influenza virus, HIV has a tendency to undergo frequent mutations, especially in its *env* gene. These mutations are expressed as altered envelope proteins gp120 and gp41. In one patient, California researchers isolated dozens of variants of HIV over a period of a year. The possibility of the existence of multiple variants requires a vaccine to elicit different antibodies to be effective or to be directed at a single protein essential to viral replication or infection. In this context, it is also noteworthy that HIV exists as three main groups (M, N, and O), and many subgroups (or clades) as well.

Economic Issues

Another problem facing vaccine researchers is the overall "deflation factor." After years and years of trying, the pharmaceutical companies are feeling the pressures of defeat. The original estimate of candidates for a vaccine in developed countries has dwindled, partly because fewer individuals consider themselves at risk for HIV infection and because HAART drugs have lifted the cloud of doom over those infected. Thus, the market for vaccines will mainly come from developing countries, a fact that means reduced profits.

Fears of regulation by governments and lawsuits from people claiming injury from the vaccine have further let the steam out of the vaccine development effort (sick individuals can accept that a drug does not work or has side effects, but healthy individuals take exception to a vaccine that makes them ill). The investment community has become somewhat disillusioned by the failures, and that pessimism is fueled by the deflated profits anticipated from reduced use of a vaccine. Indeed, investing in a vaccine normally brings less profit than investing in a drug because a vaccine is used only a few times, while a drug is used innumerable times over the course of an illness. Moreover, cost of development remains high because the science continues to be tough, as demonstrated by NIH's 1994 decision to halt trials of two vaccines because of disappointing results.

The economic consideration is also related vaccine effectiveness, especially since a flawed vaccine may be preferable to no vaccine. An NIH statistical analysis made in 1992 emphasizes this view: The analysis indicated that over a ten-year period, a 60% effective vaccine introduced in 1992 would prevent nearly twice as many HIV infections as a 90% effective vaccine introduced in 1997.

Lack of Animal Models

A major problem attending vaccine development is the fact that HIV has a restricted host range (humans); animals do not display the symptoms of AIDS, nor do most animal species harbor the virus. Researchers are intrigued by this observation and are interested in determining the basis of resistance because they could possibly fashion a mechanism for human resistance. For vaccine developers, though, the problem has a substantial practical implication because a useful animal must be found for vaccine testing. Without an animal model, researchers cannot predict whether an experimental vaccine might work in humans.

Through the early 1990s, the only animal available for vaccine testing was the chimpanzee. These animals can be infected with HIV, but they do not display significant symptoms of AIDS, even after years of infection. However, they do mount an antibody response within three to nine months after infection with experimental AIDS vaccines. Chimpanzees are an endangered species, and by federal law they may not be imported (Figure 9.8). In the United States, only about 1500 chimpanzees are available for all biomedical research, and most are committed to other projects. Moreover, chimpanzees cost about $50,000 each. Another primate, the gibbon, can also be infected with HIV, but it is rarer than the chimpanzee.

A possible solution to the animal model problem may lie in the Indian rhesus macaque monkey, a much more common species of primate. Rhesus macaque monkeys cannot be infected with HIV, but they develop an AIDS-like illness when infected with simian immunodeficiency virus (SIV) or with the hybrid virus HSIV.

Still another proposed solution to the animal model problem was the so-called human mouse. This animal is a special breed of mouse born without a functioning immune system and genetically altered to include elements of the human immune system by implanting thymus and lymph node tissue from human

FIGURE 9.8

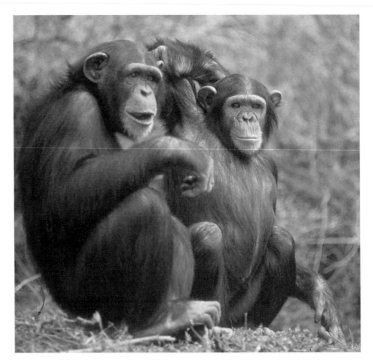

Chimpanzees, which are considered an endangered species, are among the few animals available for testing of AIDS vaccines.

fetuses. However, enough deficiencies in this animal model were encountered to abandon it. But hopes for a rodent model continue, and researchers are using genetic engineering techniques to produce mice and rats whose T-lymphocytes have human CD4 receptors and coreceptors, and whose cells produce some of the unique proteins and other factors that human cells supply when HIV replicates itself (Box 9.1).

But even if researchers succeed in building or locating an animal that supports HIV replication, there remains the problem of locating an HIV strain whose replication in animals mimics its replication in humans. As noted above, HIV does not replicate well in chimpanzees and other animals, so inoculating an animal with a candidate vaccine and then challenging the animal with HIV has not provided a rigorous test of whether the vaccine is likely to help humans. That concept appeared to change in 1999 when scientists at Emory University reported that an HIV-infected chimpanzee developed an AIDS-like illness in which the T-lymphocyte population was virtually depleted in 6 months as the viral load skyrocketed. Although this potentially lethal strain was equally devastating in other chimpanzees, some investigators pointed out that the strain is excessively virulent for testing purposes, since the same T-lymphocyte depletion in humans takes years to accomplish. Meanwhile, proponents of the strain voiced their opinion it would make the chimpanzee challenge model more persuasive. The debate remains unresolved.

The Human Mouse

Investigators seeking an AIDS vaccine and wishing to determine drug effectiveness are seriously hampered by the lack of a good animal model. Vaccine developers need to know whether an experimental vaccine can elicit antibody production in a test animal, and drug producers require a small-animal model to bridge the gap between laboratory cultures and human trials.

The search for a good animal model frustrated researchers until 1988, when two laboratory teams from California transplanted components of the human immune system into mice and produced what the media immediately labeled "the human mouse." The mice involved had been identified five years previously as having severe combined immunodeficiency (SCID), an immune disorder in which no B- or T-lymphocytes are produced. The animals had essentially no immune system. One team performing the research was led by Michael McCane, an immunologist at Stanford University. McCane's group took thymus, lymph node, and liver tissue from an aborted human fetus and

placed it under the capsulelike membrane surrounding the mouse's kidney. A week later, they injected fetal human immune system cells into the experimental mice, hoping that the immature cells would home in on the thymus, develop into mature T-lymphocytes, and circulate to the lymph nodes. Two weeks after the transplant, the mice could fight off infection when inoculated with *Pneumocystis carinii*. They had apparently acquired an immune system—and, experiments showed, it was an immune system of *human* cells. The researchers even located antibody-producing B-lymphocytes in their prized mice.

The second team, working independently, successfully transplanted white blood cells from adult human tissues into SCID mice. They demonstrated the animals' immune functions by injecting tetanus toxoid into the animals and showing that the mice could produce antibodies against the toxin.

The implanted white cells would conceivably protect the mice for life. The researchers hope that the lessons learned from the mice will protect human lives, as well.

Vaccine Trials

At the beginning of the twenty first century, over 30 groups were actively working in laboratories around the world to develop an AIDS vaccine (11 were in the United States). Each group consists of industrial, university, and government scientists, combining their resources and talents.

To determine the efficacy of candidate vaccines, the FDA requires a procedure similar to that used for drug testing. First, there is preclinical testing in animals, intended to assess whether a promising vaccine is biologically active and safe enough to be tested in people. Next comes the Phase I trial, in which the vaccine is tested in relatively few individuals (perhaps 25) to determine safety in humans. In the Phase II trial, several hundred persons are enlisted to assess side effects and effectiveness as an immunizing agent. And finally, thousands of volunteers participate in the Phase III trial to certify safety and effectiveness.

Once vaccine trials get to Phase III stage and involve thousands of volunteers, four questions about the candidate vaccine must be answered: How strong is the evidence that the vaccine offers any protection? How likely is it that the trials can prove whether the vaccine will work in the general public? Is it ethical to spend millions of dollars for such trials rather than using the money to encourage behavioral changes known to protect people? And is the government marching ahead with the trial for the sake of appearing to make progress rather than because the products look promising?

Issues to Consider

During vaccine trials, a number of technical, social, and ethical concerns can be expected to surface. For example, volunteers can only participate in a single trial because once they are inoculated with a particular vaccine, they have been "used," and injections with other vaccines would not give reliable results. Thousands of volunteers are needed for trials, and the requirement for one-time participation shrinks the pool of available participants considerably. Attracting volunteers may also be difficult because few animal studies will have been performed before human studies begin. Therefore, volunteers might be reluctant to participate in a vaccine trial.

Another dilemma confronting volunteers in a vaccine trial is the possibility of improved vaccines. It may happen, for instance, that a volunteer vaccinated with a candidate vaccine may be unable to mount an immune response at some time in the future when injected with an improved vaccine. Moreover, once volunteers have been immunized, they will test positive whenever an HIV antibody test is performed. This positive result may suggest falsely that they have been infected by HIV, and they may suffer the discrimination associated with HIV carriers. (To prevent this possibility, volunteers are given notarized documents explaining their participation in the vaccine trial.) Also, for the volunteers, an HIV antibody test will be useless as a diagnostic measure should infection occur at a later time.

An ethical problem is how to test a vaccine's effectiveness while counseling persons on measures to avoid HIV (Figure 9.9). When a person volunteers to be in a vaccine trial, the doctor is ethically obliged to counsel the person on HIV-prevention measures. In the event that such measures are followed, how could researchers determine whether failure to contract HIV was due to the vaccine or the counseling? In the past, for trials of a measles vaccine, by contrast, it was assumed that a certain percentage of volunteers would be unavoidably exposed to measles over the course of the trial. However, that assumption could not apply to an AIDS vaccine trial because changes in high-risk behaviors might also limit exposure to the virus and account for failure to develop the disease.

Ethical questions also abound when vaccine trials are conducted in poor countries. For example, how can it be determined that participants are fully aware of what the trials involve and whether they truly give their consent? Also, should vaccines tested in a particular country use the same subtypes (or clades) of viruses pres-

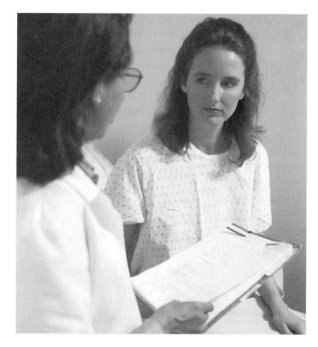

FIGURE 9.9
A potential test patient being counseled before entering a vaccine's test trials.

ent in that country? Another thorny issue is what to do if volunteers in poor countries become infected during the vaccine trials—should they be given state-of-the-art drugs even if the country cannot afford them? Or should they be administered the highest level of care attainable in that country? One obvious solution is to conduct initial trials in developed countries, as a 1993 document from an international medical group recommended; but officials in developing countries than wonder why they are being treated paternalistically. To help resolve the issue, the UNAIDS has decided to let each country answer the question for itself.

A further consideration is the excessively long incubation period before AIDS develops in an HIV-infected individual. This period can be ten years or longer in some persons. Thus, with disease as the clinical endpoint, the value of a vaccine cannot be statistically measured until an extraordinary amount of time has passed (during which many volunteers would probably leave the study and the costs would become astronomical). Time is less of a consideration if a therapeutic vaccine is tested. In this case, the reduced amount of virus in the body (the viral load) can be measured as a test of the vaccine's effectiveness. That analysis can be accomplished in three years according to public health estimates, and far fewer people would be required since fewer would be lost. With less dangerous diseases, a vaccine's effectiveness can be tested by inoculating the vaccinated volunteers with doses of the pathogenic agent. It is unlikely that this practice will be followed in AIDS vaccine development because HIV is too deadly. Thus, another measure of a vaccine's success will be unavailable to researchers.

There are also a series of commercial product liability concerns that must be considered by vaccine manufacturers as well as by potential vaccinees (Healthline 9.3). To minimize liability concerns, a researcher needs to practice good science, good medicine, and good ethics. For instance, the reason for undertaking a clinical study of an AIDS vaccine with human volunteers should be scientifically sound, especially since good animal models are currently lacking. The clinical trial should be designed and carried out to yield useful scientific information consistent with the protection of human subjects. Moreover, the selection and screening of potential vaccinees should be scientifically appropriate. The plan for the vaccine trial should be submitted for rigorous scientific review by an institutional review board that includes medical practitioners and ethicists. And the basic parameters of informed consent and medical ethics must be followed throughout the trial.

The Race to Vaccine

On May 25, 1961, President John F. Kennedy stood before a special joint session of Congress and challenged the United States to send an astronaut to the moon by the end of the decade. Scientists and engineers were astonished by Kennedy's audacity, for at that time, the United States had not even carried out a manned spaceflight, let alone seriously considered a moonshot. Nevertheless, the American scientific community shifted its resources into high gear the next day as the campaign for the moon began. And on July 20, 1969, astronaut Neil Armstrong made the historic first footprints of a human being on the moon.

Now we fast-forward to May 18, 1997 and the commencement speech at Baltimore's Morgan State University. President Bill Clinton is at the podium addressing 850 graduates and proclaiming a new national goal: an AIDS vaccine by 2007. "If the twenty-first century is to be the Century of Biology," he says, "let us make an AIDS vaccine its first great triumph." He indicates that to spearhead the initiative, the U.S. government will create a new $30 million AIDS vaccine laboratory at the NIH; other countries will be enlisted in the effort to develop a vaccine; and the pharmaceutical industry will be challenged to make an AIDS vaccine a major priority. "There are no guarantees," President Clinton adds, but he expresses confidence in the collective wisdom of the world's scientists. And so, with great fanfare, the race for an AIDS vaccine begins in earnest.

We now fast-forward one more time, to 2002. The Vaccine Research Center at the NIH is in full operation, and several candidate vaccines are being considered for clinical trials (a primary focus of the center is to move basic research results more aggressively into clinical trials). The Bill and Melinda Gates Foundation has awarded a $100 million grant to the International AIDS Vaccine Initiative, a New York-based nonprofit organization that sponsors trials of AIDS vaccines as rapidly as possible after development (the World Bank and the British government also supplied funds). And there is a new excitement in research laboratories as scientists gradually render obsolete the notion of a traditional vaccine and refocus on a vaccine that will provide both antibody- and cell-mediated immunities. They are striving for even partial success within the 2007 timetable, mindful that such a breakthrough would open new research avenues for the future.

There is a also a new spirit of cooperation among academic and industrial scientists, a cooperation fostered by new leadership. The Vaccine Research Center is headed by Gary Nabel, a molecular biologist with extensive experience in vaccine development. Nabel works with Nobel laureate David Baltimore, head of NIH's influential eleven-member AIDS Vaccine Research Committee. Baltimore was appointed in 1998 and charged with reinvigorating AIDS vaccine development by coordinating the direction for all AIDS vaccine research. The committee reports to the NIH Office of AIDS Research (headed by Neal Nathanson) and advises all NIH directors. It has succeeded in encouraging a host of new AIDS vaccine projects sponsored by universities, governments, nonprofit organizations, and industrial corporations.

Among the notable cooperative efforts are the Waterford Project and EuroVac. The Waterford Project is a privately funded venture linking Robert Gallo's Institute of Human Virology with researchers at Harvard University and the University of California to seek a vaccine combining the work of various researchers. For example, the group is working on a linking to a DNA molecule the genes that encode gp120 molecules and CD4 receptors and packing the new DNA into *Salmonella* cells for delivery as a vaccine to the body tissues. EuroVac is a similar effort, but it combines the talents of AIDS research groups in Europe. Moreover, several pharmaceutical firms have reentered the vaccine race with vigor—Merck & Company with its multiple gp120 vaccines is an example. Government guarantees of vaccine purchases have created incentives for these giant corporations.

Since 1997, the community of AIDS vaccine researchers has been heartened by these advances, as well as by the increase in federal funding for vaccine development, which is now over $250 million per year. It might also be possible for the public to be more involved: In his 2001 book *Shots in the Dark*, science writer Jon Cohen recounts the March of Dimes campaign that supported polio vaccine development and calls for a "March of Dollars" to spark the AIDS vaccine race. Engaging ideas like this reflect the spirit of scientists and spur the search for an AIDS vaccine. Indeed, during his 1997 speech, President Clinton remarked " . . . with the strides of recent years, it is no longer a question of *whether* we can develop an AIDS vaccine; it is simply a matter of *when*. And it cannot come a day too soon."

LOOKING BACK

The development of vaccines for viral diseases was an outgrowth of the cultivation of viruses in tissue cultures. Early vaccines, such as the first polio vaccine, were composed of whole viruses, but subsequent vaccines contained only fragments of viruses or microorganisms capable of antibody production. A sterilizing vaccine induces an immune response that will later provide protection against establishment of a pathogenic organism in the body. A therapeutic vaccine, by contrast, prevents infection from progressing to disease—for example, HIV infection to AIDS.

Most efforts to develop an AIDS vaccine have focused on chemical subunits of the virus such as the glycoproteins of the viral envelope or the proteins of the capsid. To increase the immune response, protein subunits such as gp120 are bound to adjuvants such as alum or to other viruses such as cowpox or canarypox viruses. Research is also being performed on the V3 loops of the gp120 molecules, where antibodies are believed to bind.

Antibodies produced against CD4 molecules can also be used in a vaccine because they induce the production of other antibodies, which react with HIV as CD4 molecules might react. A whole-virus vaccine involving SIV or inactivated HIV is favored by some researchers because it would reduce the time and money invested in vaccine development. However, the safety of using whole viruses in a vaccine remains an issue to be addressed. Some intriguing work has been done with plasmids, the loops of DNA found in bacterial cells. When bound to HIV genes and injected into cells, a DNA vaccine stimulated the cells to produce proteins that act as immune stimulants in the body.

Vaccine development is hampered by the complexity of HIV's structure and replication, including the fact that viruses may penetrate cells before antibodies can neutralize them. Lack of appropriate animals for testing purposes, the possible development of enhancing antibodies, viral mutations, and deleterious reactions associated with carrier proteins in vaccines are other problems that researchers must contend with.

Procedures similar to those for drug testing are employed with vaccine trials, and periods of many years are anticipated before final vaccine approval. Researchers must address the problems of locating volunteers and conducting scientifically valid trials while counseling volunteers on AIDS-prevention techniques. In addition, it is unethical to inoculate vaccinees with doses of infectious HIV to test a vaccine's effectiveness. Commercial product liability concerns also need to be considered. Despite these drawbacks, the scientific community and the public remain optimistic that an AIDS vaccine will be developed during the next ten years.

REVIEW

This chapter has explored the development of a vaccine to prevent AIDS. To test your knowledge of this topic, select the phrase that best completes each of the following statements. The correct answers are listed in Appendix A.

_C_ 1. All the following statements are true except
   a. Certain vaccines contain whole viruses.
   b. A subunit vaccine is known as a second-generation vaccine.
   c. Developing a vaccine against HIV infection is an unrealistic expectation.
   d. All vaccines currently in use stimulate the human immune system.

_B_ 2. Among the major subunits being considered for use in an AIDS vaccine are
  a. fragments of the RNA of HIV.
  b. gp120 and gp41.
  c. the *nef* and *rev* genes.
  d. segments of proviral DNA.

_A_ 3. In subunit vaccines, the immune-stimulating agents are made more attractive to macrophages by
  a. binding the agents to adjuvant.
  b. converting the agents to DNA molecules.
  c. binding the agents to glucose molecules.
  d. converting the agents to RNA molecules.

_D_ 4. A viable-vector vaccine utilizes HIV genes linked to
  a. viral capsids.
  b. p17 protein associated with reverse transcriptase.
  c. envelope proteins of HIV and SIV.
  d. canarypox viruses cultivated in the laboratory.

_a_ 5. A therapeutic vaccine is one that
  a. prevents an infected person from progressing to disease.
  b. contains whole active viruses.
  c. cannot be taken by infected individuals.
  d. is used only in animals.

_a_ 6. Possible solutions to the problem of the lack of a suitable animal model for vaccine testing may involve any of the following except
  a. using antihuman antibodies.
  b. developing a mouse with a human immune system.
  c. using rhesus macaque monkeys.
  d. using test tube cultures of human cells.

_d_ 7. Liposomes have found value in vaccine technology as
  a. immune-stimulating reagents for viral subunits.
  b. substitutes for reverse transcriptase molecules.
  c. enzymes to produce subunits from macromolecules.
  d. adjuvants to enhance immune system stimulation.

_a_ 8. The whole-virus vaccine developed by Salk's group contains
  a. HIV particles without envelopes.
  b. envelope subunits rearranged to form whole viruses.
  c. normal HIV particles minus reverse transcriptase.
  d. normal HIV particles minus the protein capsid.

_a_ 9. The propagation of viruses for vaccine use depends heavily on the
   a. ability to cultivate viruses in tissue culture.
   b. identification of growth genes in the virus.
   c. action of enzymes similar to reverse transcriptase.
   d. formation of ISCOMs by the viruses during cultivation.

_a_ 10. Among those who would probably be candidates for an AIDS vaccine are all the following except
   a. children between the ages of 5 and 15.
   b. persons who use injection drugs.
   c. individuals who practice anal intercourse.
   d. allied health science professionals.

_b_ 11. A vaccine containing subunits is considered safer than one containing whole viruses because
   a. subunits do not stimulate an antibody response.
   b. subunits do not infect cells or replicate in the body.
   c. whole viruses may induce antibody production.
   d. whole viruses may lack the protein necessary for immune system stimulation.

_a_ 12. A vaccine composed of attenuated viruses
   a. has viruses that multiply in the body.
   b. contains virus inactivated with chemicals.
   c. cannot be used to induce immunity.
   d. is in the developmental stage for AIDS.

_d_ 13. Aluminum sulfate and mineral oil have both been used in vaccines to
   a. produce segments of DNA from proviral DNA.
   b. inhibit reverse transcriptase activity.
   c. bind viruses to the CD4 receptor sites of cells.
   d. make subunits more attractive to macrophages.

_b_ 14. Mutations that occur in a virus tend to
   a. enhance the effectiveness of the immune response.
   b. limit the usefulness of a vaccine.
   c. enhance the binding activity of envelope proteins.
   d. limit the type of adjuvant that can be employed.

_b_ 15. All the following are ethical or social concerns that may surface during vaccine trials except
   a. volunteers can only participate in a single trial.
   b. multiplying viruses will be used in the AIDS vaccine.
   c. counseling must be given to all recipients of the vaccine.
   d. participating in a vaccine trial will prompt a positive test for HIV antibodies.

Baltimore, D., and C. Heilman. 1998. "HIV vaccines: prospects and challenges." *Scientific American*, July.

Bloom, B. 1996. "A perspective on AIDS vaccines." *Science* 272: 1888–1890.

———. 1998. "The highest attainable standards: Ethical issues in AIDS vaccines." *Science* 279: 186–189.

Bolognesi, D. P. 1988. "Natural immunity to HIV and its possible relationship to vaccine strategies." *Microbiol. Sci.* 5(1): 236–241.

Caldwell, M. 1993. "The long shot." *Discover*, August.

Cimons, M. "New prospects on the AIDS vaccine scene." *ASM News* 68(1): 19–22.

Cohen, J. 1996. "A shot in the dark." *Discover*, June.

———. 1999. "Glimmerings of hope from the well." *Science*, 285: 656–658.

———. 2000. "AIDS vaccines show promise after years of frustration." *Science* 291: 1689–1670.

———. 2001. "Deep denial." *The Sciences*, January/February.

———. 2002. *Shots in the Dark: The Wayward Search for an AIDS Vaccine.* New York: W. W. Norton.

Cowley, G. 1994. "Will we ever have a vaccine?" *Newsweek*, June 27.

Green, J. 1995. "Who put the lid on gp120?" *New York Times Magazine*, March 26.

Klinman, D. M., et al. 1992. "Comparative immunogenicity of gp120-derived proteins and their induction of anti-V3 loop region antibodies." *J. AIDS* 5: 1005–1008.

Koff, W. C. 1991. "Advances in AIDS vaccine development." *ASM News* 57: 73–77.

Letvin, N. L. 1998. "Progress in the development of an HIV-1 vaccine." *Science* 280: 1875–1878.

Weiss, R. S. 2001. "Waiting for a vaccine." *Science* 292: 862–864.

Williams, P. 1990. "New optimism arising among AIDS vaccine researchers." *ASM News* 56: 9–10.

AIDS in Perspective

LOOKING AHEAD

The epidemic of HIV infection and AIDS has many implications of a nonbiological nature that affect society in numerous ways. This chapter places the AIDS epidemic in the perspective of society and explores certain implications of the epidemic. On completing the chapter, you should be able to . . .

- Describe how social institutions are touched by the AIDS epidemic and explain some of the effects of the epidemic on society.
- Summarize why HIV infection and AIDS are unique problems in the workplace and indicate the steps for developing an AIDS policy in business settings.
- Discuss some legal issues affecting AIDS patients, including discrimination and confidentiality, and identify some economic consequences of the AIDS epidemic.
- Understand the economic impact of the AIDS epidemic on the United States and the world, especially the alarming trends in Africa.
- Appreciate the special problems that the AIDS epidemic poses to health care and medical professionals.
- Identify some special needs of the AIDS patient during care in the hospital and at home.
- Describe some future expectations for the development of the AIDS epidemic and specify certain lessons learned from the epidemic.

INTRODUCTION

In the 1990s, the *New York Times* reported the story of Ellen Ahlgren, a 71-year-old resident of Northwood, New Hampshire. Mrs. Ahlgren learned that thousands of babies infected with HIV were living out their short lives in cold and sterile hospital cribs and decided to do something to help them—she would make quilts for them. Together with several other women in her

New England town, Mrs. Ahlgren sewed about a dozen quilts and sent them to Boston City Hospital.

The response from hospital administrators was so gratifying that the circle of quilters, begun in 1988, soon expanded. A series of fliers distributed around New England spread the word, and within weeks, Mrs. Ahlgren was even receiving quilts in the mail. An article in *Quilters Newsletter* magazine brought hundreds of letters and many offers of help. Today, Mrs. Ahlgren's modest group has become a nationwide organization called ABC Quilts. More than 1000 persons aged 9 to 90 are sewing quilts in 44 states, all doing their share to help the children with AIDS. As of September, 2002, ABC Quilts has provided 450,000 quilts. Another group called Quilts for Kids was founded in 1990.

If future historians were to judge the worth of our society by our response to the AIDS epidemic, they would doubtlessly find many positives as well as many negatives. Certainly, Mrs. Ahlgren's work would be among the positives, as would the efforts of tens of thousands of other volunteers who have come forward to give of themselves in a time of crisis. On the negative side is the discrimination shown to AIDS patients in employment, housing, and medical care; the deferral of services to AIDS patients; and the moral judgments verbalized by some who pontificate on what people do rather than who they are.

In this closing chapter, we place the AIDS epidemic in perspective and examine how it has influenced society. The epidemic has affected the way people live, where they work, how they interact with other people, where their money is spent, and how they receive health care. As a disease of troubling social complexity, AIDS manages to touch all people in one way or another, and all people are called on to react to it either directly or indirectly. It is also clear that the AIDS epidemic will continue well into the twenty-first century. Therefore, a look into the future is the logical way to close this story of AIDS, much as a look at the past opened the story many pages ago.

AIDS and Society

When the bubonic plague swept across Europe in the 1300s, it profoundly changed the way people lived. The massive death toll, for example, contributed to the end of feudalism because landowners had to pay high wages to for work from the decimated peasantry. Moreover, the authority of the clergy, already in decline, deteriorated further because the Church was helpless in the face of disaster, and with many priests and monks dying, a new order of reformers arose. Medical practices became more sophisticated; new standards of sanitation were imposed; and a 40-day period of detention (a quarantine) before vessels could dock at a port was instituted.

In many ways, the AIDS epidemic has also changed modern society. Reaching into virtually all social institutions (e.g., family, community, business, government, school), the AIDS epidemic has stimulated changes that have endured (Figure 10.1). A generation ago, for instance, it would have been unthinkable to exercise free expression about homosexuality, condom use, and sexual practices such as anal intercourse. Today, these subjects are discussed openly. Indeed, social taboos have lifted to the point that in 1991, the New York City Board of Education voted to distribute free condoms in the public schools to help prevent the spread of HIV.

Because HIV travels directly from person to person, the AIDS epidemic is a universal problem. As such, it touches highly industrialized as well as developing countries and affects the life of virtually every human being. Who, for instance, in urban business centers has not known an HIV-infected coworker? Which educational institution has not been required to develop a policy on AIDS? How many times has the average health care worker needed to use gloves, masks, or other protective devices in the course of a day's employment? And which funeral directors have been reluctant to provide a dignified burial to a person recently deceased from AIDS?

The AIDS epidemic has also compelled individuals to make new judgments or has served to reinforce old outlooks on many practices taking place in society. It has heightened the awareness of homosexuality, developing tolerance and understanding in some individuals but aversion and repulsion in others. It has engendered a fresh look at the epidemic of drug addiction and stimulated compassion in the form of needle exchange and drug treatment programs, while hard-

FIGURE 10.1

One of the social effects of the AIDS epidemic has been free expression regarding condom use. Posters and advertisements like these were much less visible a generation ago.

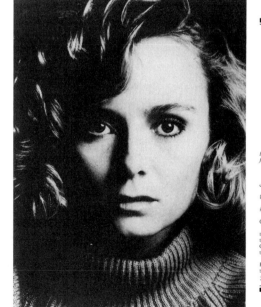

AIDS in Perspective

ening the stance of others that drug addiction is a punishable crime. It has increased attention on the plight of the poor and homeless, but it has also encouraged others to castigate those who take resources from social programs seen as more worthy of support.

Debates stimulated by the AIDS epidemic continue unabated in the media as well as in social gatherings. For instance, the issue of mandatory premarital testing has not yet been settled, and needle exchange programs still stimulate controversy. A lively debate continues on the extent of sex education and AIDS education in the schools, not to mention whether condoms should be freely distributed in these settings. Public health and health care professionals are not united on the nature and course of HIV therapies, nor do they agree on the usefulness of vaccines.

Debate also continues among ethicists who address the thorny issues surrounding therapy and vaccine use. For instance, ethicists argue about the high cost of using drugs in underdeveloped nations, and whether this obstacle to equitable care is tolerable. They point out that the complexity of the HAART regimen often precludes its use, and they question the ethics of physicians who prescribe less complicated but also less effective regimens. They wonder aloud whether rich countries should be permitted to test new drugs in poor countries that could not afford the drugs if they were found to be effective. They debate the use of placebos in controlled experiments (when some patients are purposefully denied therapy), and they press for new statistical designs that gauge a study's success while it is in progress, rather they at its conclusion.

In the inner city, the stigma of AIDS continues without any foreseeable end. No decline in the infection rate has been observed in U.S. minority populations, and for intensely poor and alienated ghetto dwellers, AIDS is just another force over which they have no control. Treatments are generally too little and too late for the poor, and infected individuals may not even be inclined to ask for assistance. Poor women, for example, may not wish to seek help for fear of losing their children to foster care. In the inner city, the AIDS epidemic has superimposed itself on the epidemics of drug addiction, welfare dependency, crime, teenage pregnancy, and homelessness, and on the general social decay. None of these epidemics can be interrupted without attention to all.

But the AIDS epidemic has also served as a catalyst to bring the positive side of the human spirit to the fore. Volunteers have emerged to service AIDS hotlines, develop educational materials, and give comfort to AIDS patients. In the hospitals, many doctors, nurses, and other professionals take pride in their work with HIV-infected persons (Figure 10.2). Business organizations have generously supplied funds to assist education, treatment, and prevention campaigns; a number of grassroots organizations have sprung up to act as advocates of persons with AIDS; and since 1990, the U.S. government has been spending more than $2 billion annually on AIDS-related programs. Many see the collective action as evidence that humans function best when they are profoundly challenged.

FIGURE 10.2

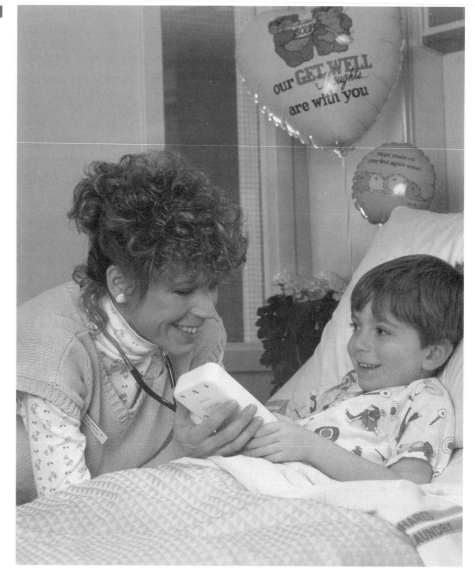

In many cases, the AIDS epidemic has served to bring the positive side of the human spirit to the fore. Many physicians and nurses take pride in giving comfort to AIDS patients. At a center for children in Albany, New York, a nurse cares for a young patient infected with HIV.

AIDS in the Workplace

Until well into the twenty-first century, successful management of the consequences of the AIDS epidemic in the workplace will be an ongoing challenge for the business community. Included under the general heading "business" are both managers and employees in public and private sectors, as well as members of state agencies, labor unions, educational institutions, law enforcement agencies, and health care establishments.

HIV infection and AIDS pose a particular problem in the workplace because the disease strikes the majority of people in their economically most productive years. And although individuals with HIV infection may be asymptomatic for ten or more years, their blood and body fluids are infectious. This presents special risks for workers in occupations where routine exposure to body fluids occurs.

Public health epidemiologists point out that in the United States, most future cases of AIDS will occur in persons currently employed in the workforce. As new treatments come into use, these workers will remain on the job longer. Indeed, as the years unfold, having employees and coworkers with HIV infection or AIDS will become a more common experience in both large and small businesses.

The challenge of managing AIDS in the workplace should elicit compassion for those with HIV infection and AIDS and prompt education and training to eliminate fear among coworkers. Aspects of a business's policy should address transmission methods for HIV, safe work practices, unique aspects of the work environment, protection for workers in these environments, and laws against discrimination. Basically, the major way to allay workers' fears is to educate workers through a consistent, well-thought-out approach for dealing with HIV infection and AIDS.

Developing an AIDS policy need not be a difficult proposition if established methods are followed. A person or task force should determine the organization's point of view, use medical facts to substantiate recommendations, take legal and cost issues into account, and consider organizational values and civic responsibilities. Existing policies can be factored in, and consistent style should be utilized. The policy may be AIDS-specific or more general in approach, as we explore next.

An AIDS-specific policy should seek to inform all employees about AIDS and recognize that persons with HIV infection and AIDS pose significant and sensitive issues in the workplace. Guidelines for handling such issues should include a commitment to a healthy and safe work environment, a statement that AIDS is to be treated the same as any other illness with regard to employee policies and benefits, and the assurance that employees with AIDS may continue to work with reasonable accommodation, as long as they are medically able. The guidelines should also call on coworkers to extend compassion or risk dismissal. Statements could reinforce the belief that all workers should be educated about AIDS and include an invitation to employees to contact their supervisor in confidence if they are concerned about or affected by AIDS (Healthline 10.1).

Healthline 10.1

1 **Q** Our business wants to establish a policy on AIDS. How should we proceed?

A Establishing a policy on AIDS is a good more for any business. A group should be formed for this purpose, and it should include representatives from all segments of the business. The policy should take the form of a statement encompassing such things as the business's point of view on AIDS, some pertinent medical facts, certain legal and economic issues, laws on discrimination, and safe work practices. Representatives from a local health department or AIDS education center can be contacted for input.

2 **Q** What should I do if I feel I am the subject of discrimination at work because of my HIV infection?

A The issue of AIDS discrimination is handled primarily at the local and state levels. If you believe you have been discriminated against, you should contact a lawyer or the state office of human rights. At the latter, your complaint will be handled by a person trained in dealing with human rights violations. You may be entitled to relief from the source of the discrimination as well as monetary compensation for any damages arising from the discrimination.

3 **Q.** What recourse do I have if the results of my HIV test are made known without my consent?

A Confidentiality is an essential tenet of any HIV testing program. If confidentiality has been breached, you may have grounds for a lawsuit or other legal action. State and local laws usually protect confidentiality. You should seek legal assistance or contact the state office of human rights for help.

A more general policy can be developed on the supposition that there is no medical reason to treat AIDS differently from other major illnesses. To this end, a policy statement addressing AIDS, cancer, heart disease, and other serious health problems should be prepared. Such a policy should indicate that employees with life-threatening illnesses will be allowed to continue their normal pursuits, as long as they can meet performance standards and do not pose a health threat to others. The policy should request managers to protect the confidentiality of employees with HIV and encourage employees to work with personnel relations experts on their concerns. Reasonable accommodations should be made for affected employees, and coworkers should be requested to exercise sensitivity and be responsive to those employees' physical and mental needs. A statement attesting to the therapeutic value of continued employment should be included in the policy.

Each of the two policy approaches has its advantages. The general approach projects the notion that AIDS is no different from other major illnesses and avoids possible discrimination in favor of AIDS. Also, it is likely to be read carefully by a broader range of people, because more individuals will be affected. By comparison, the AIDS-specific policy addresses the issues associated with AIDS directly and enhances employee education about the disease. Employees have little question about where the company stands on this single topic and can act accordingly. Experience indicates that companies are less likely to follow this approach, however, and usually opt for the more general life-threatening illness policy.

But suppose a company chooses to avoid publishing any policy. This approach may reflect management's view that HIV infection and AIDS could not occur in its employees. It may also indicate that frank talk about transmission methods is too sensitive an issue, that open talk about AIDS will condone the methods by which it is transmitted, or that discussions of AIDS will indicate that someone in the company has the disease. Such views are generally cast in a negative light, and management is often seen as burying its head in the sand until the problem goes away (the so-called ostrich mentality, Figure 10.3). Workers usually appreciate insights into contemporary issues such as AIDS and welcome a firm stand taken by the company. To be productive, employees need to know the rules of the workplace, including the rules on AIDS.

FIGURE 10.3

Some companies choose to avoid developing an AIDS policy, hoping that the epidemic will not affect their businesses. Such an attitude is like the ostrich's practice of burying its head in the sand until danger passes.

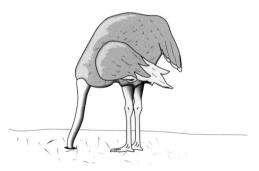

The CDC's encouragement that U.S. worksites implement AIDS-related policies has apparently borne fruit. By the end of the 1990s, a survey indicated that over half of worksites had AIDS policies in place and nearly 20 percent were offering AIDS education programs.

Legal Issues

In 1987, the U.S. Supreme Court rendered a landmark decision in the case of *School Board of Nassau County v. Arline.* The suit involved a teacher named Gene Arline who was dismissed from her teaching job in Nassau County, Florida, because she had tuberculosis. Arline contended that by dismissing her, the school board violated her rights under the 1973 Federal Rehabilitation Act. This statute protects handicapped persons against discrimination based on, among other things, the erroneous perceptions of employers. The Supreme Court, in a 7 to 2 decision, agreed with Arline and ruled that she was a handicapped person. It also emphasized that employers cannot distinguish between physical impairment and contagiousness, because they both stem from the same handicap. In so doing, the justices reaffirmed and protected the employment rights of any individual who has had, or presently has, a contagious disease. Although the decision applied to tuberculosis, it also applied by inference, to HIV infection and AIDS.

A second decision of importance was rendered in 1988 in the case of *Chalk v. U.S. District Court.* That year, the U.S. Supreme Court judged that a person suffering from AIDS was a handicapped person under the Federal Rehabilitation Act. The suit was brought by Vincent Chalk, a California teacher assigned to a nonteaching position when school officials learned he had AIDS (Figure 10.4). Finding in Chalk's favor, the Supreme Court reaffirmed the notion that the decision in *Nassau v. Arline* applies to AIDS as well as tuberculosis. The court also concluded that an employer cannot defend against a claim by asserting that employees do not want to work with persons with AIDS. An easily transmitted secondary infection would be the only defense considered in such an instance.

A further clarification came in 1997. That year, the U.S. Supreme Court ruled that a person with HIV infection should be afforded the same rights as one with AIDS. The case was brought by an HIV-positive woman named Sidney Abbott, who was refused treatment for a cavity at the office of a Maine dentist (the dentist insisted that the treatment be performed at a maximum-containment facility at a local hospital; the dentist's services would be free, but the hospital charges would be the patient's responsibility). Abbott's lawyer argued that she was protected from discrimination under provisions of the 1990 Americans with Disabilities Act, and the Court agreed. Justice Anthony Kennedy, writing for the majority, indicated that HIV infection satisfies the statutory and regulatory definition of physical impairment, especially since having the diseases impairs the reproductive process (Abbott testified that she feared passing the disease to her child if she conceived) and because HIV infection commonly leads to terminal disease. The decision has far-reaching ramifications since it suggests that a person with HIV infection has a disability even though no one can see signs of the disease.

FIGURE 10.4

Vincent Chalk, the California teacher whose suit affirmed the U.S. Supreme Court's decision that persons with AIDS are to be treated the same as and to have the same rights as any handicapped persons.

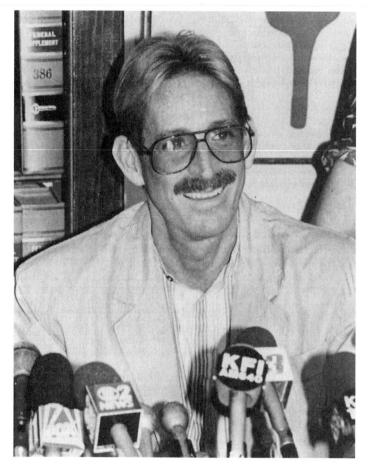

The Supreme Court decisions in the three cases mandate that AIDS be treated as a handicap, not only by public institutions but also by private businesses that receive federal assistance. Such private businesses include those having substantial contracts with the federal government and those receiving financial assistance from federal agencies. They also encompass institutions receiving Medicaid or Medicare money. Any such institutions or businesses cannot discharge an employee unless the employee's disease is contagious and poses an actual danger to others, and unless a reasonable accommodation would fail to eliminate the transmission danger (Figure 10.5).

The issue of "reasonable accommodation" for AIDS patients has stimulated a certain level of discussion, because having AIDS is synonymous with being handicapped, and federal law requires these accommodations. For the AIDS patient, reasonable accommodations include such things as released time for doctor's appointments or other medical care, rest periods during the workday if medically necessary, physical restructuring of the work area (e.g., ramps

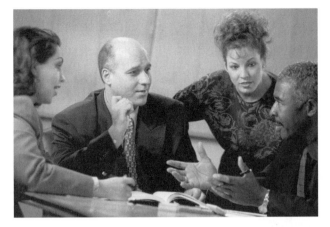

for wheelchair access), and the development of part-time work schedules to meet the individual's needs. According to law, the accommodations need not impose undue financial and administrative burdens on the employer. But to avoid extending such accommodations, the employer must show that they would create an imminent and substantial risk to the safety or health of the employee or others. Added expense, a change of schedule, or hiring additional employees are not considered undue burdens. In essence, the law has made it clear that the employer must cooperate as long as the AIDS patient can do the job.

Although the issue of discrimination has been addressed in federal law, it is spoken to primarily in state law. In New York, for example, the state Division of Human Rights handles all discrimination complaints from AIDS patients arising from violations of human rights law. Most complaints involve employment, housing, commercial space, and credit. After investigating a case, the division may recommend a hearing, while processing AIDS cases as soon as possible and preserving testimony on tape. If employment discrimination is proven, individuals are entitled to reinstatement of employment, back pay, admission to health care, and monetary compensation. Punitive damages and reimbursement for attorney's fees may also be awarded.

Confidentiality is essential when dealing with AIDS, particularly with respect to HIV testing. The individual states are largely responsible for confidentiality laws. In 1989, for example, the New York State legislature enacted one of the more comprehensive confidentiality laws. The law requires the written consent of the participant for any HIV-related testing. (The consent must be on a state-authorized form, and precounseling and postcounseling are required.) It also specifies that anyone wishing to be tested must be informed that anonymous testing is available. (Organ and blood donors are excepted.) Finally, it restricts disclosure of test results when providing health and social services (but permits disclosure in certain specified categories).

But confidentiality laws can sometimes appear too restrictive. In 1996, for instance, an individual in New York was identified as the source of HIV infection in 20 or more women he named as sex partners. The state legislature immediately investigated the effects of New York's confidentiality laws. Two years later, it established a state registry and began requiring physicians to report the names of HIV-positive individuals. Trained health workers now ask (but do not require) the individuals listed in the registry to name their sexual and/or needle-sharing partners, and they notify the named contacts that they may have been exposed to HIV. Although confidentiality is a key provision of the law, AIDS activists voice the concern that the list could fall into the hands of insurance companies, employers, or others who could discriminate against the infected patient. Supporters of the law maintain that if they are located, individuals can be treated at an early stage of the disease and increase their chances of survival.

Other legal issues arising from the AIDS epidemic involve laboratory and hospital care. It is important that managers take precautions to protect themselves against legal action for negligence, libel and slander, failure to obtain consent, breach of confidentiality, failure to warn, or failure to maintain a safe workplace. Negligence can be charged, for example, if a hospital mistakenly supplies units of HIV-positive blood for transfusion. A slander case could arise if a patient receives a positive result from an AIDS test that later is revealed to be false. (The patient could prove that the test was unreliable or improperly performed.) Failure to obtain consent may violate a state law if a patient is tested covertly.

Result reporting may be the basis for other legal problems. Positive test results should be reported to the physician whose duty is to inform the patient and health authorities according to state law (Figure 10.6). The reporting must be done according to standard protocols established by local authorities. Breach of confidentiality can be charged if the patient's consent forms are not filled out. Informing other people in a patient's life is also a delicate matter that could result in a breach of confidentiality by the physician. What position should the physician take, for example, if the HIV-positive patient refuses to inform a regular sex partner of the test results? And what of the doctors, nurses, and laboratory technicians who are not warned that a particular patient may have AIDS? Can they cite the manager for failure to maintain a safe work environment?

Ultimately, the managers of laboratory and hospital facilities must ensure that their policies fall in the mainstream of acceptable procedures. Currently, most institutions utilize the CDC's guidelines for preventing HIV transmission as their blueprint. Furthermore, institutions generally have legal staffs to advise management and to keep it abreast of federal, state, and local laws as well as the standards for health care in sister institutions.

Economic Issues

In 1984, Congress made the first annual appropriation of funds to study and deal with AIDS. The amount was $61 million. By 1989, the annual appropriation had

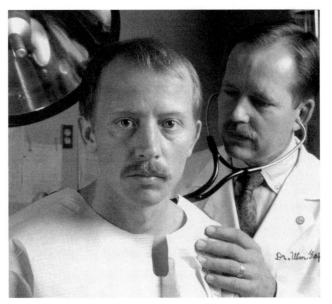

FIGURE 10.6
Part of the physician's responsibility is to inform a patient of positive HIV test results in a dignified and confidential matter. Failure to do so may be the basis for a legal judgment against the physician.

grown to $1.3 billion (an astonishing increase of 2000 percent), and by 2001, it was over $2.5 billion.

There is little doubt that the AIDS epidemic has had a heavy impact on the world's economy and will continue to do so for years. The costs can be direct as well as indirect. The annual federal expenditure of more than $2.5 billion is an example of a direct cost, as is the estimated $120,000 to care for an AIDS patient over the course of the illness (Healthline 10.2). Indirect costs arise from such things as implementing universal precautions in hospitals (e.g., disposable gloves, masks, protective wear), employing infection control procedures, mandating blood-screening, improving laboratory precautions, and establishing educational campaigns. For the "worried well" patient, indirect costs arise from counseling expenses, testing procedures, loss of time at work, and infections that may occur while the person is stressed.

There is also a significant indirect social cost when productive members of a society become ill and die. A common method of calculating the indirect costs of a disease is to estimate the wages lost to disability and premature death. For AIDS, the CDC evaluated the economic loss to society from the first 10,000 cases. It found that an estimated 8387 years of work valued at $189 million were lost to disability, and that $4.6 billion in earnings were lost because of premature death. These figures, it should be emphasized, were for only 10,000 cases. By contrast, the HAART drugs apparently pay for themselves: In 2001, researchers reported that the drug cocktails give HIV patients an additional two or three years of life expectancy, during which the patient's contributions to society exceed the average $15,000 cost of the drugs.

1 **Q** I have heard many figures quoted on the costs for caring for an AIDS patient over the course of the disease. How are these figures generated?

A Estimating costs for health care for an AIDS patient is a difficult matter because hospital costs, including pharmaceutical and laboratory costs, vary. Physician costs are another variable. The opportunistic diseases contracted, the number of hospital stays, the quality of medical care, and general health of the individual at the outset are other factors to be considered. Even the geographic location where the care is administered is a factor in the final determination.

2 **Q** I'm somewhat confused about Medicare and Medicaid. Exactly what is Medicare?

A In the United States, Medicare is a federally sponsored health care program for persons over 65 years of age. It is part of the Social Security system. Hospital and physician costs are covered, and no limits exist on the financial assets of the recipient.

3 **Q** How about Medicaid?

A Medicaid is also a federally sponsored program under the auspices of Social Security Administration. In contrast to Medicare, however, Medicaid is for persons of all ages, as long as their income is below a certain level. Hospital and physician costs can be covered under Medicaid, depending on what a person applies for. It is necessary, however, that a person's available assets be expended before Medicaid benefits will be available.

Other economic costs arise from the increasing numbers of cases of pediatric AIDS. Newborns with AIDS are commonly the offspring of poor, ill, or drug-addicted parents. More than $200,000 per year may be required to care for these newborns, and an orphan life may follow for those who survive (Figure 10.7). Sociologists have estimated, for example, that in this generation in New York City 50,000 to 100,000 children will lose one or both parents to AIDS. By 2001, an estimated 20,000 orphans were available in the city for adoption or foster care, a fearsome legacy of AIDS.

Some economists would argue that spending more than $2.5 billion in federal funds annually is too high a price to pay for AIDS. Funding proponents suggest, however, that the United States spends approximately $500 billion per year on medical care, and the expenditure for AIDS is a small fraction of this amount. Moreover, as an infectious disease, AIDS has potential to spread to a great portion of the population if left unchecked. Disorders such as heart disease and cancer do not have a similar infectious potential.

Another reason offered for appropriating the necessary funds for AIDS is the disease's concentration in young and middle-aged adults. These individuals usually fund the health care system (and the economy in general), in contrast to children and elders who seek assistance from it. Moreover, in many nations, AIDS robs the country of its young, educated, professional class of individuals that form the key underpinning of the society. Such a loss further weakens an economy that could already be fragile. Proponents of funding also point out that knowledge generated from AIDS research has many corollary benefits. Learning about HIV, for example, helps us understand how certain other retroviruses cause leukemia, and understanding the details of Kaposi's sarcoma gives insight on how other cancers may be initiated in the body.

On a global basis, it is imperative that wealthy nations become involved in the plight of poorer nations because AIDS is a worldwide disease that is continuing to spread. At the end of 2001, for example, sub-Saharan Africa was home to an estimated 28.5 million of the world's 40 million people infected with HIV. In countries of this region, the disease has a destabilizing effect as it undermines whole economies, strains medical resources, and contributes to political upheavals and war. Eventually, according to historians, the wealthier nations will be drawn into these political and social traumas. Indeed, one estimate suggests that by 2004, AIDS will be the largest epidemic in human history and could account for more deaths worldwide than the bubonic plague (the Black Death) of the 1300s.

These alarming statistics have not been lost on the world community. In 2002, the United Nations established the Global Fund to Fight AIDS, Tuberculosis, and Malaria. Treating established

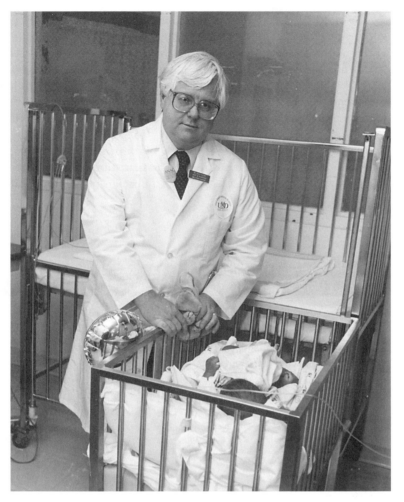

FIGURE 10.7
Cases of pediatric AIDS impose a substantial economic burden on society because health care costs tend to be much higher for children than for adults. James Oleske is the medical director of the pediatric AIDS unit at Children's Hospital in Newark, New Jersey. By 1994, there were more than 300 infants and children under his care.

cases of these diseases is a priority of the fund, as is the more traditional effort of prevention. Supporters of treatment point out that when people know that drugs are available, they will submit to testing and preventive counseling. Moreover, they will be inclined to practice safer sex, while feeling less stigmatized if they are infected with HIV. Treatment also lowers viral loads and reduces the possibility of HIV spread.

Private donors and pharmaceutical companies have also joined the effort: The Bill and Melinda Gates Foundation has contributed $100 million to the fund, and this sum has been matched by Merck & Company. Furthermore, Merck has promised to sell two of its protease inhibitors to poor countries at about a tenth of the U.S. price. Bristol-Myers has also announced lower prices for its drugs and has waived its patent rights in South Africa to stimulate the production of generic equivalents in that country.

As of 2001, the AIDS epidemic was consuming about $20 billion each year within the United States, including about $2.5 billion for antiretroviral drugs (Table 10.1). Outside the United States, overall spending was a fraction of the U.S. figure, a mere $1.8 billion. The disparity was addressed that year by a UNAIDS team of epidemiologists, who worked to determine what it would take to slow the spread of HIV in the future. The team developed figures showing that worldwide spending needed to increase to $3.2 billion in 2002 and continue to increase in the years thereafter, reaching a peak of $9.2 billion in 2005. The $9.2 billion in 2005 would be apportioned as $4.8 billion for prevention programs and $4.4 billion for treatment of infected patients and support for their families. Included in the projection were funds to purchase 6 billion condoms per year,

TABLE 10.1 Spending (in Millions) for the Leading Antiretroviral Drugs in the United States for the Years 1999-2000	
Drug	**Cost**
Reverse transcriptase inhibitors	
Combivir (lamivudine plus zidovudine)	$478.40
Zerit (d4T;stavudine)	$315.90
Epivir (3TC;lamivudine)	$260.20
Sustiva (efavirenz)	$178.60
Viramune (nevirapine)	$108.10
Ziagen (abacavir)	$107.50
Videx (ddl;didanosine)	$78.60
Retrovir (AZT;zidovudine)	$55.00
Hivid (ddC;zalcitabine)	$9.70
Rescriptor (delavirdine)	$7.40
Retrovir IV	$0.70
Total	$1,600.10
Protease inhibitors	
Viracept (nelfinavir)	$440
Crixivan (indinavir)	$234
Norvir (ritonavir)	$101
Fortovase (saquinavir soft capsules)	$80
Invirase (saquinavir hard capsules)	$30
Total	$933

SOURCE: Chemical Market Reporter, April 17, 2000.

screen 35 million pregnant women for HIV, treat 900,000 pregnant women to prevent HIV passage to their newborns, distribute sterile needles and syringes to 3 million injection drug users, and conduct education programs for 6 million prostitutes (sex workers).

AIDS and Medical Professionals

Many Americans were shocked during the 1980s when several surgeons announced that they would no longer perform complex operations on patients who tested positive for HIV infection or had AIDS. In a day when vaccines and antibiotics control the transmission of nearly all the infectious diseases, doctors had come to assume that both they and their patients were fully protected—that is, until the advent of the AIDS epidemic.

AIDS taxes to the limit the compassion and selflessness that should distinguish the health profession from other callings. It has imposed on the healing arts a number of other stresses that weigh heavily on the day-to-day practice of giving health care. Though the vast majority of health professionals have acted responsibly, it appears that some physicians and nurses have not shown the courage that society has come to anticipate from them.

Caring for an AIDS patient can be a stressful experience for many reasons. The AIDS patient is often young and desperate and may be about the same age as the health care provider. Such a patient, in contrast to an elderly patient, would not normally be expected to die soon, and it may be difficult to discuss diagnoses and prognoses with the patient. In the cases of homosexual men, there is usually no legal spouse, and the patient may wish a lover or friend to make responsible decisions in case of his incapacitation. Legal empowerment may also be a problem, and parents may insist on considerable input. Moreover, the health care professional may face the ethical dilemma of when to use or withhold life-sustaining treatment, especially in view of the patient's relative youth.

Having to observe universal precautions is another burden imposed by the AIDS epidemic (Figure 10.8). There are restrictions to observe (e.g., how to dispose of needles), barrier devices to be used (e.g., gloves, masks, goggles), and procedures for handling body fluids and tissues (e.g., blood). Added to these are the exaggerated fears arising from occupational exposures to infected tissues. Such fears are ill-founded because the overwhelming evidence indicates that health professionals have an extremely small chance of contracting HIV during their normal duties. Through June 2001, for instance, only 57 cases of HIV infection arising from occupational transmission had been documented in the United States (of over 750,000 AIDS cases to that date).

There is also the ethical question of whether doctors and dentists who have HIV infection should inform their patients of their health condition. In 1991, both the American Medical Association (AMA) and the American Dental Association (ADA) suggested that their infected members should inform patients of their situation or cease practicing. The recommendations, which are nonbinding but influential, followed the revelation by the CDC that a Florida dentist had

The exposure to potentially infected blood places extraordinary stress on surgeons and other medical professionals. The need to observe universal precautions adds to that stress.

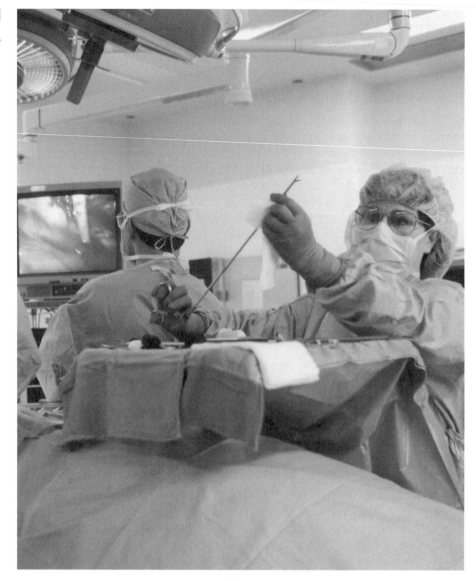

apparently transferred HIV to several patients during dental procedures. HIV-positive dentists were cautioned to avoid performing invasive techniques such as tooth removal, teeth cleaning, or orthodontia. It should be noted, however, that compliance with the recommendations was voluntary and that not all state health organizations agreed with the AMA and the ADA.

Practicing in a rural area can also pose an ethical dilemma for medical professionals. It may be uneconomical, for instance, for a local hospital to obtain the sophisticated machinery to test the T-lymphocyte counts of AIDS patients. A machine for doing such counts costs up to $100,000, and a rural physician may be denied the diagnostic information available to urban counterparts. For rural patients, it may be difficult to obtain transportation to health care facilities; support groups may be few and far between; educational programs may be lacking; and confidentiality may be problematic since everyone in a small town is well-known.

Caring for the AIDS Patient

The AIDS patient requires special sensitivity from caregivers because of the unique aspects of the disease associated with its transmissibility and prevalance in certain groups in the population. Typically, an AIDS patient will experience multiple hospitalizations for the treatment of opportunistic diseases. In between hospitalizations, however, the AIDS patient may be cared for at home.

On these bases, two broad aspects of care emerge. In the hospital setting, medical care for the AIDS patient will depend on the type and severity of the opportunistic disease present. Another type of care, emotional care, can be equally important, because a potentially fatal disease has been contracted, often in the patient's prime of life (Figure 10.9). Moreover, the patient may be aware that transmission could have occurred to a loved one. And there is the possibility that the patient may feel stigmatized because he or she practices a homosexual lifestyle or is a drug addict. Added to these is the possibility that the patient may

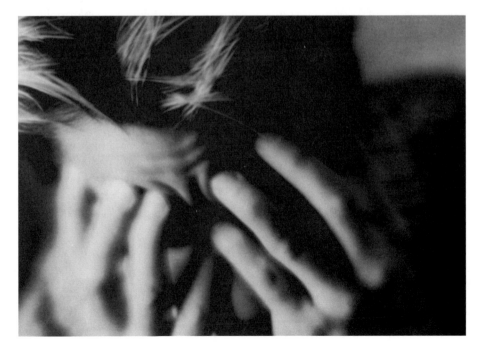

FIGURE 10.9
For AIDS patients, emotional care may be as important as medical care. The patient is often in the prime of life, and the disease is potentially fatal. Caregivers must therefore be prepared to deal with mental trauma as well as physical trauma.

need to be isolated because of the presence of a potentially transmissible opportunistic disease, such as tuberculosis. In such a case, other patients in the hospital, especially those with compromised immune systems, may be susceptible to the opportunistic disease. If the patient does not understand the need for isolation, the feelings of being an outcast will exacerbate the emotional turmoil.

It is therefore important that the medical professional provide social and environmental stimulation to supplement medical care. Frequent office visits, for example, will assure the patient that health care providers have not withdrawn from fear and will increase the patient's self-esteem. Talking as well as touching can communicate acceptance and personal concern. If a patient is ambulatory, a conscious effort should be made to encourage use of common patient areas. During times of confinement, an abundance of reading material and easy access to radio and television will increase contact with the outside world and help alleviate the feeling of isolation. Visits from professional counselors and spiritual advisers help support the patient's emotional needs as well.

For the AIDS patient, there are minute-by-minute vacillations of mood and disposition. On any given day, emotions may include guilt, anger, self-pity, sorrow, determination, hope, and faith. Meditation, prayer, or other spiritual constructs can help keep the patient more centered and help reduce stress. Some patients keep themselves busy by participating in AIDS-related service projects, such as visiting schools to talk with young people about HIV infection. One patient calls it her way of "hanging onto life."

Education and Terminology

The medical professional must also assume the role of educator. Not only does the patient need authoritative information but the patient's family and friends must know exactly what is taking place to be able to cope. It is surprising how ignorant people can be of a situation until it "hits home." In this respect, AIDS is like any other disease. Fear can quickly add to the stress of the situation, and the health care provider should be ready to correct misinformation while providing useful insights within the limits of what is known.

Sometimes, terminology can make an important difference. For example, it is well to remember that persons with AIDS are "AIDS patients" rather than "AIDS victims." No crime has been committed, so the term "victim" should be avoided. Furthermore, there are no "innocent victims" of AIDS, because this term would imply that there are "guilty," and there are none. Neither is there any "blame" to be assessed, because there was no intention to harm. There are only sick men, women, and children, all of whom need help.

Home Care

In the home setting, the AIDS patient needs compassionate care between episodes of opportunistic disease, during times of illness not appropriate for hospital treatment, and in the terminal stages of the disease if the patient desires to remain at home. Under these circumstances, the health care provider can help the AIDS patient avoid exposure to opportunistic diseases, maintain a program of exercise and nutrition, and alleviate the concerns of family and friends. In addition, the caregiver can provide emotional support and assist the patient in the final days.

In day-to-day activities, the AIDS patient needs to follow good hygienic practices to preclude exposure to opportunistic microorganisms. Frequent hand-washing with antimicrobial soap is an example of such a hygienic practice. Avoiding certain animal pets, staying away from crowds, following disinfection practices when house-cleaning, and cooking foods thoroughly are other examples of healthful practices (although different circumstances apply to each). Consulting with a nutritionist to devise a high-quality diet to maintain good health is well advised. Avoiding ill persons is also recommended, because the AIDS patient has a compromised immune system.

The issue of sexual activity raises practical, social, and ethical dilemmas that can best be solved through love and understanding. Though sexual intercourse can transmit HIV, barrier protections such as condoms can substantially reduce the risk of infection and should be given serious consideration.

The emotional stresses in home care can increase when household members harbor fears about the risks of caring for the AIDS patient. Professional assistance by trained counselors and support groups can help those affected express and alleviate their fears. It is comforting to know, for example, that virtually no cases of HIV infection or AIDS have occurred in persons who gave home care to an AIDS patient and did not engage in risky behaviors. Once again, complete authoritative information is essential to understanding.

Providing good-quality care and comfort to the AIDS patient at home demands nothing more than love and common sense. The patient may need to be bathed, helped with walking or eating, or have dressings changed. Visiting nurses and healthcare professionals can guide caregivers who are unsure of themselves. Perhaps the patient will appreciate transportation to a support group of peers or desire to have a prescription filled or simply enjoy having someone to talk to. Filling these needs can be as valuable as injecting an antibiotic.

When the end is near, the AIDS patient will appreciate help putting things in order. An attentive ear will help the patient talk out whether medical intervention is desired during the final hours and, if so, how much. The physician should be involved in these discussions so that no uncertainty lingers. Patients will also be thankful for help in completing final tasks and specifying funeral rites. Perhaps the greatest kindness that one can perform is helping to bring a friend's life to a dignified end.

The Future of AIDS

In the June 25, 1990 issue of *Newsweek* magazine, a reporter wrote the following: "A sense of crisis is hard to sustain. It thrives on earthquakes and tornadoes, plane crashes and terrorist bombings. But forces that kill people one at a time have a way of fading into the psychic landscape."

So it has been with AIDS. While the 1980s witnessed screaming headlines about the crisis wrought by HIV, the new century appears to be a time in which news about the AIDS epidemic is usually buried somewhere in the middle of the newspaper or discussed on the late news just prior to the sports and weather. Even the familiar red ribbons, worn to express concern about AIDS, have become scarcer. The fickle beacon of prime-time publicity that highlights certain causes seems ready to move on.

But the sad fact is that the AIDS epidemic is far from over (Figure 10.10). Indeed, in the minds of many public health officials, the new century will be more difficult than the previous one. For example, 6 to 8 million people worldwide were believed to be infected by HIV in 1990, but that number is now 36 million. Moreover, an estimated 700,000 persons worldwide had died of AIDS by 1990; by December 2001, the UNAID estimate was 24.8 million or more. And just as interest in AIDS wanes, the disease is making a bold new move in the United States as it tightens its grip on the poor and minorities (especially among injection drug users), while leaving middle-class heterosexuals relatively unscathed. In the United States, AIDS has become the primary cause of death in women between 25 and 44 years of age.

The Complexity of AIDS

AIDS was easily the most complex disease of the twentieth century. Ironically, the century opened with a strikingly similar disease, tuberculosis. In the early 1900s, tuberculosis was responsible for one death in seven from all causes. The disease primarily affected young adults, and it often incubated in the patient long before symptoms manifested themselves. Tuberculosis seemed to be "someone else's disease," because it occurred in underprivileged classes and people from lower socioeconomic groups. But it occasionally affected the better-known; it claimed the lives of the composer Chopin and the poet Keats. In recent decades, drug therapy has brought tuberculosis under a measure of control. In many cases, the tubercle bacilli remain in the body, but their multiplication is retarded by the drug and the severest effects of the disease are not experienced.

Though fading from media headlines, the AIDS epidemic is far from over. For example, over 40 million people worldwide were believed to be infected by the human immunodeficiency virus as of 2002.

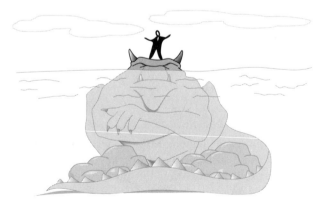

AIDS in Perspective

Many epidemiologists foresee a similar pattern for HIV infection and AIDS. Rather than remaining an acute disease with clear symptoms of illness, AIDS is undergoing an evolution to a chronic disease, that is, a disease persisting over a long period of time with few symptoms and no crisis period. According to this model, HIV would remain in the body, kept under control by drugs, and the infected person could look forward to a reasonably normal life. Diabetes is another chronic disease in today's society. How people live with tuberculosis and diabetes is how they may one day live with AIDS.

Before AIDS joins the ranks of chronic diseases, however, we can expect many more bits of knowledge that add to our understanding of the disease. For example, Kaposi's sarcoma is now thought to be a disease linked to AIDS only by coincidence. A separate virus, a herpesvirus, may be the cause. We can also expect new insights into the wasting syndrome that often characterizes AIDS, and we may possibly see a connection between the wasting and a specific parasitic infection influenced by a deteriorating immune system. Researchers will also continue to unlock the secrets of the immune system and may discover chemical substances that retard HIV replication.

Other advances in HIV and AIDS research concern the modalities used in treatment. One need only look to 1996 and the emergence of HAART treatment regimen for an example (Chapter 8). The multidrug therapies, despite their drawbacks, slowed the growth of the U.S. AIDS epidemic as the death rate in patients declined sharply. Development of the protease inhibitors exemplified the potency of molecular medicine: Beginning some years earlier, researchers deciphered the structure of protease, analyzed the dynamics of its action, and developed drugs targeted against it. The successful use of rational treatments bodes well for the future of investigator-driven basic science and the ability of applied and pure scientists to work in harmony. Of course, many challenges remain, including how to simplify regimens, how to reduce costs, how to cope with drug resistance, and how to target other weak points of HIV.

The development and use of new drugs reinforces the need for early diagnosis because early intervention is essential for precluding the development to AIDS. It is clear that the window of opportunity for controlling HIV infection is a relatively narrow one and that therapy should begin early after exposure. New and improved diagnostic tests focusing on HIV antigens can also be expected (Chapter 7). These tests will expand the window of opportunity by making an earlier diagnosis of HIV infection possible.

We can also look ahead to vigorous new efforts to develop an AIDS vaccine (Chapter 9). The commitment of significantly increased resources has raised hopes of developing a vaccine before the first decade of the twenty-first century ends. Unfortunately, it now appears that a vaccine having modest efficacy will be the goal, considering the many setbacks already encountered. Nevertheless, having a less than perfect vaccine may be preferred to having no vaccine; it can serve as a jumping-off point for research on an improved preparation. Scientists can then continue to seek answers to the nagging problems of eliciting a completely protective immune response while addressing the difficult issues surrounding testing of candidate vaccines and trying to understand the body's unusual reaction to HIV.

1 **Q** Will AIDS be as serious a health problem in ten years as it is today?

A Unfortunately, AIDS will continue to be a serious health problem until well into the twenty-first century. For example, the World Health Organization estimated in 2002 that over 35 million people are infected by HIV and 5 million more people became infected with AIDS. Concern about transmission of HIV, especially to health care workers, will continue to be acute, and universal precautions will continue to be recommended. AIDS education campaigns will also be expanded, especially among injection drug users.

2 **Q** Will AIDS still be a life threatening-illness in ten years?

A In ten years, HIV infection and AIDS may be diseases that can be managed. By using drugs and other therapies, it may be possible to control these diseases, much as diabetes can be controlled today. The patient with HIV infection or AIDS may then be able to lead a fairly normal life as long as the medical recommendations are followed. AIDS may become a chronic disease rather than the acute disease we have known it as.

3 **Q** What will future treatments for HIV infection and AIDS consist of?

A It is very possible that in the future patients with AIDS will be treated with a variety of regimens. For example, drug therapy may be supplemented with immune-enhancing therapy to restore immune system functions; gene therapy may be available as well. A patient may also receive behavioral therapy to prevent further transmission of HIV and psychological therapy to help him or her cope with the infection and better understand it so that he or she can more actively participate in the healing process.

Furthermore, the future holds new treatment modalities that focus on varying aspects of the patient and the disease. For cancer therapy, it is not unusual for a person to undergo radiation treatment, chemotherapy, and even surgery. For HIV infection and AIDS, a patient may undergo chemotherapy for controlling HIV, immune-enhancing treatments to restore the immune system, behavioral therapy to alter high-risk behavior patterns, and psychological therapy to restore the "thinking well" pattern.

But accompanying these advances are a number of lingering questions. For example, how do HIV proviruses integrate into human DNA, and once there, how do they force the host cells to follow their commands? Why are there apparently no individuals who are naturally immune to HIV? Why do infection rates vary so substantially from country to country? Why is HIV-1 so much more dangerous than HIV-2? What roles do sexually transmitted diseases play in AIDS development? What are the precise functions of HIV's genes? Which is the ideal drug therapy, and when is the most effective time to use it? And will we ever have an AIDS vaccine? The daunting tasks of finding answers to these questions will require the best minds and huge investments.

The Lessons of AIDS

We will not really know what the AIDS epidemic is like until current events become history (Healthline 10.3). Our descendants will someday pass judgment on where our society stood tall and where it erred. But we need not wait that long to understand some of the lessons the AIDS epidemic has taught us. It has revealed, for instance, that scientists do not have an answer for everything, nor are they as all-knowing as we sometimes perceive them to be. Perhaps it is well to remember that scientists seeking research funding are somewhat like a set of wheels in which the squeaky wheel gets the oil of public support. Retrovirologists did not begin "squeaking" until the early 1980s, and so there were no quick fixes for HIV when it arrived in our midst.

But that observation leads to another lesson because we have seen how scientists can gear up for action when a crisis presents itself. Once it was clear that an epidemic of infectious disease was sweeping across the world, scientists moved quickly to identify the responsible virus, develop a diagnostic test, and make available a set of useful therapies. Though some may argue that the pace of discovery was painfully slow, others will note that it was relatively rapid. For comparison's sake, they will point to the bacteria. These microbes were identified as causes of disease in the 1880s, but antibiotics did not become available until the 1940s, some 60 years later. By contrast, the human immunodeficiency virus was identified in 1984, and AZT was already in use by 1987, only 3 years afterward.

The AIDS epidemic has also demonstrated that humans can act with compassion, intelligence, and selflessness to overcome the fear that accompanies the influx of a new disease. How dangerous and insidious this fear can be is illustrated by the following story adapted from an ancient legend:

> One day on a road in the English countryside, a clergyman happened to meet Plague. "Where are you bound?" asked the clergyman. "To London," responded Plague, "to kill a thousand." They chatted for a few moments, then went their separate ways. Some weeks later, the two chanced to meet again on the same road. As they conversed, the clergyman inquired, "I may have misunderstood, but I recall you were going to kill a thousand. How is it that two thousand died?" "Ah yes," replied Plague. "I killed only a thousand. Fear killed the rest."

In the early and mid-1980s, a climate of fear marked the emerging AIDS epidemic. There was fear of the virus, fear of the disease, fear of the AIDS patient, and a general fear of the unknown. Mean-spirited and irrational responses often could be traced to these fears. The late 1980s and the 1990s, by contrast, were a time of understanding and compassion, of knowledge and coping, of wisdom and generosity. Leaders have come forward to wage the fight against HIV; adequate financial resources have been made available by government and industry; legal protection has been extended where necessary; and accurate, timely surveillance has been implemented to track the epidemic and project its future course. And fear has waned.

Probably the primary reason for the passing of fear has been education (Figure 10.11). Educational campaigns launched in the 1980s have generally been well funded and well managed, and they have usually reached the populations at which they were directed. The concern in future years is that AIDS will primarily affect groups removed from education (such as injection drug users). In general, however, education has done much to set society on a course where it can effectively deal with the AIDS epidemic. In 1920, in *The Outline of History*, the noted author H. G. Wells wrote: "Human history becomes more and more a race between education and catastrophe." Indeed, education prompted a certain author to write this book.

LOOKING BACK

The epidemic of HIV infection and AIDS has affected contemporary society profoundly, touching everyone in the world in some way. It has compelled individuals to make new judgments or has reinforced old outlooks on many practices, while stimulating many debates and bringing the positive side of the human spirit to the fore.

FIGURE 10.11

Educational campaigns will continue to be the greatest deterrent to the spread of HIV. Here a young student participates in an AIDS lesson in an elementary school.

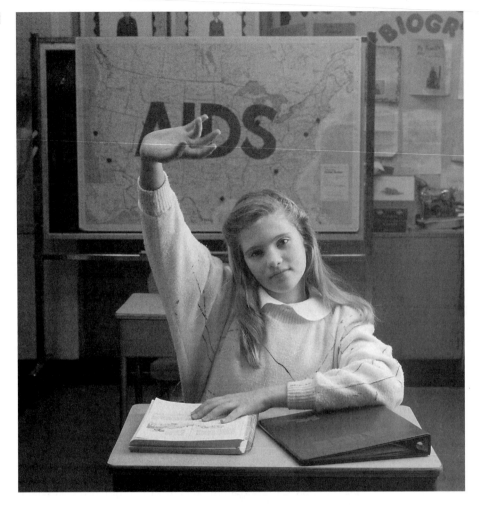

In the workplace, the AIDS epidemic can be managed successfully if a policy is developed and promulgated by employers. The policy could be AIDS-specific or more general in scope, each type having advantages. Workers appreciate knowing the position an organization takes. According to federal and state laws, HIV infection and AIDS are treated as handicaps, and the rights of handicapped workers are set forth, including the employer is responsibility to provide reasonable accommodations. Discrimination and confidentiality are legal issues arising from the AIDS epidemic, as are issues that involve hospital and home care.

The economic burdens of HIV infection and AIDS are substantial, in both direct and indirect forms. In the United States, federal expenditures for AIDS care and research now exceed $2.5 billion annually, and the costs of dealing with pediatric AIDS cases are particularly high because of the large number of children orphaned by the epidemic. On a worldwide basis, the AIDS epidemic is exacting a heavy toll in African nations, where an estimated 28.5 million people are infected with HIV.

The AIDS epidemic presents ethical dilemmas for medical professionals who do not wish to expose themselves to HIV-contaminated tissues. Moreover, there are special concerns in caring for AIDS patients, such as patients' legal empowerment and, in many cases, their relative youth.

The AIDS epidemic is expected to expand during the twenty-first century, but in the United States and certain other parts of the world, HIV infection and AIDS are increasingly coming under control and are being viewed as chronic rather than acute diseases. In the future, the disease could be managed much as tuberculosis and diabetes are managed today. As the years pass, more knowledge will come to the fore about AIDS, new treatments will be devised, and a vaccine will become available. Education will continue to be the chief factor in allaying fear of HIV infection and AIDS.

REVIEW

Having finished this chapter, you should feel confident in discussing some of the implications of the AIDS epidemic in society. To test your knowledge, place a T to the left of the statement if it is true or an F if it is false. Appendix A contains the correct answers.

__F__   **1.** It is generally advantageous for a business to have an unstated policy regarding AIDS.

__T__   **2.** According to decisions by the U.S. Supreme Court, a person suffering from AIDS is considered to be handicapped.

__F__   **3.** The guidelines issued by the CDC are rarely utilized by laboratory or hospital facilities in the development of safety policies.

__F__   **4.** The 2001 federal expenditure for AIDS research and care of patients was less than $10,000 per year, and it is becoming less each year.

__T__   **5.** Federal law requires that employers make reasonable accommodations for AIDS patients, including time off for doctor's appointments and rest periods during the workday.

__T__   **6.** Observing universal precautions is one of the multiple burdens imposed on members of the health care system by the AIDS epidemic.

__F__   **7.** An AIDS-specific policy developed by businesses for use in the workplace projects the idea that AIDS is no different from other major illnesses such as cancer or heart disease.

_F_   **8.** In future years, it is very likely that all persons infected with HIV will develop AIDS and can expect to die.

_F_   **9.** HIV infection and AIDS are generally not a problem in the workplace because most people affected are not in their economically productive years.

_F_   **10.** By 1996, the AIDS epidemic was virtually over.

_T_   **11.** One of the ethical dilemmas that medical professionals must consider is whether to perform surgery on a patient whose HIV status is uncertain.

_F_   **12.** The knowledge generated from AIDS research has no application in any other field of medicine.

_T_   **13.** It is illegal to inform others of a patient's HIV status without the patient's consent.

_T_   **14.** The development of new drugs for treating HIV infection and AIDS will require that diagnosis be performed as soon as possible because early intervention can preclude disease development.

_T_   **15.** One of the lessons of the AIDS epidemic is that scientists do not have a ready answer for every medical problem that may face society.

FOR ADDITIONAL READING

Aggleton, P., and H. Homans, eds. 1988. *Social Aspects of AIDS*. New York: Falmer Press.

Bateson, M. C., and R. Goldsby. 1988. *Thinking AIDS*. Reading, MA: Addison-Wesley.

Beardsley, T. 1998. "Coping with HIV's ethical dilemma." *Scientific American,* July.

Binswanger, H. P. 2001. "HIV/AIDS treatment for millions." *Science* 292: 221–223.

Cowley, G. 1993. "The future of AIDS." *Newsweek,* March 22.

Ezzell, C. 2000. "AIDS drugs for Africa." *Scientific American*, November.

Finkbeiner, A. K. 1994. "Into the valley of death." *The Sciences*, March/April.

France, D. 2001. "The HIV disbeliever." *Newsweek*, August 28.

Griffith, J. L. 1989. "How to protect your lab on legal issues." *Medical Laboratory Observer*, February.

Kramer, L. C. 1990. "Legal and ethical issues affect conduct toward AIDS sufferers." *Occupational Health and Safety,* January.

Paul, W. E. 1995. "Reexamining AIDS research priorities." *Science* 267: 633–637.

Puckett, S. B., and A. R. Emery. 1988. *Managing AIDS in the Workplace.* Reading, MA: Addison-Wesley.

Schwartlander, B., et al. 2001. "Resource needs for HIV/AIDS," *Science* 292: 2423–2436.

Sesser, S. 1994. "Hidden death." *The New Yorker,* November 19.

Answers to Review Questions

Chapter 1

1. F (1981); 2. F (Kaposi's sarcoma); 3. T; 4. F (blood);
5. T (but not exclusively); 6. F (Luc Montagnier); 7. T;
8. F (decreased); 9. F (pandemic); 10. F (100,000); 11. T;
12. F (monkeys); 13. F (milder); 14. T; 15. F (Africa)

Chapter 2

1. e; 2. e; 3. b; 4. a; 5. c; 6. d; 7. a; 8. d; 9. b; 10. e;
11. d; 12. c; 13. a; 14. c; 15. a.

Chapter 3

1. K; 2. J; 3. N; 4. O; 5. O; 6. H; 7. L; 8. M; 9. D;
10. P; 11. Q; 12. B; 13. C; 14. M; 15. G; 16. H; 17. A;
18. O; 19. E; 20. H; 21. C; 22. I; 23. C; 24. F; 25. N.

Chapter 4

1. AIDS-dementia complex; 2. Walter Reed; 3. Kaposi's
sarcoma; 4. cytomegalovirus; 5. *Pneumocystis carinii;*
6. 10 years; 7. HIV infection; 8. lymphadenopathy;
9. 6000; 10. 800; 11. *Candida albicans;* 12. gastrointestinal system; 13. HIV wasting syndrome; 14. pentamidine
isethionate; 15. cats.

Chapter 5

1. b; 2. c; 3. c; 4. a; 5. d; 6. d; 7. a; 8. d; 9. a; 10. b;
11. a; 12. c; 13. a; 14. a; 15. b.

Chapter 6

1. F; 2. T; 3. T; 4. F; 5. T; 6. F; 7. T; 8. F; 9. T; 10. T;
11. F; 12. F; 13. F; 14. T; 15. T.

Chapter 7

1. ELISA; 2. false negative; 3. electrophoresis;
4. T-lymphocytes; 5. viral load; 6. serological; 7. western
blot analysis; 8. false positive; 9. antigens; 10. polymerase
chain reaction; 11. Food and Drug Administration;
12. radioimmunoprecipitation assay; 13. serum;
14. mother; 15. gene probe; 16. 6 to 10 weeks;
17 .99 percent; 18. primer DNA; 19. ELISA; 20. military.

Chapter 8

1. L; 2. D; 3. F; 4. K; 5. C; 6. H; 7. D; 8. G; 9. F;
10. O; 11. M; 12. D; 13. B; 14. A; 15. O; 16. E; 17. F;
18. I; 19. G; 20. J; 21. N; 22. A; 23. E; 24. P; 25. G.

Chapter 9

1. c; 2. b; 3. a; 4. d; 5. a; 6. a; 7. d; 8. a; 9. a; 10. a;
11. b; 12. a; 13. d; 14. b; 15. b.

Chapter 10

1. F; 2. T; 3. F; 4. F; 5. T; 6. T; 7. F; 8. F; 9. F; 10. F;
11. T; 12. F; 13. T; 14. T; 15. T.

A Suggested Format for a 10-Session Course: The Biological Basis of AIDS

A ten-session program highlighting the biological basis of AIDS can be developed using this book as a text. The ten sessions may be offered over a period of ten weeks or at briefer intervals. Each session could encompass 60 to 90 minutes of instruction and discussion, and sessions could be supplemented by myriad videos, brochures, pamphlets, and other educational materials available from numerous sources. A suggested format for such a course follows.

Session Number	Subject Matter	Chapter Number
1	Introduction to HIV infection and AIDS, including overview of the epidemic's development and current statistics	1
2	Structure and replication of HIV relative to other viruses; significance of key functional components of HIV; introduction to control and prevention of viral disease and viruses	2
3	Development and operation of the human immune system; mechanisms of HIV interference with the immune function; implications of HIV interference	3
4	Pathology of HIV infection and AIDS; signs and symptoms; stages of disease and descriptions of opportunistic diseases; pediatric AIDS	4
5	Epidemiology and transmission of HIV by various modes; high-risk behaviors and groups affected; how AIDS is not transmitted and why	5

(continued)

Session Number	Subject Matter	Chapter Number
6	Methods for avoiding exposure to HIV, including methods for personal protection, protection of health care workers, and protection of public safety workers; AIDS education in schools	6
7	Diagnosis of HIV infection and AIDS; indirect antibody tests and direct antigen tests; implications of HIV testing	7
8	Treatments for HIV infection and AIDS; modes of activity of treatments, including therapeutic methods for opportunistic diseases; drug development and testing	8
9	Prospects for an AIDS vaccine; different strategies for vaccine development and testing; problems in vaccine development	9
10	AIDS in broad perspective; the social, legal, economic, and accessory implications of the AIDS epidemic; AIDS in the future	10

Pronunciation Guide

Chapter 1

amyl   a'mil
cytomegalovirus   si'to-meg"ah-lo-vi'rus
dengue   den'ge
Kaposi's sarcoma   kap'o-seez sar-ko'mah
lymphadenopathy   lim-fad"e-nop'ah-thee
mitogen   mi'to-jen
Montagnier   mon-tan-ya'
Pneumocystis carinii   nu"mo-sis' tis car-in'e-e
pneumocystosis   nu"mo-sis-to'sis

Chapter 2

acyclovir   a-si'klo-veer
attenuated   ah-ten'u-a-ted
azidothymidine   az'i-do-thi'mid-een
deoxyribonucleic   de-ox"e-ri"bo-nu-kla'ik
encephalopathy   en-sef"ah-lop'ah-thee
genome   je'nome
glycoprotein   gli"ko-pro'teen
ischohedron   i-ko"sah-heed'ron
polymerase   pol-im'er-ase
protease   pro'te-ase
syncytium   sin-sish'e-um

Chapter 3

apoptosis   a-pop'to-sis
Candida albicans   kan'dee-dah al'bi-kanz
Cryptococcus neoformans   krip"to-kok'us ne-o-form'anz
cytomegalovirus   si'to-meg"ah-lo-vi'rus
lymphocyte   lim'fo-site
lymphokinase   lim'fo-ki-nase
lymphopoietic   lim"fo-poi-et'ik

phagocytosis   fag"o-si-to'sis
Pneumocystis carinii   nu"mo-sis' tis car-in'e-e
syncytium   sin-sish'e-um
Toxoplasma gondii   toks"o-plaz'mah gon'de-e

Chapter 4

Candida albicans   kan'dee-dah al'bi-kanz
candidiasis   kan"de-di'ah-sis
Cryptococcus neoformans   krip"to-kok'us ne-o-form'anz
cryptosporidiosis   krip"to-spor-id'e-o'sis
Cryptosporidium coccidii   krip"to-spor-id'e-um
   kok-sid'e-e
cryptococcosis   krip"to-kok-o'sis
cytomegalovirus   si'to-meg"ah-lo-vi'rus
dementia   de-men'she-ah
encephalopathy   en-sef"ah-lop'ah-thee
Histoplasma capsulatum   his"to-plaz'mah cap-su-lat'um
Isospora belli   i-sos'po-rah bel'li
Kaposi's sarcoma   kap'o-seez sar-ko'mah
lymphadenopathy   lim-fad"e-nop'ah-thee
Mycobacterium avium-intracellulare
   mi"ko-bak-te're-um ave'e-um in"tra-sel-u-lar'e
opportunistic   op"or-tu-nis'tik
pentamidine isethionate   pen-tam'i-deen i-se-thi'o-nate
Pneumocystis carinii   nu"mo-sis' tis car-in'e-e
Toxoplasma gondii   toks"o-plaz'mah gon'de-e
toxoplasmosis   toks"o-plaz-mo'sis

Chapter 5

chancroid   shank'roid
chlamydia   klah-mid'e-ah
clitoris   klit'o-ris

columnar   co-lum′nar
Cryptosporidium   krip″to-spor-id′e-um
cytomegalovirus   si′to-meg″ah-lo-vi′rus
epidemiologist   ep′i-de″me-ol′o-jist
Isospora   i-sos′po-rah
Kaposi's sarcoma   kap′o-seez sar-ko′mah
Legionella pneumophilia   lee-jen-el′ah mu-mof′I-lah
pentamidine isethionate   pen-tam′i-deen i-se-thi′o-nate
proboscis   pro-bahs′kis
urethra   yu-re′thra

Chapter 6

candidiasis   kan″de-di′ah-sis
chlamydia   klah-mid′e-ah
lymphogranuloma   lim″for-gran-yu-lo′mah
nonoxynol   no-noks′i-nol
paraphernalia   par″ah-fer-nal′e-ah
trichomoniasis   trik″o-mo-ni′ah-sis

Chapter 7

electrophoresis   e-lek″tro-for-e′sis
immunofluorescence   im″yu-no-floor-es′ens
isothiocyanate   i″so-thi″o-si′ah-nate
polymerase   pol-im′er-ase
radioimmunoprecipitation
   ra′de-o-im″yu-no-pre-sip″i-ta′shun

Chapter 8

acyclovir   a-si′klo-vir
amantadine   ah-man′tah-deen
atovaquone   a-tov′a-quon
azidothymidine   a′zi-do-thi′mi-deen
bisheteroarylpiperazine   bis-het-er-o-aryl-pip-er-a-zine
castanospermine   kas″ta-no-sper′meen
clotrimazole   clo-tri′mah-zole
Crixivan   cri-vax′in
cytomegalovirus   si′to-meg″ah-lo-vi′rus
delavirdine   del-a-vir′deen
deoxyadenosine   de-ox″e-ah-den′o-seen
deoxycytidine   de-ox″e-ci′ti-deen
deoxyguanosine   de-ox″e-gwan′o-seen
deoxythymidine   de-ox″e-thi′mi-deen
didanosine   di-dan′o-seen
dinitrochlorobenzene   di-ni-tro-klor″o-ben′zeen
efavirenz   eh-fa-vir′enz

erythropoietin   e-rith″ro-poi′e-tin
foscarnet   fos-car′net
fluconizole   flu-kon′ah-zole
fullerens   ful′er-eenz
ganciclovir   gan-si′klo-vir
heteropolyanion   het″er-o-pol″e-an-i′on
hydroxynaphthoquinon   hi-drok′si-naf″tho-qwin-on
hypericin   hy″per-i′cin
Indinavir   in-din′a-vir
interferon   in″ter-fer′on
Invirase   in′vir-ase
isoniazid   i″so-ni′ah-zid
ketoconazole   ke″to-kon′ah-zole
lamivudine   lam-iv′u-deen
leucovorin   loo″ko-vor′in
miconazole   mi-kon′ah-zole
nevirapine   ne-vir′a-peen
Norvir   nor′vir
pentamidine isethionate
   pen-tam′i-deen i-se-thi′o-nate
phosphonoformate   fos″fo-no-for′mate
placebo   plah-se′bo
Pneumocystis carinii   nu″mo-sis′ tis car-in′e-e
protease   pro′te-ase
ribavirin   ri″bah-vi′rin
rifabutin   rif-a-bu′tin
ritonavir   ri-ton′a-vir
saquinavir   sa″quin′a-vir
stavudive   sta″vyu-deen
syncytium   sin-sish′e-um
thalidomide   thal-id′o-mide
thimosins   thi′mo-sinz
thrombocytopenia   throm″bo-si′to-pe′ne-ah
trimethoprom-sulfamethoxazole
   tri-meth′o-prim sul′fah-meth-oks′ah-zol
trimetrexate   tri-meh-trex′at
zalcitabine   zal-cit′a-been
zidovudine   zi-do′vyu-deen

Chapter 9

adjuvant   ad′ju-vant
attenuated   ah-ten″yu-a′ted
azidothymidine   a′zi-do-thi′mi-deen
genome   je′nome
idyotype   id′e-o-tipe
macaque   ma-cak′
vaccinia   vak-sin′e-ah

Glossary

This glossary contains concise definitions of approximately 200 terms related to the biology of AIDS. The number in the parentheses refers to the chapter in which the term is discussed most completely.

acquired immune deficiency syndrome (AIDS) as defined by the CDC, a disabling or life-threatening illness caused by the human immunodeficiency virus (HIV) and characterized by HIV encephalopathy, HIV wasting syndrome, or certain diseases due to immunodeficiency in a person with laboratory evidence for HIV infection or without certain other causes of immunodeficiency (4).

acyclovir an antiviral drug commonly used to treat herpes simplex infection (8).

adjuvant a substance such as aluminum sulfate that is chemically bound to subunits in a vaccine to make the subunits more attractive to phagocytes and thereby enhance the immune process (9).

AIDS-dementia complex a severe brain infection caused by HIV and accompanied by mental and physical deterioration (4).

AIDS-related complex a pre-AIDS condition in which the patient experiences lymphadenopathy, constant fever, fatigue and night sweats, extensive diarrhea, and other severe symptoms that accompany the destruction of T-lymphocytes (4).

AL 721 an anti-HIV drug composed of several lipids and currently under study (8).

alpha interferon a form of interferon produced by genetic engineering and used against Kaposi's sarcoma (8).

amphotericin B an antifungal drug used to treat serious fungal diseases such as cryptococcosis (8).

ampligen a drug consisting of double-stranded RNA that may stimulate immune system activity to destroy HIV (8).

anal intercourse sexual activity in which the penis of the insertive partner is placed into the rectum of the receptive partner (5).

antibodies proteins derived from B-lymphocytes and plasma cells that combine chemically with antigens and microorganisms containing antigens to effect neutralization; antibodies are an essential feature of specific resistance against infectious disease (3).

antibody-mediated immunity immunity in which antibodies provide the actual mode of defense, in comparison with cell-mediated immunity in which cells function as defenders (3).

antigen a substance, usually a large protein or polysaccharide, that stimulates the activity of the immune system; antigens are interpreted as nonself in the immune process (3).

antisense molecule an anti-HIV synthetic RNA molecule used as a drug; the molecule unites with and neutralizes the messenger RNA molecule coded by proviral DNA following entry of HIV into the host cell (8).

antiseptic a chemical used to kill pathogenic microorganisms on a living object, such as the surface of the human body (6).

apoptosis the natural mechanism by which a cell dies at the end of its life cycle (3).

attenuated viruses viruses able to multiply in the body but at a rate so low that disease is not established; used in first-generation vaccines (9).

autoclave a laboratory instrument used to sterilize instruments or materials by means of pressurized steam (6).

azidothymidine (AZT) an anti-HIV compound closely related to deoxythymidine that interferes with the production of proviral DNA by taking the place of deoxythymidine in the nucleic acid and bringing chain elongation to an end; also known as zidovudine and Retrovir (8).

bacteriophage a type of virus that attacks and replicates within bacteria (2).

B-lymphocyte an essential cell of the immune system that dominates antibody-mediated immunity; when stimulated by lymphokines, B-lymphocytes convert to antibody-producing plasma cells (3).

budding the process by which HIV passes through the membrane of a host cell at the completion of the replication process; while passing through, the HIV nucleocapsid takes on a portion of the cell membrane as an envelope (2).

bursa of Fabricius the lymphoid organ of the gastrointestinal tract of the embryonic chick where B-lymphocytes are formed (3).

Candida albicans a yeastlike fungus that lives benignly in many individuals but causes thrush and esophageal infection in AIDS patients (4).

candidiasis an opportunistic disease in AIDS patients in which *Candida albicans* multiplies in the oral cavity and esophagus causing tissue erosion, inflammation, and difficulty in swallowing and eating; also known as thrush (4).

capsid the layer of protein that surrounds the nucleic core of a virus such as HIV (2).

capsomeres the protein subunits of the capsid of a virus (2).

castanospermine an anti-HIV drug that apparently prevents syncytium formation by infected host cells (8).

CD4 a protein molecule on the surface of a T-lymphocyte or brain cell that serves as the attachment point for HIV; each CD4 molecule contains 433 amino acids (2).

cell-mediated immunity immunity in which cells provide the actual mode of defense, in comparison with antibody-mediated immunity, in which antibodies function as defenders (3).

Centers for Disease Control and Prevention (CDC) a major agency of the United States Public Health Service charged with protecting the health of the U.S. populace by providing leadership and direction in the prevention and control of infectious disease and other preventable conditions (1).

chemokine a small hormonelike protein that is secreted by certain body cells such as phagocytic cells and that acts as a chemical messenger (2).

compound Q a substance that is isolated from the root of the Chinese cucumber and has been demonstrated to destroy HIV-infected macrophages under laboratory conditions (8).

condom a soft, stretchable sheath placed over the penis during sexual activity to form a barrier between semen and the internal tissues of the sexual partner (6).

coreceptors protein molecules involved in viral binding to cells (2).

cryptococcosis an opportunistic disease in AIDS patients in which *Cryptococcus neoformans* multiplies in the lungs and brain causing headaches, stiff neck, and paralysis (4).

Cryptococcus neoformans a fungal parasite often located in the lungs as a benign inhabitant but that causes severe lung and brain infections in AIDS patients (4).

cryptosporidiosis an opportunistic disease in AIDS patients in which *Cryptosporidium coccidi* multiplies in the intestinal tissue and causes severe diarrhea, dehydration, and emaciation (4).

Cryptosporidium coccidi a protozoal parasite that is a benign inhabitant of the intestine in many individuals but causes severe diarrhea in AIDS patients (4).

cytomegalovirus (CMV) a virus that exists benignly in many individuals but causes disease of many internal tissues in AIDS patients (4).

cytomegalovirus disease an opportunistic disease in AIDS patients in which the cytomegalovirus multiplies aggressively in lung, liver, kidney, and other tissues, causing multiple forms of disease (4).

cytotoxic T-lymphocyte a T-lymphocyte that is activated by the lymphokines of helper T-lymphocytes; once

activated, the cells enter the circulation and move to the antigen site, where they attack antigen-infected cells; the cytotoxic T-lymphocyte is a host cell for HIV (3).

dextran sulfate   an anti-HIV agent that apparently blocks viral binding to host cells and prevents syncytium formation (8).

dideoxycytidine (ddC)   an anti-HIV drug similar to AZT but containing cytosine where AZT contains thymine; the mode of action of ddC is similar to that of AZT, but the side effects are believed less severe (8).

dideoxyinosine (ddI)   an anti-HIV drug similar to AZT but containing inosine where AZT contains thymine; the mode of action of ddI is similar to that of AZT, but the side effects are believed less severe (8).

disinfectant   a chemical used to kill pathogenic microorganisms on a lifeless object such as a tabletop (6).

DNA polymerase   a portion of the reverse transcriptase molecule that synthesizes DNA, using viral RNA as a template, and also synthesizes a second DNA strand complementary to the first strand (2).

DNA vaccine   a noninfectious vaccine comprising plasmids modified to carry one or more protein-encoding genes (9).

electrophoresis   a laboratory procedure in which an electrical current is used to separate a mixture of proteins in a gel (7).

entry inhibitors   molecules that prevent HIV infection by preventing formation of cell receptor sites so that the virus particle can not enter the cell (8).

env gene   the gene that codes for HIV envelope proteins (2).

envelope   a flexible lipid-bilayer membrane that surrounds the capsid of many viruses; the envelope can contain projections called spikes (2).

enzyme-linked immunosorbent assay (ELISA)   a serological test in which enzyme-linked substances are used to test for the presence of HIV antibodies; the test is used to indirectly identify HIV (7).

epidemiologist   one who discovers that an epidemic is in progress, defines the circumstances under which it spreads, and makes recommendations on controlling the epidemic in a population (5).

epidemiology   the study of the various factors that influence the frequency and distribution of diseases in a community (5).

erythropoietin   a protein hormone produced synthetically and by kidney cells, used to promote red blood cell production in the bone marrow of AIDS patients (8).

false negative   a result of a laboratory test that suggests that HIV is not present in the body when in fact it is present (7).

false positive   a result of a laboratory test that suggests that HIV is present in the body when in fact it is not present (7).

fast-track procedure   a procedure in which a treatment investigational new drug (IND) is released for patient use during a Phase II trial (8).

first-generation vaccine   a vaccine composed of whole microorganisms or their toxins (9).

Food and Drug Administration (FDA)   an agency of the U.S. federal government that tests drugs to ensure their safety and effectiveness (8).

fusion inhibitors   a class of drugs designed to interfere with the fusion of a virus with its host cell (8).

gag gene   one of the nine HIV genes; codes for the viral capsid proteins (2).

ganciclovir   an antiviral drug commonly used to treat cytomegalovirus (CMV) infections of the eye and other organs (8).

gene probe   a single-stranded molecule of DNA that can recognize and bind to a complementary DNA segment on a large DNA molecule (7).

gene probe test   a laboratory test in which a gene probe is used to bind with proviral DNA from HIV if the proviral DNA is present; the test is used to directly identify HIV (7).

genome   an accumulation of genetically functional nucleic acids at the core of HIV and other viruses (2).

glycoprotein   any protein molecule containing one or more carbohydrate groups (2).

glycoprotein (gp) 41   a glycoprotein molecule having a molecular weight of 41 kilodaltons and found in the envelope spikes of HIV; the gp41 molecule makes the connection between HIV and host cell after the reaction between gp120 and CD4 has taken place (2).

glycoprotein (gp) 120   a glycoprotein molecule having a molecular weight of 120 kilodaltons and found in the envelope spikes of HIV; the gp120 molecule unites with the CD4 molecule of the host cell during the adsorption phase of viral replication (2).

glycoprotein (gp) 160 a forerunner of gp120 and gp41 molecules in HIV that can stimulate antibody production when used in an AIDS vaccine (9).

half-life the period of time required for half the original amount of drug in the blood to disappear (8).

helix the tightly wound coil form taken by many viruses, including the virus of rabies (2).

helper T-lymphocyte a T-lymphocyte that releases lymphokines after being activated by an antigen-bearing macrophage; lymphokines stimulate other cells of the immune system; the helper T-lymphocyte is a host cell for HIV; also called CD4 or T4 cell (3).

hemophiliac a person whose blood system lacks a certain clotting factor and, therefore, has difficulty in forming a blood clot; hemophiliacs have been exposed to HIV via infusions of clotting factors derived from human blood that was infected (5).

heterosexual a male or female who prefers a sexual partner of the opposite gender (5).

Histoplasma capsulatum a fungus that lives benignly in many individuals but causes severe lung disease in AIDS patients (4).

HIV encephalopathy a condition due to HIV and characterized by disabling cognitive and/or motor dysfunction interfering with activities of daily living or loss of behavioral developmental milestones in a child, progressing over weeks to months, in the absence of concurrent illness or condition other than HIV infection that could explain the findings (4).

HIV infection the condition wherein HIV exists as a provirus in the nucleus of its host cells and the infected person has mild nonspecific symptoms such as fatigue, mild fever, and swollen lymph nodes (4).

HIV wasting syndrome a condition due to HIV characterized by involuntary loss of more than 10 percent of baseline body weight plus either chronic diarrhea or chronic weakness and documented fever in the absence of concurrent illness or condition other than HIV infection that could explain the findings (4).

homosexual a male who prefers a sexual partner of the same gender; a female homosexual is referred to as a lesbian (5).

HPA 23 heteropolyanion 23, an anti-HIV drug that is believed to inhibit reverse transcriptase activity (8).

HTLV-III/LAV the name used for the AIDS virus before 1986 and before the name human immunodeficiency virus (HIV) was introduced; the acronym stands for human T-cell lymphotropic virus type III/lymphadenopathy-associated virus (1).

human immunodeficiency virus (HIV) the RNA-containing particle of nucleic acid and protein that is regarded as the cause of HIV infection and AIDS; the virus replicates inside host cells of the immune system and brain and brings about their destruction (2).

hypericin an antiviral drug for possible use against HIV (8).

icosahedron a geometric shape with 20 triangular faces; the form taken by many viruses, including, for a time, HIV (2).

idiotype the region of an antibody molecule that binds to an antigen molecule in an antigen-antibody reaction; currently under study for use in an AIDS vaccine (9).

immune system a complex set of cells, chemical factors, and processes in which blood cells called lymphocytes respond to and eliminate foreign agents or substances in the body's tissues (3).

inactivated viruses viruses unable to multiply in host cells because of some chemical or physical treatment; used in certain vaccines (9).

indinavir (Crixivan) an anti-HIV compound that acts as a protease inhibitor to block the final steps of HIV synthesis in the host cells (8).

indirect immunofluorescence assay (IFA) a laboratory test for HIV antibodies in which fluorescent-tagged substances unite with HIV antibodies if the latter are present on the surface of a carrier particle (7).

integrase an enzyme that incorporates proviral DNA in the DNA of the host T-lymphocyte (2, 8).

interferon an antiviral substance produced by human cells on exposure to viruses (8).

interleukin-2 a lymphokine that activates natural killer cells (8).

isoniazid a chemotherapeutic agent effective against tuberculosis (8).

Kaposi's sarcoma a cancerous condition often associated with AIDS, in which slow-growing tumors in the blood vessel linings cause red to violet patches on the skin surface that eventually become purplish-brown nodules; in AIDS patients, nodules also form in the internal organs (4).

liposomes artificial membranes composed of lipidlike substances and used as adjuvants in vaccines (9).

lymphadenopathy   swelling of the lymph nodes, adenoids, and other tissues of the immune system (4).

lymph nodes   pockets of white blood cells prevalent in the neck, armpits, groin, and other body regions; cells of the immune system inhabit the lymph nodes (3).

lymphocyte   a type of leukocyte that functions in the immune system (3).

lymphopoietic cells   forerunner cells of the immune system that can become B-lymphocytes or T-lymphocytes (3).

lysogeny   the phenomenon in which a virus remains in the cell cytoplasm as a fragment of DNA and fails to replicate in or destroy the cell (2).

lytic cycle   the process wherein a virus replicates within a host cell and destroys the host cell during the process (2).

M group (of HIV-1)   one of three major groups of HIV-1 viruses, it cause 99 percent of the world's AIDS cases (8).

macrophage   a large amoeboid cell that phagocytizes antigens and sets the immune process into motion (3).

major histocompatibility (MHC) proteins   proteins present on the surface of body cells that are unique for that particular individual and act as recognition sites during the immune process (3).

microorganism   a microscopic form of life, including bacteria, viruses, fungi, protozoa, and some multicellular parasites (4).

Morbidity and Mortality Weekly Reports (MMWR)   a weekly publication of the Centers for Disease Control that summarizes contemporary health problems in the United States and presents cumulative statistics on certain infectious diseases (1).

Mycobacterium avium-intracellulare   a small bacterial rod that causes severe lung disease in AIDS patients (4).

Mycobacterium tuberculosis   a small bacterial rod that causes tuberculosis (4).

N group (of HIV-1)   one of three major groups of HIV-1 viruses (2).

nanometer   a unit of measurement equivalent to one billionth of a meter; the unit is abbreviated as nm and is used to measure the dimensions of viruses (2).

natural killer cell   a type of T-lymphocyte that attacks tumor cells (3).

needlestick   the pricking of one's finger with a contaminated needle while performing a medical procedure (6).

nef **gene**   the "negative regulatory factor gene," which codes for a protein that enhances the movement of genetic messages in the cytoplasm of the host cell (2).

nonnucleoside analogs   a group of drugs that target and react with reverse transcriptase (8).

nonoxynol-9   a spermicidal cream used with a condom to inactivate HIV (6).

nonreactive   testing negative in a serological test (7).

nonspecific resistance   protection against all foreign organisms not just specific ones (3).

nucleoside   a molecule consisting of deoxyribose and a nitrogenous base; nucleosides are building blocks of DNA and RNA (8).

O group (of HIV-1)   one of three major groups of HIV-1 viruses (2).

opportunistic organism   an organism that may exist in the body but cause no harm because the body's natural defense keeps it under control; when the defense is compromised, the organism seizes the "opportunity" to infect (4).

pandemic   an epidemic of worldwide scope (1).

parallel-track procedure   one in which patients are enrolled in a clinical trial even though they are ineligible for controlled clinical trials of experimental drugs (8).

parasite   a type of heterotrophic organism that feeds on live organic matter such as another organism (2).

pediatric AIDS   AIDS in a baby or a young child (5).

pentamidine isethionate   a drug available in injectable and aerosolized form for use against *Pneumocystis carinii* pneumonia (8).

peptide T   a peptide consisting of eight amino acids and currently under study as an anti-HIV agent (8).

phosphonoformate   an antiviral drug active against cytomegaloviruses; also known as Foscarnet (8).

plasma cells   highly active antibody-producing cells that are derived from B-lymphocytes (3).

Pneumocystis carinii   a protozoal parasite that is a benign inhabitant of the lungs in most individuals but causes a severe pneumonia in AIDS patients (4).

Pneumocystis carinii pneumonia   an opportunistic disease in AIDS patients in which protozoa multiply furiously in the lungs, take up most of the air spaces, and severely reduce the ability of the body to exchange gases with the external environment (4).

pneumonia   a microbial disease of the bronchial tubes and lungs; may be caused by various bacteria, viruses, fungi, and protozoa (1).

pol **gene**   the gene that codes for HIV viral enzymes (2).

polymerase chain reaction (PCR)   a procedure in which a small amount of DNA is amplified by encouraging copying of the DNA using specific enzymes, a piece of primer

DNA, and a series of DNA building blocks; the gene probe test can then be utilized to identify the DNA (7).

postexposure prophylaxis preventive measures taken after exposure to a causative agent (8).

protease an enzyme that cleaves the proteins of potential HIV particles and prepares the proteins for union into the viral capsid (2, 8).

protease inhibitor a synthetic anti-HIV drug that unites with and neutralizes the enzyme protease, which is used in synthesis of the HIV capsid (8).

protein (p) 17 a protein of the HIV capsid currently under study for use in a vaccine (9).

provirus a double-stranded DNA molecule derived from the activity of reverse transcriptase and incorporated into the genetic material in the nucleus of a host cell (2).

pyrimethamine an antimicrobial drug used to treat infections by *Toxoplasma gondii* (8).

radioimmunoprecipitation assay (RIPA) a laboratory test for HIV antibodies in which radioactive-tagged HIV antigens unite with HIV antibodies if the latter are present (7).

reactive testing positive in a serological test (7).

retrovirus a virus such as HIV whose RNA is used as a template for the synthesis of DNA mediated by the enzyme reverse transcriptase (2).

rev gene "regulator of the expression of viral protein" gene, which shifts the balance from production of viral regulatory proteins to proteins that make up virus particles (2).

reverse transcriptase the enzyme of certain viruses (such as HIV) that uses RNA as a template to synthesize a complementary molecule of DNA (2).

reverse transcriptase inhibitors a chemical that prevents the action of reverse transcriptase (8).

ribonuclease a portion of the reverse transcriptase molecule that destroys the RNA after it has been used as a template for DNA synthesis (2).

ritonavir (Norvir) an anti-HIV compound that acts as a protease inhibitor to block the final steps of HIV synthesis in the host cells (8).

saquinavir (Invirase) an anti-HIV compound that acts as a protease inhibitor to block the final steps of HIV synthesis in host cells (8).

second-generation vaccine a vaccine composed of microbial subunits obtained from broken microorganisms (9).

semen the mixture of sperm cells and glandular fluids that is ejaculated from the male reproductive system during sexual activity (5).

sensitivity refers to the probability that a serological test such as ELISA will give a positive result when the serum contains the antibodies sought (7).

seroconvert to test positive in a serological test (7).

serological test any laboratory test used to detect antibodies in the serum (7).

seronegative lacks the antibodies sought in a serological test (7).

seropositive has the antibodies sought in a serological test (7).

serum the clear fluid portion of the blood that has no blood cells or clotting agents (1).

simian refers to a monkey or monkeylike animal such as a chimpanzee (1).

simian AIDS AIDS in monkeys or monkeylike animals.

slim disease an alternative expression for AIDs based on the extensive wasting syndrome that occurs; the term is commonly used in Africa (5).

soluble CD4 a synthetic drug consisting of free (soluble) CD4 molecules intended to unite with HIV in the bloodstream and prevent HIV attachment to host cells (8).

specific resistance resistance founded in the immune system and directed at neutralizing a specific microorganism or compound (3).

specificity refers to the probability that a serological test such as ELISA will give a negative result when the serum lacks the antibodies sought (7).

spikes projections of the viral envelope that assist the union of the virus with its host cell (2).

sterilization the removal of all life forms, with particular reference to bacterial spores (6).

sterilizing immunity the action of a vaccine that prevents infection (9).

subunits concentrated suspensions of viral or bacterial fragments used in a vaccine to stimulate an immune response (9).

subunit vaccine a vaccine containing parts of microorganisms such as capsid proteins or purified spike glycoproteins (9).

sulfamethoxazole a sulfur-containing drug that when combined with trimethoprim, can be used to treat *Pneumocystis carinii* pneumonia (8).

suppressor T-lymphocyte a T-lymphocyte that dampens the activity of the immune system by affecting the cytotoxic T-lymphocytes (3).

syncytium a giant, multinucleated, functionless cell mass; the infection of host cells by HIV marks the cell surface with gp120 molecules that encourage cells to bind together and form a syncytium (2, 3).

T4 cell an alternative term for helper T-lymphocyte (3).

T8 cell an alternative term for suppressor T-lymphocyte (3).

tat gene (transactivator gene) a proviral gene that appears to be involved in the activation of HIV from the latent proviral state to the state of replication (2).

therapeutic immunity the action of a vaccine that prevents disease (9).

third-generation vaccine a vaccine composed of microbial subunits obtained synthetically by genetic engineering techniques (9).

thrombocytopenia a side effect associated with AZT use in which an allergic reaction to the drug occurs and the body's blood platelet count and ability to form blood clots are reduced (8).

thrush an infection of the mouth (and, possibly, esophagus) caused by the fungus *Candida albicans* and accompanied by milky white flakes on the tongue and other parts of the oral cavity; also known as candidiasis (4).

thymus a flat, bilobed organ that lies in the neck below the thyroid, the T-lymphocyte is produced in this organ (3).

T-lymphocyte an essential cell of the immune system that dominates cell-mediated immunity and functions as a helper, cytoxic, or suppressor T-lymphocyte; certain T-lymphocytes are host cells for HIV; also called T-cells (2).

Toxoplasma gondii a protozoal parasite that is a benign inhabitant of the blood in many individuals but causes severe infection of the brain in AIDS patients; domestic housecats harbor *T. gondii* (4).

toxoplasmosis an opportunistic disease in AIDS patients in which *T. gondii* multiplies in brain tissue, causing lesions, cerebral swelling, and seizures; in patients without AIDS, toxoplasmosis is a mild mononucleosislike disease (4).

treatment IND an investigational new drug used for treatment of a disease; often released to physicians while drug trials are ongoing (8).

trimethoprim a drug that when combined with sulfamethoxazole, can be used to treat *Pneumocystis carinii* pneumonia (8).

trimetrexate an anticancer drug also used to inhibit *Pneumocystis carinii* (8).

tuberculosis a bacterial disease of the lungs caused by *Mycobacterium tuberculosis* accompanied by progressive deterioration, difficult breathing, blood in the sputum, and eventual suffocation (4).

universal precautions recommendations published by the CDC to protect health care workers from infection by patients, as well as the reverse, and to prevent the spread of HIV among patients through contaminated devices or surfaces (6).

urethra the thin tube that carries semen and urine through the penis and out to the exterior (5).

V3 loop a loop of HIV amino acid that help the virus to attach to the CD4 receptor site (2).

vaginal intercourse sexual activity in which the penis of the insertive male partner is placed into the vagina of the receptive female partner (5).

viable-vector vaccine a vaccine consisting of nonpathogenic viruses whose DNA contains a segment that will code for HIV proteins (9).

vif gene regulatory gene necessary for the reverse transcription of RNA to DNA (2).

virion a completely assembled virus outside its host cell (2).

viruses particles of nucleic acid (either DNA or RNA) surrounded by a protein sheath and, sometimes, a membranous envelope; neither prokaryotic nor eukaryotic; highly infectious (2).

vpr gene regulatory gene that encodes viral protein R, which assist transport of viral DNA into the host cell nucleus (2).

vpu gene regulatory gene that encodes viral protein U, which breaks down the CD4 receptor protein, a protein that prevents HIV from budding out of the cell (2).

Walter Reed classification system a seven-stage classification system that charts the course of disease development from exposure to HIV through to AIDS (4).

western blot analysis a serological test in which standardized HIV proteins are used to test for the presence of HIV antibodies separated from one another by gel electrophoresis; the test is used to identify HIV indirectly (7).

whole-virus vaccine a vaccine containing entire virus particles that have been killed (9).

World Health Organization (WHO) a specialized agency of the United Nations that works to promote physical, mental, and social health in peoples of the world (5).

zidovudine an alternate name for azidothymidine (8).

Index

PHOTO CREDITS